Health
Matters

Health Matters

The Exercise and Nutrition Health Education Curriculum
for People with Developmental Disabilities

by

Beth Marks, RN, Ph.D.

Jasmina Sisirak, M.P.H.

and

Tamar Heller, Ph.D.

Rehabilitation Research and Training Center on Aging
with Developmental Disabilities
Department of Disability and Human Development
University of Illinois at Chicago

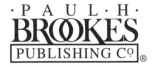

·P·A·U·L·H·
BROOKES
PUBLISHING CO.®

Baltimore · London · Sydney

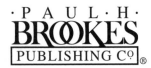

Paul H. Brookes Publishing Co.
Post Office Box 10624
Baltimore, Maryland 21285-0624
USA

www.brookespublishing.com

Manufactured in the United States of America by Versa Press, East Peoria, Illinois.

The information provided in this book is in no way meant to substitute for a medical or mental health practitioner's advice or expert opinion. Readers should consult a health or mental health professional if they are interested in more information. This book is sold without warranties of any kind, express or implied, and the publisher and authors disclaim any liability, loss, or damage caused by the contents of this book.

Every effort has been made to ascertain proper ownership of copyrighted materials and obtain permission for their use. Any omission is unintentional and will be corrected in future printings upon proper notification.

Purchasers of *Health Matters: The Exercise and Nutrition Health Education Curriculum for People with Developmental Disabilities* are granted permission to print and photocopy the Instructor References, Participant Handouts, and Testing Procedure Manual contained in the Software from a microcomputer located within the Purchaser's own facilities in the course of the Purchaser's service provision to families, students, or other individuals. Printed copies may only be made from an original CD-ROM. None of the forms may be reproduced to generate revenue for any program or individual. Photocopies may only be made from an original book or CD-ROM. *Unauthorized use beyond this privilege is prosecutable under federal law.* You will see the copyright protection notice at the bottom of each photocopiable or printable page, and a licensing agreement accompanies the CD-ROM included with this book.

Funded by U.S. Department of Education, Office of Special Education and Rehabilitative Services, National Institute on Disability and Rehabilitation Research, Grants H133B980046 and H133B031134; Centers for Disease Control and Prevention's Disability and Health Branch, Grant C CRS514155; the National Institute on Aging, Grants P50 AG15890-12 and P30 AG22849-01; and The Retirement Research Foundation. The contents of this curriculum do not necessarily represent the policy of the U.S. Department of Education and should not be viewed as an endorsement by the Federal government.

Library of Congress Cataloging-in-Publication Data

Marks, Beth.
    Health matters : the exercise and nutrition health education curriculum for people with developmental
    disabilities / by Beth Marks, Jasmina Sisirak, and Tamar Heller.
        p.   cm.
    Includes bibliographical references and index.
    ISBN-13: 978-1-55766-999-5
    ISBN-10: 1-55766-999-6
    1. Developmentally disabled—Health and hygiene.   2. Health education.   3. Health promotion.
    4. Nutrition.   5. Exercise.   I. Sisirak, Jasmina.   II. Heller, Tamar.
    III. Title.
    RC570.2.M37   2010
    362.196'8—dc22   2008050522

British Library Cataloguing in Publication data are available from the British Library.

2020	2019	2018	2017				
10	9	8	7	6	5	4	3

Contents

Contents of the CD-ROM

About the Authors

Beth Marks, RN, Ph.D., Research Assistant Professor, Department of Disability and Human Development, University of Illinois at Chicago, 1640 West Roosevelt Road, Chicago, Illinois 60608

Dr. Marks is also Associate Director for Research in the Rehabilitation Research and Training Center on Aging with Developmental Disabilities at the University of Illinois at Chicago and President of the National Organization of Nurses with Disabilities. She directs research activities related to health promotion and health advocacy, primary health care, and occupational health and safety for persons with disabilities. Dr. Marks has developed and implemented community-based surveys related to health and safety for people with disabilities and has written publications and presented papers in the area of disability, health, and community engagement in the United States and internationally. She has coedited a special issue for *Nursing Clinics of North America* titled *Promoting Health across the Lifespan for Persons with Developmental Disabilities* and a feasibility study report, *Advancing Nursing Education at Bel-Air Sanatorium and Hospital in Panchgani, Maharashtra, India,* through The Global Health Leadership Office/WHO Collaborating Center at the University of Illinois at Chicago.

Jasmina Sisirak, M.P.H., Associate Project Director, Department of Disability and Human Development, University of Illinois at Chicago, 1640 West Roosevelt Road, Chicago, Illinois 60608

Ms. Sisirak's research interests consist of nutrition, health literacy, and health promotion for persons with intellectual and developmental disabilities. She coordinates several health promotion projects in the Rehabilitation Research and Training Center on Aging with Developmental Disabilities and has written publications and presented papers in the area of disability, health, and nutrition. Ms. Sisirak received her bachelor of science degree in dietetics at Southern Illinois University and her master of public health at the University of Illinois at Chicago. Currently, she is a doctoral candidate in Community Health Sciences in the School of Public Health at the University of Illinois at Chicago.

Tamar Heller, Ph.D., Professor, Head of the Department of Disability and Human Development, University of Illinois at Chicago, and Director of the Institute on Disability and Human Development, the University Center of Excellence in Developmental Disabilities, 1640 West Roosevelt Road, Chicago, Illinois 60608

Dr. Heller also directs the Rehabilitation Research and Training Center on Aging with Developmental Disabilities and projects on family support and health promotion interventions for individuals with disabilities, including the Special Olympics Research Collaborating Center.

Dr. Heller has written more than 150 publications and has presented numerous papers at major conferences on family support interventions and policies, self-determination, health promotion, and aging of people with developmental disabilities. She has coedited two books (*Health of Women with Intellectual Disabilities*, Blackwell Publishing, 2002; *Older Adults with Developmental Disabilities: Optimizing Choice and Change*, Paul H. Brookes Publishing Co., 1993) and edited special issues of *Technology and Disability, American Journal on Mental Retardation, Journal of Policy and Practice in Intellectual Disabilities,* and *Family Relations.* She is the president of the board of the Association of University Centers on Disabilities. In 2005 she was a delegate to the While House Conference on Aging. As a cofounder of the national Sibling Leadership Network, she is a member of its steering committee. Her awards include the 2009 Autism Ally for Public Policy Award of The Arc/The Autism Program of Illinois; the 2008 Lifetime Research Achievement Award, International Association for the Scientific Study of Intellectual Disabilities, Special Interest Group on Aging and Intellectual Disabilities; and the 2009 Community Partner Award of Community Support Services.

Preface

Health Matters: The Exercise and Nutrition Health Education Curriculum for People with Developmental Disabilities is based on the successful outcomes of the innovative Health Promotion Program for Adults with Developmental Disabilities (DD) at the University of Illinois at Chicago (UIC), a 12-week exercise program that includes exercise, nutrition, and health education components. The goals of the program are to 1) improve fitness; 2) increase knowledge about healthy lifestyles; and 3) teach family, staff, and friends how to support participants to achieve these goals.

The benefits of health promotion activities have been well documented for the general population; however, individuals with developmental disabilities are often not included in health promotion activities. For people with disabilities, changes in lifestyle and environmental conditions may have the same potential to improve physical, mental, and social functioning and prevent the onset of lifestyle-related conditions as they do in the general population. Health promotion programs designed for adults with disabilities are therefore necessary.

UIC HEALTH PROMOTION PROGRAM

In order to better understand ways to promote healthy lifestyles among adults with DD, the UIC Health Promotion Program has been evaluated through several research projects since 1998. The projects have been conducted at UIC in the Department of Disability and Human Development by the Rehabilitation Research and Training Center on Aging with Developmental Disabilities (RRTCADD), Center on Health Promotion for Persons with Disabilities, and the UIC Midwest Roybal Center for Health Promotion and Behavior Change. Funding has been provided by the National Institute on Disability and Rehabilitation Research, Centers for Disease Control and Prevention, National Institute on Aging, and The Retirement Research Foundation.

The principal investigators and co-investigators for the UIC university-based health promotion program for adults with DD (1998–2003) were Tamar Heller, Ph.D., James H. Rimmer, Ph.D., and Beth Marks, RN, Ph.D. Todd Creviston, M.S., and Kelly Hsieh, Ph.D., served as project coordinators. The principal investigators and co-investigators for the UIC community-based health promotion program for adults aging with DD (2003–2008) were Beth Marks, RN, Ph.D., and Tamar Heller, Ph.D. Jasmina Sisirak, M.P.H., served as project coordinator.

Research participants enrolled in both the center-based (1998–2003) and the community-based (2003–2008) Health Promotion Program to participate in a comprehensive program consisting of exercise activities, nutrition and cooking classes, and health education classes with peer support. The classes consisted of the following activities:

1. The exercise classes included 1 hour of physical activity 3 days per week to improve fitness. Emphasis was placed on flexibility, cardiovascular endurance, balance, and muscle strength. Participants were taught how to properly use the equipment and exercise safely.

2. The nutrition and cooking classes were held 3 days per week for 1 hour. The lessons consisted of tips on healthy eating and food preparation, examination of eating routines and food labels, shopping tips, and the selection of healthy foods from restaurant menus.

3. The health education classes met 3 days per week for 1 hour. The lessons consisted of activities helping participants to understand their attitudes toward health, exercise, and food; find exercises that they like to do and set goals; gain skills and knowledge about exercises and healthy eating; support each other during the course of the class; and identify in their community where they could exercise regularly.

The center-based UIC Health Promotion Program for Adults with DD was tested on 62 adults age 30 years and older with Down syndrome from six agencies providing day and residential services in Illinois. The intervention group included four groups of 37 participants, and the control group included 25 persons (Heller, Hsieh, & Rimmer, 2004; Rimmer, Heller, Wang, & Valerio, 2004). The project produced the evidence-based curriculum *Exercise and Nutrition Health Education Curriculum for Adults with Developmental Disabilities, First Edition* (Heller, Marks, & Ailey, 2001). The results demonstrated the following for participants following the intervention:

• Greater life satisfaction

• Increased exercise knowledge

• More positive attitudes toward exercise

• Increased confidence in ability to exercise

• Fewer socioemotional barriers preventing participants from exercising

• Improved cardiovascular fitness

• Increased muscle strength and endurance

With the aim of increasing the UIC Health Promotion Program's generalizability in the community, we developed the Face-to-Face and Web-Based Train-the-Trainer Health Promotion Program (2003–2008), led by staff in community-based organizations (CBOs). This community-based research study documented the effectiveness of disability support programs (DSPs) in CBOs in teaching adults aging with DD to complete more physical activity and eat healthier foods in their home and workplace. The program continues to provide CBO staff 6–8 hours of training on how to 1) develop a 12-week physical activity and health education program personalized to their clients' needs, 2) teach adults with DD about physical activity and nutrition using this curriculum, and 3) support individuals with DD to make long-term lifestyle changes.

The community-based UIC Health Promotion Program for Adults with DD demonstrated the capacity of DSPs to change health-related behaviors and improve the health status of their clients and of themselves (Marks, Sisirak, et al., 2008; Marks et al., 2007). This program was tested on four groups of 91 participants from four different vocational and residential agencies in Illinois and New Mexico. The intervention group included four groups of 51 participants, and the control group included 40 persons. Results showed significant changes in psychosocial health status, including decreased perceived pain, increased self-efficacy, and increased social/environmental supports. Staff participants after the program had significantly higher outcome expectations of exercise and nutrition for themselves. In addition, staff had significantly more support for nutrition following the program and a higher intake of fruits and vegetables.

CURRICULUM PREMISES

The curriculum incorporates the following concepts that affect a participant's ability to change health behaviors: self-efficacy (Bandura, 1982, 1986), social support (including paid and unpaid caregiver support), self-advocacy, choice-making, and leadership development. This builds on other curricula, such as the RRTCADD's *Person-Centered Planning for Later Life: A Curriculum for Adults with Mental Retardation* (Sutton, Heller, Sterns, Factor, & Miklos, 1993) and *Making Choices as We Age: A Peer Training Program* (Heller, Preston, Nelis, Pederson, & Brown, 1995). An emphasis is placed on knowledge related to the benefits of exercise and good nutrition, available exercise and nutrition options in the community, personal choices regarding one's preferred lifestyle, and support from friends and relatives.

The following premises are incorporated in the curriculum:

- People with disabilities have a right to receive education and services that promote their health.
- People can contribute to their own well-being by becoming knowledgeable about their health and health resources and by becoming active participants in health promotion activities.
- Health promotion is not a form of social control but must be based on the needs and lifestyle preferences of individuals.
- Support from caregivers and increased access to exercise activities promote exercise adherence.

CURRICULUM DESIGN

Motivating people to change their behavior can be viewed as a process or continuum related to a person's readiness to change. The curriculum is based on Bandura's Social Cognitive Theory (Bandura, 1977, 1982, 1986) and the five stages of change in the Transtheoretical Model (TTM) of Behavior Change: precontemplation, contemplation, preparation, action, and maintenance (Prochaska & DiClemente, 1992; Prochaska et al., 1994). The Social Cognitive Theory and the TTM provide a framework for structuring activities for service providers and participants so that they learn strategies for modifying or changing health behaviors in a cyclical manner rather than in a simple linear process and strategies for improving participants' self-confidence to change behavior.

Bandura's Social Cognitive Theory

The curriculum uses concepts from Bandura's Social Cognitive Theory (Bandura, 1977, 1982, 1986) to support behavior change. With the Social Cognitive Theory, behavior change is seen as a function of 1) setting personal goals based on one's attitudes toward a change in behavior, 2) understanding the tasks required to achieve those goals, and 3) having self-efficacy expectations (self-confidence) in being able to achieve the goals (Bandura, 1977, 1982, 1994). In other words, individuals are more likely to change their health-promoting behaviors if they believe that 1) their current behaviors pose threats to personally valued goals, such as health; 2) health promoting behaviors will help reduce the threat (attitudes); and 3) they are personally capable of adopting the new behaviors (self-efficacy expectations). Self-efficacy is documented as a major predictor of adherence to preventive health programs (O'Leary, 1985) and to exercise and fitness involvement (McAuley, Lox, & Duncan, 1993). Bandura also emphasizes the informative and motivational role of reinforcement and the role of observational learning through modeling the behavior of others; thus, environmental cues, such as support from others, play an important role.

Transtheoretical Model of Behavior Change

The TTM approaches behavior change across five stages (precontemplation, contemplation, preparation, action, and maintenance), in which one becomes increasingly more motivated and ready to modify or change a particular behavior. In the precontemplation stage, people are often unaware or under-aware of the need to change their behavior. As people move into the contemplation stage, they become increasingly aware that they should change their behavior and start to assess the impact of their behavior. As people gain a greater appreciation of the pros and cons related to specific behaviors, people are more inclined to take action. However, behavior changes will be more successful if people make plans to change a specific behavior and develop goals in the preparation stage. In the action stage, people change their behaviors and are engaging in new behaviors. The maintenance stage is a time in which people identify strategies and supports to maintain healthy behaviors.

By using both the TTM and the Social Cognitive Theory, people begin to understand the processes of modifying, changing, and maintaining changes in health behaviors. As you use the curriculum with your health promotion classes, you may see participants going through these five stages at different rates. In fact, people often move back and forth between stages a number of times before they maintain their behavior change goal. In addition, people use different processes (or activities) to move from one stage of change to another, so it is important to target the right activity (processes) at the right time (stages). In using this model, you can tailor your activities to match a person's stage of readiness to change his or her behavior. For example, for people who are not interested in becoming more active, you may find that encouraging a step-by-step movement along the continuum of change may be better than encouraging them to move directly into action.

Each stage is part of a continuum of readiness to change and includes specific topics designed to provide participants with options for changing their behavior. The five Units in this curriculum incorporate the five stages of change. The model in Figure 1 provides a visual representation of the five stages of change that are used in each of the units.

Unit 1 *Precontemplation Stage*—People are often unaware or under-aware of the need to change their behavior. The lessons focus on increasing the participants' understanding of health, exercise, and nutrition, along with making decisions about one's health.

Unit 2 *Contemplation Stage*—People are aware that they should change their behavior and are seriously thinking about change but have not made a commitment to take action. In this section, participants consider lifestyle change and assess their exercise and nutrition behaviors.

Unit 3 *Preparation Stage*—People are ready to take action and change a specific behavior. The lessons focus on setting goals and examining barriers and influences that may affect their ability to exercise or eat a more nutritious diet.

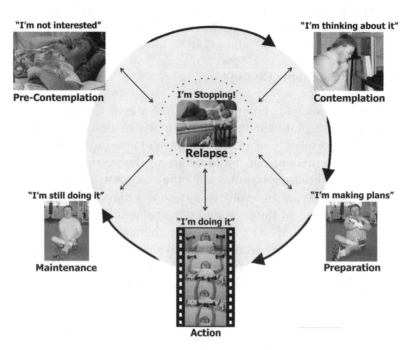

Figure 1. Becoming physically active and choosing healthy foods: Stages of behavior change.

Unit 4   *Action Stage*—People are taking action and have changed their behavior(s). Participants are exercising and trying to include healthy foods in their diets. In this section, classes focus on reinforcing participants' new behaviors to maintain their exercise and nutrition goals.

Unit 5   *Maintenance Stage*—People are considering ways to prevent relapse. The lessons in this section focus on reviewing what participants have learned and different ways to maintain their program. After the 12-week structured program of classes aimed at teaching and supporting people to feel more confident to engage in regular physical activity and make healthy food choices, people are encouraged to continue with classes as a part of lifelong learning. The Lifelong Learning Lessons in Appendix A feature 22 supplemental lessons developed with participants in the UIC Health Promotion Program to complement the 36 lessons that make up the core program to sustain long-term adoption of healthy lifestyles.

REFERENCES

Bandura, A. (1977). *Social learning theory.* Upper Saddle River, NJ: Prentice Hall.

Bandura, A. (1982). Self-efficacy: Toward a unifying theory of behavior change. *Psychological Review, 84,* 191–215.

Bandura, A. (1986). *Social foundations of thought and action: A social cognitive theory.* Upper Saddle River, NJ: Prentice Hall.

Heller, T., Hsieh, K., & Rimmer, J. (2004). Attitudinal and psychological outcomes of a fitness and health education program on adults with Down syndrome. *American Journal on Mental Retardation, 109*(2), 175–188.

Heller, T., Marks, B., & Ailey, S. (2001). *Exercise and nutrition health education curriculum for adults with developmental disabilities.* Rehabilitation Research and Training Center on Aging with Developmental Disabilities, University of Illinois at Chicago.

Heller, T., Preston, L., Nelis, T., Pederson, E., & Brown, A. (1995). *Making choices as we age: A peer training program.* Chicago & Cincinnati: University of Illinois at Chicago and University of Cincinnati.

Marks, B., Sisirak, J., Heller, T., & Riley, B. (November 6, 2007). *Impact of a train-the-trainer program on the psychosocial health status of staff supporting adults with intellectual and developmental disabilities.* Paper presented at American Public Health Association, 135rd annual meeting & exposition, Washington, DC.

Marks, B., Sisirak, J., & Hsieh, K. (2008). Health services, health promotion, and health literacy: Report from the State of the Science in Aging with Developmental Disabilities Conference. *Disability and Health Journal, 1*(3), 136–142.

McAuley, E., Lox, C., & Duncan, T.E. (1993). Long-term maintenance of exercise behavior in middle-aged adults. *Journal of Gerontology: Psychological Sciences, 48*, 672–681.

O'Leary, A. (1985). Self-efficacy and health. *Behavior and Research Therapy, 23*, 437–451.

Prochaska, J., & DiClemente, C. (1992). Stages of change in the modification of problem behaviors. In M. Hersen, R. Eisler, & P. Miller (Eds.), *Progress in behavior modification* (pp. 184–218). Sycamore, IL: Sycamore.

Prochaska, J.O., Velicer, W.F., Rossie, J.S., Goldstein, M.G., Marcus, B.H., Rakowski, W., et al. (1994). Stages of change and decisional balance for 12 problem behaviors. *Health Psychology, 13*, 38–46.

Rimmer, J., Heller, T., Wang, E., & Valerio, I. (2004). Improvements in physical fitness in adults with Down syndrome. *American Journal on Mental Retardation, 109*(2), 165–174.

Sutton, E., Heller, T., Sterns, H.L., Factor, A., & Miklos, S. (1993). *Person-centered planning for later life: A curriculum for adults with mental retardation.* Akron, OH: University of Illinois at Chicago and University of Akron, Rehabilitation Research and Training Center on Aging with Mental Retardation.

Acknowledgments

We would like to acknowledge the initial work conducted by the dedicated program staff of the University of Illinois at Chicago Health Promotion Program. The exercise classes were instructed by Todd Creviston, M.S.; Don Smith, M.S.; Francis Gando; and Irene Valerio under the direction of James H. Rimmer, Ph.D. Sandra Gomez, M.S., RD, LD, taught the nutrition classes under the direction of Carol Braunschweig, Ph.D. Beth Marks, RN, Ph.D.; Sarah Ailey, RN, Ph.D.; Kelly Hsieh, Ph.D.; Jasmina Sisirak, M.P.H.; and Joanne Lee taught the health education classes under the direction of Tamar Heller, Ph.D. In addition, Allison Brown, Ph.D., assisted with developing and pilot-testing the psychosocial assessments, and two nursing students from the Netherlands, Karin Bruijnis and Marleen Haveman, provided assistance in the exercise, nutrition, and health education classes.

The work of persons with disabilities and staff supporting persons with intellectual and developmental disabilities in community-based agencies has been invaluable in the creation of this curriculum.

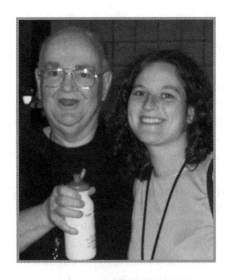

Section I

Introduction to the Curriculum

Improved health education and health literacy is a critical component for people to gain control over their health and manage chronic conditions (World Health Organization [WHO], 2001). Persons with low health literacy have higher utilization of treatment services, increased hospitalization and emergency services, and lower utilization of preventive services, resulting in higher health care costs (Marks, Sisirak, & Hsieh, 2008). Using this curriculum as a component of your health promotion program can be a means to improve health literacy skills and a sense of personal empowerment among adults with DD, that is *to say his or her own word, to name the world, and to gain control over one's own health* (WHO, 1972). People with limited or inaccurate knowledge about the body and the causes of disease may not understand the relationship between lifestyle factors (e.g., diet and exercise) and health outcomes and recognize when they need to seek care. Having health literacy skills allows people to share personal and health information with health care providers; engage in self-care and chronic disease management; adopt health-promoting behaviors, such as exercising and eating a healthy diet; and act on health-related news and announcements. In turn, these outcomes impact health outcomes, health care costs, and quality of care.

CURRICULUM FORMAT

The curriculum was developed as a 12-week program with three 1-hour lessons per week. Each lesson covered a specific topic. The lessons were designed to build upon each other with some intentional overlapping of the content. This allowed participants to continuously review materials throughout the program.

The overall format of this curriculum encourages instructors to reproduce the parts they need to teach a specific lesson. In addition, a CD-ROM with color versions of the instructor references and participant handouts that accompany each lesson is available in the back of the book. While not required, we encourage duplication of the handouts so that each participant can make a personalized notebook out of the handouts. Personalizing each notebook encourages ownership and engagement in the exercise and health education program.

The Personal Notebook can include a goals worksheet that can be used to develop goals with each participant during the first class session of the program. Most lessons contain participant handouts that can be included in the Personal Notebook. The Physical Activity Observation Sheet (PAOS) that appears in Lesson 1 can be used to determine a participant's readiness for physical activity before each session. PAOS can also be used as a teaching and motivational tool for participants. The PAOS form can be used before every exercise class. Using PAOS with participants is a useful way to engage participants into a discussion about key concepts related to exercise and physical activity.

USING THE CURRICULUM TO START YOUR EXERCISE AND NUTRITION HEALTH EDUCATION PROGRAM

A variety of activities are included in the curriculum that can be modified to fit your teaching style and the needs of your participants. After the program is over, people can begin a Lifelong Learning Course or continue to do the activities that they tried during the course of the health education program. In Appendix A, we have included 22 additional lessons that were developed in response to requests from people with DD to have more information regarding issues related to health, physical activity and nutrition after the 12-week program was completed. We recommend using parts of the curriculum to provide health education for caregivers and other support persons. Here are some suggestions on using the curriculum:

- The curriculum is for people with DD.
- The curriculum can be completed at the community activity center, home, school, or work.
- The curriculum can be completed morning, afternoon, or early evening.
- The recommended class size is 6–10 participants.
- We recommend having at least two instructors for the classes.
- Although not empirically tested, this curriculum has been used with high school students, transition-age adolescents, and older adults with a range of physical, psychological, and intellectual disabilities because its design encourages trainers to customize the program and workbooks for each trainee.

TIPS FOR STARTING A HEALTH PROMOTION PROGRAM

A health promotion program should include a variety of activities that people enjoy doing (Rimmer, 2000). For example, on Monday, Wednesday, and Friday, a person in the program may want to walk briskly for 30 minutes, lift weights for 20 minutes, and do flexibility exercises for 10 minutes. Riding a stationary bike, swimming, dancing, or doing an aerobic activities video can be substituted for walking. See Appendix B for a glossary of terms used throughout the curriculum and Appendix C for an exercise workout overview. Appendix D provides an overview of Universal Design strategies.

Prior to starting a program, you should follow the testing procedures for psychosocial and physical fitness that are found in the Testing Procedure Manual in Appendix E. You should also consider the following steps:

1. *Obtain permission from a health care provider for each participant* (Rimmer, 2000). Make sure that participants can safely begin exercising and will not aggravate any existing health conditions by regular exercise activity. The health care provider may recommend specific tests depending on the person's age and physical condition to determine any limitations in doing physical activities.

2. *Encourage participants to do physical activities throughout the day.* Incorporate physical activity into daily routines throughout the day. When added to a structured health promotion program, this can increase a person's fitness level and allow the participant to consume more calories if he or she is trying to lose weight.

3. *Make sure that your program is based on sound and tested theory.* For example, the Transtheoretical Model of Behavior Change (Prochaska & DiClemente, 1992; Prochaska et al., 1994) and Bandura's Social Cognitive Theory (Bandura, 1982, 1986) can offer a framework for structuring activities for participants and service providers to learn the processes of modifying or changing health behaviors and improving one's self-confidence to change one's behavior. Find activities that fit the needs and interests of the individuals in the class. Make sure that the activity is accessible for all or most of the class.

4. *Teach participants to exercise a minimum of 3 days per week for at least 30 minutes.*

5. *Keep the program fun and rewarding.* People must have fun doing the exercise activity in order to continue with their exercise program. Expose people to a variety of activities that they can do with their friends and/or family members and/or by themselves.

6. *Foster fitness among staff members and caregivers.* People are more likely to engage in exercise activities if they see people around them participating in exercise programs. Mounting evidence suggests that sustainable health promotion programs include supportive environments and attitudes. Having "buy-in" from all program partners, including people with disabilities, service providers, family members, and community partners, is a critical component for long-term success.

TEACHING APPROACHES

Implementation of the curriculum emphasizes two primary concepts based on primary health care: 1) maximum individual involvement in the planning and implementation of exercise and nutrition goals and 2) health promotive rather than curative activities. In addition, strategies from McElmurry, Newcomb, Lowe, and Misner's *Primary Health Care Curriculum Grade K–8 for Urban School Children* (1995), such as problem-solving techniques, conflict resolution, role playing, and using open-ended questions are used to teach this curriculum. These strategies may be used to facilitate the learning process in each of the classes, depending on the group and the individual style of the instructor.

Problem-Solving Techniques

Problem solving is a strategy that is not directly addressed in the curriculum but is recommended for the instructor as an underlying approach in each of the lessons (McElmurry et al., 1995). The problem-solving or decision-making approach provides participants with the skills and attitudes necessary to become lifelong learners. In order for problem solving to work in the classroom, instructors may consider the following techniques:

- Have objectives that can be accomplished through the use of each lesson.
- Set the tone for the progress of the class by ensuring that participants are relaxed and the atmosphere is calm, nonthreatening, and nonjudgmental.
- Practice the principles and reinforce them with participants at every opportunity.

Conflict Resolution

Conflict is defined as a clash of opinions, needs, or wants between individuals or groups (McElmurry et al., 1995). The result of a conflict may be positive or negative. When handled correctly, conflict can lead to growth within individuals or groups. It can help participants see that their needs and wants may be different from those of others and that this may result in disagreements. Conflict resolution is another strategy used throughout the curriculum as an underlying approach to teaching the content of each lesson. Conflict resolution can help people understand that the person with whom they disagree has the right to his or her own needs and wants. Moreover, each person has the right to be accepted regardless of his or her point of view. Lastly, conflict resolution can help participants identify positive ways of resolving conflict such as demonstrating a willingness to discuss the situation to clarify the problem and trying to search for a solution that is agreeable to each person.

Role Playing

Role playing may also be used by the instructor to teach the curriculum content. Using role playing introduces the content through the participants' actual health experiences (McElmurry et al., 1995). Initially, ask for volunteers or select participants who are likely to talk and role-play and who can follow general instructions related to the role or situation for the first few lessons. In the role-playing exercises, have participants look for specific points or identify with the feelings of the character in the role play. Participants' interest, involvement, and learning is easier when they have a specific task. Encourage people to express themselves freely. Address all remarks to each character by name.

Using Open-Ended Questions

Use open-ended questions to encourage group participation in the discussion. Focus the discussion on the feelings, thoughts, and actions of the characters and on the purposes and consequences of their actions. Help participants relate their experiences to situations that they might have or will encounter. After participants have completed the role play, commend everyone for their efforts. Discuss what you thought was good about the role play and then suggest areas for improvement. Make sure that each participant has an opportunity to participate in a role-play situation.

ADDITIONAL CONSIDERATIONS

In using this curriculum with a variety of participants, you may consider some additional teaching considerations, including Universal Design strategies, field trip activities, newsletters and cameras, and lifelong learning lessons. An overview of each of these approaches is provided below.

Universal Design Strategies

Through a joint project with Easter Seals, creative teaching strategies and solutions incorporating principles of universal design were developed for use with people who have severe/profound intellectual disabilities, a variety of physical disabilities, and/or unique learning styles. These Universal Design strategies can be found in Appendix D.

Field Trip Activities

You may find it useful to combine the field trip activities in the health education curriculum with your structured exercise classes, depending on group dynamics among the participants and group structure (e.g., time constraints, staff participant ratio). The field trip activities are designed to integrate both the health education and exercise classes into an activity that will give participants opportunities to experience being physically active and making healthy food choices in their community. Lessons can be taught with or without the field trip activities.

Incorporating Newsletters and Cameras

Newsletters and cameras (digital and videos) can be used in every class as a way of including participants and having active involvement. Weekly newsletters can be used to summarize weekly class activities for participants and to encourage involvement of support persons by having participants share their newsletters. The newsletters should include the following new items: 1) health, exercise, and nutrition related information; 2) new types of exercises; and 3) summaries of class discussions. Users can use the prewritten newsletters provided in the curriculum or make their own newsletters.

Lifelong Learning Lessons

The lifelong learning lessons were developed based on our teaching experiences with participants in the community-based UIC Health Promotion Program for Adults with DD.

Based on participants' interest in ongoing health education, 22 lessons were created as a way of initiating and encouraging lifelong learning related to health and the adoption of healthy lifestyles. These lessons are designed to complement the 36 lessons that are taught in the program to sustain long-term adoption of healthy lifestyles. Specifically, the aim of the classes is to reinforce the information presented during the core program and to provide ongoing support for people to continue developing new skills and greater confidence to engage in regular physical activity and make healthy food choices.

Classes in the lifelong learning series can be taught based on individual needs and interest, and the topics have been arranged based on the core themes used in the lessons for the 12-week program. These themes are divided into four primary topics: 1) advocacy and social support, 2) exercise and physical activity, 3) nutrition, and 4) general health. Six of the nutrition lessons were developed through a project funded by Special Olympics International (SOI). Through the SOI project, these lessons were developed as a part of the *Learning Through Pictures: Nutrition and Physical Activity Education Curriculum for Adults with I/DD* (Sisirak & Marks, 2005).

EVALUATING CHANGES IN PARTICIPANTS

The exercise and nutrition curriculum was designed to foster responsible, positive attitudes toward healthy behaviors for people with developmental disabilities. Although these are long-term goals that may be difficult to assess, we can evaluate growth toward these goals. Program evaluation is an important step from program initiation to program completion. It enables you to continuously improve and adapt your program to meet the needs of people with disabilities. Evaluation also provides support for broadening the program to include more people. In general, three types of program evaluation can be done: 1) goals- based evaluation (e.g., Are you meeting your objectives?), 2) process-based evaluations (e.g., What are your program strengths and weaknesses?), and 3) outcomes-based evaluation (e.g., What are the benefits to each participant?) (McNamara, 1997). Although it is good to do a mixture of all three, for the purpose of this curriculum, we will focus only on outcomes-based evaluation.

The purpose of the outcomes-based evaluation is to assess enhanced learning or change in attitudes (e.g., knowledge, perceptions, attitudes, skills), improved physical activity adherence and eating nutritious foods, and improved psychosocial and physical health. We recommend doing an evaluation at the beginning and at the end of the program. Wherever possible, peer and self-evaluation should be encouraged. Help participants learn to evaluate themselves. Peer evaluation is an important part of the curriculum. If possible, solicit information from support persons to assist in the evaluation of participant progress with the objectives.

SUMMARY

There are many benefits to beginning a health promotion program for adults with disabilities. Changes in lifestyle and environmental conditions may have the same potential to dramatically improve physical, mental, and social functioning for a person with disabilities. Using a health promotion program, such as *Health Matters,* can help improve the lives of adults with disabilities.

REFERENCES

Bandura, A. (1982). Self-efficacy: Toward a unifying theory of behavior change. *Psychological Review, 84,* 191–215.

Bandura, A. (1986). *Social foundations of thought and action: A social cognitive theory.* Upper Saddle River, NJ: Prentice Hall.

Marks, B., Sisirak, J., & Hsieh, K. (2008). Health services, health promotion, and health literacy: Report from the State of the Science in Aging with Developmental Disabilities Conference. *Disability and Health Journal, 1*(3), 136–142.

McElmurry, B., Newcomb, B.J., Lowe, A., & Misner, S.M. (1995). *Primary health care curriculum Grade K–8 for urban school children.* Chicago: University of Chicago, College of Nursing, Global Health Leadership Office.

McNamara, C. (1997). *Basic guide to program evaluation.* Retrieved July 3, 2008, from http://www.mapnp.org/library/evauatn/fnl_eval.htm

Prochaska, J., & DiClemente, C. (1992). Stages of change in the modification of problem behaviors. In M. Hersen, R. Eisler, & P. Miller (Eds.), *Progress in behavior modification* (pp. 184–218). Sycamore, IL: Sycamore Publishers.

Prochaska, J.O., Velicer, W.F., Rossie, J.S., Goldstein, M.G., Marcus, B.H., Rakowski, W., et al. (1994). Stages of change and decisional balance for 12 problem behaviors. *Health Psychology, 13,* 38–46.

Rimmer, J.H. (2000). Achieving a beneficial fitness: A program and a philosophy in mental retardation. *Contemporary Issues in Health, 1,* 1–36.

Sisirak, J., & Marks, B. (2005). *Learning through pictures: Nutrition and physical activity education curriculum for adults with I/DD.* Chicago: Rehabilitation Research and Training Center on Aging and Developmental Disabilities, Department of Disability and Human Development.

World Health Organization (WHO). (2001). *Health promotion: Report by the Secretariat.* Geneva: World Health Organization.

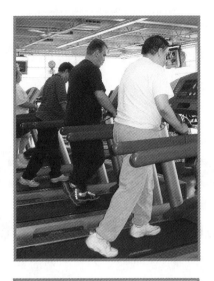

Section II

Health
Education Curriculum

Unit 1

Physical Activity and Nutrition

Making Healthy Choices

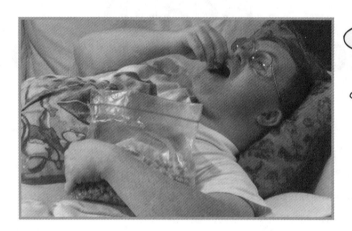

I'm not interested!

The first stage of behavior change is known as the precontemplation stage. When classes begin, people in this stage may not be interested in changing their behaviors or may be unaware or under-aware of the need to change their behaviors. It may be helpful to focus your activities on increasing participants' understanding of health and exercise and making decisions about their health.

Unit 1 Contents

Lesson 1

What Is Health?

Objectives
Participants will
• Discuss topics that the health classes will cover
• Define what health means to them
• Identify different meanings of health
• State things that may affect health

also on CD-ROM

HANDOUTS
Participant Handout(s):
Definitions of Health
What Is Healthy to Me?
Personal Notebook Cover Sheet
My Goals for the Program
Physical Activity Observation Sheet
Borg Rating of Perceived Exertion Scale

MATERIALS
Blackboard and chalk
Camera to take photos of what "being healthy" means to participants
Reminder Envelope
Three-ring binder (Personal Notebook)

Suggested Activities

INSTRUCTOR ACTIVITY	INSTRUCTOR SCRIPT/DIRECTIONS
GREET CLASS	*Hello, everyone. My name is_____.* Introduce other instructors. Have participants introduce themselves.
INTRODUCE LESSON	*This is the first class that we will have to help you make positive choices about your health. You are worthwhile people with your own ideas about what health means to you.*
DISTRIBUTE PERSONAL NOTEBOOKS	Give each participant a three-ring binder and ask them to use the **Personal Notebooks** to keep the handouts and worksheets they'll be receiving throughout the course.
	HELPFUL HINT: Prior to class, instructors may want to personalize the notebooks with each participant's photo and copy all of the handouts for the course. These handouts are located on the accompanying CD-ROM.
SAY	*This class will help you think about what is important to you and how to **manage your own health**. We all need to think about what we need or want and how to have our*

Sources:

Marks, B.A. (1996). Conceptualizations of health among adults with intellectual impairments. Unpublished doctoral dissertation, University of Illinois at Chicago. *Dissertation Abstracts International, 57–11*(B), 6877.

McElmurry, B., Newcomb, B.J., Lowe, A., & Misner, S.M. (1995). *Primary Health Care Curriculum Grade K–8 for Urban School Children.* Chicago: University of Illinois at Chicago, College of Nursing, Global Halth Leadership Office.

INSTRUCTOR ACTIVITY	INSTRUCTOR SCRIPT/DIRECTIONS
	needs met. As you learn more, you will be able to make more decisions about your health. **Learning how to take care of our health is a lifelong process.**
SAY	*This class will help you think about different ways people think about health. People think of health in many ways. Today, we will talk about what being healthy means to you.* Refer to the **Definitions of Health** handout for different examples.
ASK	*What does "being healthy" mean to you?*

DISCUSS
PARTICIPANT HANDOUTS:
  Definitions of Health
  What Is Healthy to Me?
	Review definitions of health from the **Definitions of Health** handout. Also, have participants fill out the **What Is Healthy to Me?** handout.

	• *Some people feel healthy when they are not sick or they often think of a very limited meaning, such as, "the absence of illness or disability."*
	• *Other people think they are healthy when they feel comfortable where they live and work and with their relationships.*
	• *Health can be feeling good and being able to do the things that you want to do.*
	• *Health may also include feelings of satisfaction and happiness.*
DISTRIBUTE HANDOUTS	Show participants pictures of what "being healthy" means to other people. Ask them which pictures are healthy to them.
ASK	*How do you know when you are healthy or not healthy?*
DISCUSS	*People have many ideas about the meaning of "health." What we think about health comes from our own point of view. Our minds and bodies work together to keep us healthy. We may feel healthy when we have fun with our family and/or friends. What "health" means to us depends on our needs, goals, life experiences, where we live and work, and where we have fun.*
ASK	*Do you see yourself as healthy or unhealthy?*
DISCUSS	*Knowing what health is affects how you take care of yourself.*
TAKE PICTURES	Take a photo of each participant that conveys something "healthy" or "being healthy" to him or her.
GET IN SMALL GROUPS	Divide participants into groups of two or three depending on the size of the class.
COMPLETE JOHN/JANE EXERCISE	Write this sentence on the board: *John/Jane is a healthy 45-year-old man/woman.* Have participants form a picture

INSTRUCTOR ACTIVITY	INSTRUCTOR SCRIPT/DIRECTIONS

of John or Jane and then brainstorm about him or her using the following suggestions:

- How do they look? (e.g., hair, eyes, skin, posture, weight, height, clothes)
- What do they like to do? (e.g., work, sports, hobbies)
- What do they do to stay healthy?
- What do they do to get along with people?
- How do they feel about life?
- What do they think of life?
- Do they believe in a higher power/religion?

RECORD RESPONSES

Write responses on the board. You may include such things as having energy to work and play, getting along with family and friends, having a strong body, and being able to sleep. Provide assistance as needed. (See Helpful Hints.)

DISCUSS

Review participants' responses with the class.

DISTRIBUTE PARTICIPANT HANDOUTS:
Personal Notebook Cover Sheet
My Goals for the Program
Physical Activity Observation Sheet
Borg Rating of Perceived Exertion Scale

Give participants their own **Personal Notebook Cover Sheet**. Have participants use **My Goals for the Program** to identify which goals they would like to have at the beginning of the program. The **Physical Activity Observation Sheet (PAOS)** should be used before every exercise class. Using PAOS with participants is a useful way to remind participants about key concepts related to exercise.

The **Borg Rating of Perceived Exertion Scale** is included in the Personal Notebook. Perceived exertion is how hard you feel like your body is working. It is based on the physical sensations a person experiences during physical activity, including increased heart rate, increased breathing rate, increased sweating, and muscle fatigue. Although this is a subjective measure, a person's exertion rating may provide a fairly good estimate of the actual heart rate during physical activity. Perceived exertion ratings between 12 and 14 on the Perceived Exertion Scale suggest that physical activity is being performed at a moderate level of intensity.

SUMMARIZE

People have many ideas about the meaning of "health." What we think about health comes from our own point of view. Our minds and bodies work together to keep us healthy. We may feel healthy when we have fun with our family and/or friends. What "health" means to us depends on our needs, goals, life experiences, where we live and work, and where we have fun.

It is important to know what health is because that will affect how you take care of yourself. In the next class, we will talk about the meaning of physical activity.

Evaluation

- Were participants able to describe what being healthy means to them?

Helpful Hints

You may want to ask people what they do or how they feel when they feel good (are able to work) or feel sick (are too tired to have fun) or how they feel when they have a cold or a headache.

The accompanying CD-ROM may be used to print all of the handouts for participants' Personal Notebooks. The handouts on the CD-ROM feature color versions of the illustrations and photographs.

Definitions of Health

When people define the word "health," they often settle for a very limited definition, such as "the absence of illness or disability." However, as we can see below, people define their health in many ways. In fact, people say they are healthy even though they may have a chronic disease or a disability.

ABSENCE OF SICKNESS AND PAIN

- Person appears well-nourished
- Has no aches or pains
- Does not feel sick
- Takes care of physical problems
- Does not take unnecessary risks

PHYSICAL/MENTAL/EMOTIONAL

- Likes oneself
- Eats foods that are good for oneself
- Gets enough sleep
- Is physically active
- Likes to learn new things
- Able to control and express feelings
- Sets own goals and ways to meet those goals
- Takes care of his or her body by eating healthy foods
- Takes care of his or her body by exercising regularly
- Weight is appropriate for a person's age and height

ROLES

- Has friends
- Listens to and supports others in achieving their goals
- Has a significant friend (boyfriend, girlfriend, spouse)
- Able to take care of oneself
- Shares feelings with others
- Has close relationships with others

SPIRITUAL

- Enjoys life
- Reaches personal goals
- Has enough energy to do daily activities
- Believes in a higher power and lives according to this belief

I'm healthy when I feel good.

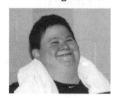

I'm healthy when I can relax.

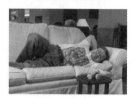

I'm healthy when I weigh what's right for me.

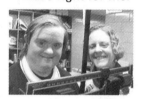

I'm healthy when I exercise.

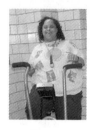

I'm healthy when I eat foods that are good for me.

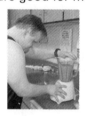

I'm healthy when I have a friend that I love.

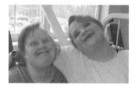

I'm healthy when I have a friend that cares for me.

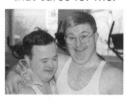

I'm healthy when I have someone special in my life.

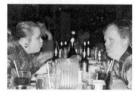

I'm healthy when I am happy.

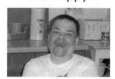

Sources:
Marks, B.A. (1996). Conceptualizations of health among adults with intellectual impairments. Unpublished doctoral dissertation, University of Illinois at Chicago. *Dissertation Abstracts International, 57–11*(B), 6877.
McElmurry, B., Newcomb, B.J., Lowe, A., & Misner, S.M. (1995). *Primary Health Care Curriculum Grade K–8 for Urban School Children.* Chicago: University of Illinois at Chicago, College of Nursing, Global Halth Leadership Office.

What Is Healthy to Me?

Circle anything that "being healthy" means to you.

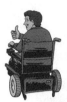

I'm healthy when I feel good.

I'm healthy when I exercise.

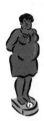

I'm healthy when I weigh
what's right for me.

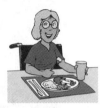

I'm healthy when I eat foods
that are good for me.

I'm healthy when I am happy.

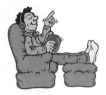

I'm healthy when I can relax.

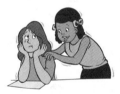

I'm healthy when I have
a friend that cares for me.

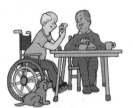

I'm healthy when I have
someone special in my life.

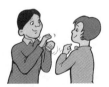

I'm healthy when I have
a friend that I love.

YOU

I'm healthy when _____

_____

Sources:

Marks, B.A. (1996). Conceptualizations of health among adults with intellectual impairments. Unpublished doctoral dissertation, University of Illinois at Chicago. *Dissertation Abstracts International, 57–11*(B), 6877.

McElmurry, B., Newcomb, B.J., Lowe, A., & Misner, S.M. (1995). *Primary Health Care Curriculum Grades K–8 for Urban School Children.* Chicago: University of Illinois at Chicago, College of Nursing, Global Halth Leadership Office.

Health Matters: The Exercise and Nutrition Health Education Curriculum for People with Developmental Disabilities
by Beth Marks, Jasmina Sisirak, and Tamar Heller

15

Unit 1

Lesson 1

What Is Health?

Personal Notebook

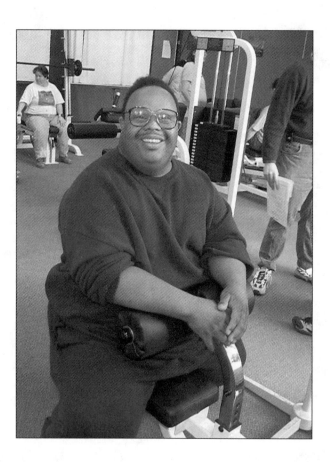

EXERCISE AND NUTRITION
HEALTH EDUCATION CLASS

My Goals for the Program

Name: _____

These are some ideas of goals that you may have as you start your health education and exercise classes. As you go through the classes, you may want to add new goals or change your old goals.

1. Help me learn new things
2. Make my body feel good
3. Make me hurt less
4. Help me get in shape
5. Improve my health
6. Make my blood pressure better
7. Make me lose/control my weight
8. Help me make healthier choices

9. Make me feel less tired
10. Make me feel happier
11. Help me meet new people
12. Make me look better
13. Lower my cholesterol level
14. Improve my strength
15. Improve my balance

Goals: _____

_____

_____

_____

_____

Steps that I will take to reach my goals: _____

_____

_____

_____

_____

   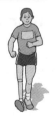

Physical Activity Observation Sheet

Date: _____   Session: _____

Interview: _____   Weight: _____

Ask the following questions (Circle yes or no):

1. Did you **sleep** last night?   Yes   No

2. Have you been **sick** today?   Yes   No

3. Did you **eat** breakfast and lunch?   Yes   No

4. Did you take your **medication(s)**?   Yes   No

5. Have your **medications changed**?   Yes   No

    Amount or type of medication: _____

    _____

6. Do you have any **pain** today?   Yes   No

    Where is your pain? _____

    _____

7. Overall, how are you **feeling** today? _____

    _____

8. In general, how does he or she **look** (e.g., pale, tired, sleepy, agitated)?

    _____

    _____

	Pre-exercise	Post-exercise
Blood pressure		
Heart rate		
Blood sugar (only if participant has diabetes)		

Physical Activity Observation Sheet

Flexibility

Completed stretches for shoulders, arms, back/torso, hamstrings, quadriceps, and calves?

(Circle response.)   Yes   No

Aerobic Training

(Circle response.)   Yes   No

Exercise modality	Exercise workload	Heart rate: _____ minutes	Heart rate: _____ minutes	Heart rate: _____ minutes	Total time	Exercise blood pressure

Targeted Heart Rate (THR) range: _____ bpm

Total exercise time: _____

Balance Training

Completed balance exercises? (Circle response.)   Yes   No

Strength Training

(Circle response.)   Yes   No

Modality	Recommended weight	Actual weight	Recommended repetitions	Actual repetitions

When 20 repetitions are done comfortably (easily), increase weight by 10%.

Borg Rating of Perceived Exertion Scale

Participants should be working at 12–13 (somewhat hard).

6	Very, very light
7	
8	Very light
9	
10	
11	Fairly light
12	Somewhat hard
13	
14	Very hard
15	
16	Very hard
17	
18	
19	Very, very hard
20	

Source: Borg, G. [1998]. *Borg's Perceived Exertion and Pain Scales.* Champaign, IL: Human Kinetics.

Lesson 2

What Is Physical Activity?

also on
CD-ROM

Objectives

Participants will

- State the meaning of physical activity
- Discuss the benefits of physical activity
- Identify different types of physical activity

HANDOUTS

Participant Handout(s):

What Is Physical Activity?

MATERIALS

Blackboard and chalk

Pens or pencils

Personal Notebooks for handouts and pictures

Suggested Activities

INSTRUCTOR ACTIVITY	INSTRUCTOR SCRIPT/DIRECTIONS
REVIEW	*In our last class, we talked about what "being healthy" means to each of us. We also learned that being healthy means different things to different people.*
INTRODUCE LESSON	*Today, we will talk about what it means to be physically active. We will also learn the benefits of physical activity and chat about types of physical activity that we can do every day.*
ASK	*What is physical activity?*
RECORD RESPONSES	List participants' contributions on the board.
DISCUSS	*Physical activity is body movement produced by your muscles.*
ASK	*Can someone show me some of the muscles that you may be using?* Participants may show their upper or lower body muscles.
ASK	*What kinds of things can one do to use these muscles?*
RECORD RESPONSES	• Walk—show leg muscles • Climb stairs—show leg muscles • Lift—show arm muscles • Reach on your toes—show calf muscles • Smile—show face muscles

INSTRUCTOR ACTIVITY	INSTRUCTOR SCRIPT/DIRECTIONS
ASK	*What is good about physical activity?*
RECORD RESPONSES	• Helps us stay healthy, keeps our heart strong, and keeps our blood pressure within normal range • Can increase our muscle strength • Reduces stress and depression, improves mood, and makes us feel good • Increases our energy • Makes you move better • Improves posture • Reduces aches and pains • Helps maintain a healthy weight • Improves immune system
ASK	*What are some examples of physical activity?*
RECORD RESPONSES	**Common chores** • Washing the dishes • Making the bed • Cleaning one's room • Shoveling snow • Pushing a stroller • Raking leaves • Wheeling self in a wheelchair • Dusting or vacuuming • Washing and waxing a car • Washing windows • Washing floors • Gardening • Climbing stairs • Walking • Mowing the lawn **Sporting activities** • Volleyball • Basketball • Riding a bicycle • Jumping rope • Running • Dancing fast • Water aerobics • Swimming laps • Golf (carrying clubs) • Racket sports • Doing exercises while watching television (e.g., riding a stationary bike; doing arm, shoulder, or other exercises with weights)
DISTRIBUTE AND DISCUSS PARTICIPANT HANDOUT: What Is Physical Activity?	Distribute the **What Is Physical Activity?** handout. Review the answers with participants: • Walking • Gardening • Running • Raking • Weight lifting • Mopping • Bowling • Dancing

INSTRUCTOR ACTIVITY	INSTRUCTOR SCRIPT/DIRECTIONS
SUMMARIZE	*Physical activity is any type of exercise or movement. It can be something that you plan to do like walking, running, or playing any sport, such as bowling or basketball.*
	Physical activity may include activities, such as yard work or household chores.

Evaluation

- Did participants discuss the meaning of physical activity?

- Did participants identify the benefits of physical activity?

- Did participants identify different types of physical activity?

Helpful Hints

Adults should engage in **moderately intense physical activities** (e.g., walking briskly, mowing the lawn, dancing, swimming, bicycling on level terrain) **for at least 30 minutes at a time on 5 or more days of the week**[1].

Sources:

[1]Prevention/American College of Sports Medicine. (2007). *Physical activity and public health guidelines.* Available online at http://www.acsm.org/AM/Template.cfm?Section=Home_Page&TEMPLATE=/CM/HTMLDisplay.cfm&CONTENTID=7764

Centers for Disease Control and Prevention (CDC). (2009). *Physical activity for everyone.* Available online at http://www.cdc.gov/physicalactivity/everyone/getactive/index.html

What Is Physical Activity?

Circle pictures of physical activity.

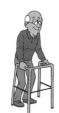

Walking

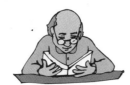

Reading

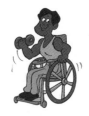

Weight lifting

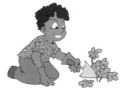

Gardening

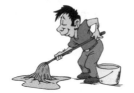

Mopping

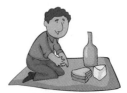

Having a picnic

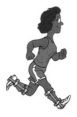

Running

Sleeping

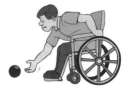

Bowling

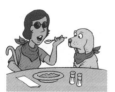

Eating

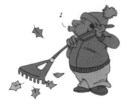

Raking

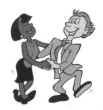

Dancing

Lesson 3

Things to Do Before We Exercise

Objectives

Participants will

- Identify appropriate clothing and shoes for exercising
- Describe the benefits of warm-ups and stretches
- Discuss the benefits of aerobic exercises and cool-downs

HANDOUTS

also on CD-ROM

Instructor Reference(s):

   Recharging Through an Exercise Program and Common Exercise Techniques

Participant Handout(s):

   What to Wear

   Tips: Warm-Ups

   Tips: Stretching

   Tips: Aerobic Exercises

   Tips: Cool-Downs

   Warm-Ups

   Stretches

💡Idea

Field Trip: Visit a store that sells recreational clothing and equipment. Participants should plan to take money for the visit.

MATERIALS

Blackboard and chalk

Pens or pencils

Camera to take photos of participants doing warm-ups and stretches

Personal Notebooks for handouts and pictures

Suggested Activities

INSTRUCTOR ACTIVITY	INSTRUCTOR SCRIPT/DIRECTIONS
REVIEW	*In our last class, we talked about physical activity as any type of exercise or movement that may include such activities as yard work or household chores. Can anyone remember some different types of physical activity?*
INTRODUCE LESSON	*Today, we are going to learn about things that we should do before we begin exercising.*
DISCUSS PARTICIPANT HANDOUT: What to Wear	*What should you wear to exercise?* Write responses on the board.
DISTRIBUTE PARTICIPANT HANDOUT	Distribute and review the **What to Wear** handout.

INSTRUCTOR ACTIVITY	INSTRUCTOR SCRIPT/DIRECTIONS
ASK	*What are some things you should do before you exercise?*
RECORD RESPONSES	You may prompt participants by suggesting stretching and doing warm-ups. Write responses on the board.
DISCUSS INSTRUCTOR REFERENCE: 　Recharging Through an 　　Exercise Program and 　　Common Exercise Techniques	Discuss the benefits of warm-ups and stretches. Discuss the benefits of aerobic exercises and cool-downs.
DISTRIBUTE AND DISCUSS PARTICIPANT HANDOUTS: 　Tips: Warm-Ups 　Tips: Stretching 　Tips: Aerobic Exercises 　Tips: Cool-Downs	Distribute and review tips for warm-ups and stretches with participants.
DISTRIBUTE AND DISCUSS PARTICIPANT HANDOUTS: 　Warm-Ups, Stretches	Distribute handouts. Demonstrate warm-ups and stretches for participants.
TAKE PICTURES	Have participants demonstrate warm-ups and stretches. Take pictures for participants to put in their Personal Notebooks.
TAKE A FIELD TRIP *(OPTIONAL)*	Field trips are extra activities that can be done to give participants opportunities to experience being physically active and making healthy food choices in their community. The lessons can be done with or without the field trip. For this field trip, take participants to a store that sells recreational clothing and equipment (e.g., Sports Authority, Target). Have participants discuss types of equipment and clothing with a sales clerk.
SUMMARIZE	Summarize the importance of warm-ups and stretches. Review how to do warm-ups, stretches, aerobic exercises, and cool-downs.

Evaluation

- Do participants understand the advantages of doing warm-ups and stretches before they do exercises?

- Do participants understand the benefits of doing cool-downs after aerobic exercise?

- Do participants know how to do warm-ups, stretches, and cool-downs?

- Can participants demonstrate how to do warm-ups and stretches?

Helpful Hints

The field trips are designed to give participants opportunities to experience being physically active and making healthy food choices in their community. Units that have field trip activities may be taught with or without the field trip.

Recharging Through an Exercise Program and Common Exercise Techniques

Warm-up exercises

- The warm-up exercises wake up our muscles, stretch our muscles and joints, and get our hearts beating faster.

- Warm-ups and stretches are done before exercising and allow us to work better.

- You may have less muscle and joint injury and soreness during and after exercises.

- Warm-ups give us time to get "psyched up" (mentally prepared) for exercising.

- These exercises help the body "loosen up" by increasing blood flow to the muscles and can prevent injury.

Stretching exercises

- These exercises provide us with a way to maintain or increase muscle strength and give our joints stability.

- Stretching helps us avoid the weakness that occurs in muscles when we are using them less because of a less active lifestyle or a painful joint.

- Stretching exercises offer a way to help relieve stiffness and prevent injuries.

Aerobic or endurance exercises

- These exercises increase the health and performance of our heart muscles and blood vessels.

- *Aerobic* means oxygen.

- Aerobic exercises make you breathe deeply.

- Aerobic exercises improve our ability to function in our daily activities.

- Examples of good aerobic workouts include regular *walking* at a comfortable pace, *bicycling,* and *swimming laps.*

Cool-down exercises

- These exercises are performed at the end of our classes.

- They help prevent blood from pooling in our legs after exercise and decrease the likelihood of feeling lightheaded or dizzy.

_____

Source: American College of Sports Medicine. (2006). *ACSM's guidelines for exercise testing and prescriptions* (7th ed.). Indianapolis, IN: Author.

What to Wear

Clothing

- Wear **comfortable** clothing.

- **Avoid tight** clothing or heavy belts around your waist.

- **Cotton** clothing is best for exercise.

- **Socks:** not too tight, natural fabrics, clean pair daily.

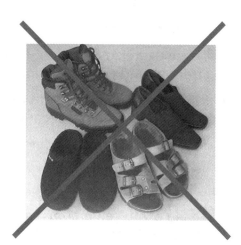

Shoes

- Try on shoes midday or later.

- Comfortable shoes with nonskid surface.

- Adequate **toe room** (finger space at end of toes).

- Snug **heels—no pinching**.

- Flexible **soles** made of rubber.

- Firm **arch supports** (lace up and rubber sole).

- Well-cushioned i**mpact points**.

- Model **specific** to your activity (e.g., running, aerobics, walking, bicycling, baseball).

- If you are experiencing any **pain** in your ankles, knees, hips, or back, you might need a shoe adjustment or a light orthotic in your shoe.

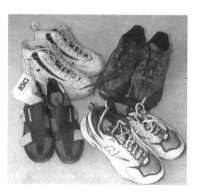

Health Matters: The Exercise and Nutrition Health Education Curriculum for People with Developmental Disabilities
by Beth Marks, Jasmina Sisirak, and Tamar Heller

Tips: Warm-Ups

Why do I warm up my muscles? Warm-ups are the most important part of any exercise program. Warm-ups tell your heart and body that something good is about to happen.

Which joints and muscles do I warm up and stretch?

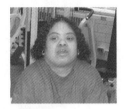
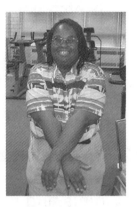

- My head and neck

- My respiratory and chest muscles

- My shoulders and arms

- My trunk and spine

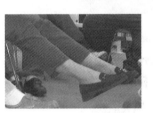

- My hips, knees, and ankles

Exercise with a slow, steady rhythm. Give your muscles time to relax between each repetition. Remember: QUALITY of the MOVEMENT is more important than QUANTITY.

- **Breathe while you exercise.** Do not hold your breath. Breathe in through your nose and out through your mouth. Counting out loud helps you breathe while you exercise.

- **How to stretch each part.** Perform the exercises gently and slowly for 5 to 10 minutes. Make each movement small and stay within a pain-free range of motion.

- A **gentle, sustained stretch** is more beneficial, rather than a bouncy movement.

- Never **force** the movements.

- **Stop if** a movement is **painful.**

- **Stretch each muscle** or joint as far as it will comfortably go and then stretch it a little further (just to where you first feel pain).

- **Hold** each stretch for **5 to 10 seconds.**

- Routines can be performed while lying, sitting, and/or standing.

Tips: Stretching

Why do I stretch? After warming up, begin stretching exercises. Stretching is best when the muscles are warm. Stretching relaxes your muscles and increases the movement in your joints.

1. **Stretch each muscle or joint as far** as it will comfortably go and then stretch it a little further (just to where you first feel pain).

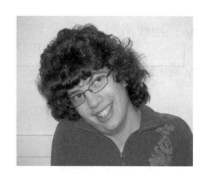

2. **Don't bounce.** A gentle sustained stretch is less stressful to your joints and more beneficial.

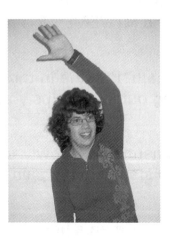

3. Stretch each muscle for **5 to 10 seconds**. Stretching should feel good. If you feel pain, stop.

4. Each stretching exercise should be done between **5 to 10 times**.

5. To maintain your flexibility, make use of the time in front of the television to do more stretching exercises.

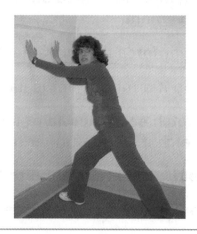

Tips: Aerobic Exercises

Why do I do aerobic exercise?
Aerobic exercises can improve your ability to function in your daily activities.

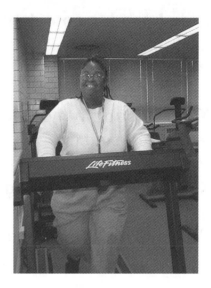

What are aerobic exercises?
Aerobic exercises can include regular *walking* at a comfortable pace, *bicycling,* and *swimming laps.*

How often should I do aerobic exercises? For the most benefit, you should do aerobic exercises for at least **30 minutes 3 to 5 times** each **week**. Every other day is ideal.

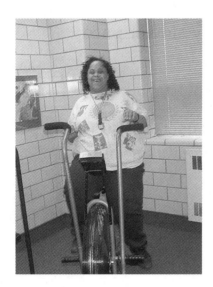

What other aerobic exercises can I do?
Aerobic dance, step aerobic classes, running, aerobic swimming, and cross-country skiing.

Tips: Cool-Downs

Why do I need to cool down at the end of my aerobic exercise?

- Helps us relax

- Keeps blood from collecting in our legs after exercise

- Keeps us from feeling lightheaded

- Prevents muscle soreness after exercise

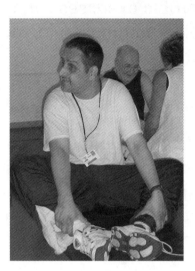

How do I cool down?

- After doing most of your strenuous exercises, take 5 extra minutes to cool down and relax.

- If you were **walking,** walk at a slower pace for 5 more minutes.

- If you were **bicycling,** cycle at a progressively slower pace for the last 5 minutes.

- In our **exercise class,** we have cooled down by using a combination of stretching, contracting our muscles, and using relaxed breathing techniques. You can practice this at home.

Warm-Ups

Basic Guidelines

- If you have pain, stop what you are doing. It should not hurt. Keep moving, but do not move as strenuously.

- Move slowly and in a way that is comfortable for you. Maintain good posture while exercising.

- Do each exercise 5 to 10 times.

- Have **FUN** and enjoy yourself!

1. SHOULDER ROLLS

Arch your torso and roll your shoulders up and back. Look down toward your navel and round your back as you bring your shoulders down and forward.

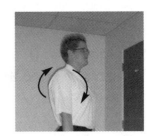

2. SHOULDER SHRUGS

Shrug your shoulders up to your ears then lower your shoulders.

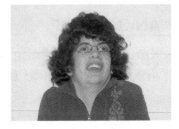

3. HEAD AND TRUNK TURNS

Gently turn your head and reach with one or both hands toward one side while looking over your shoulder. Gently turn and reach the other way.

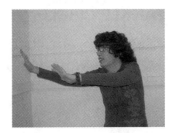

4. ARM DIAGONALS: A

Start with your arms down and crossed, hands on opposite hips. Lift your arms up and out over your head. Then close your hands and turn your arms inward. Pull your arms down and across the front of your body.

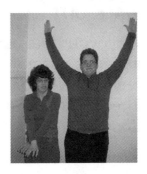

Things to Do Before We Exercise

Warm-Ups

5. ARM DIAGONALS: B

Start with your arms out straight behind your back. Slowly bring your arms to the front. Close your hands and lift your arms up and make an X over your head. Then open your hands and push your arms down and back.

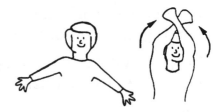

6. LEG LIFT

Straighten your knee while lifting your foot. Bend your knee and place your foot under the chair.

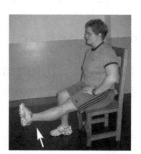

7. ANKLE PUMP

Keeping your knee straight, move your ankle toward and away from you.

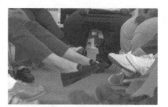

8. ANKLE CIRCLE

Keeping your knee straight, move your ankle toward and away from you in a circular motion.

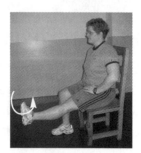

9. WALK OUT

Walk your feet out to the side of your body as far as is comfortable while keeping your feet on the floor, moving from heel to toe. Then walk back in, keeping your feet on the floor, moving from heel to toe.

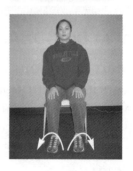

Stretches

Things to Do Before We Exercise

1. HEAD TILTS

Tilt your head sideways, bringing your ear toward your shoulder.

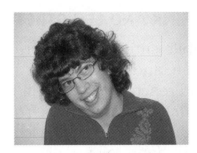

2. SIDE-TO-SIDE

Turn your head to the right and then to the left, looking over your shoulder.

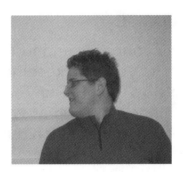

3. SHOULDER BLADE SQUEEZE

Squeeze your shoulder blades together.

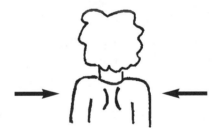

4. TRUNK SIDE BENDS

Gently lean toward your side lifting your top arm over your head and your bottom arm toward the floor.

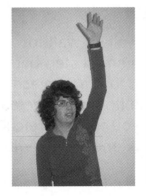
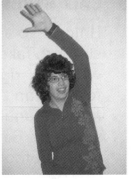

Things to Do Before We Exercise

Stretches

5. TRUNK AND LEG STRETCH

While sitting, straighten your right knee, and lift your foot. Lean forward, and reach with your left hand toward your right foot. Relax. Then straighten your left knee, and reach with your right hand toward your left foot.

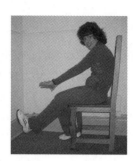

6. HEEL–TOE

Raise your toes and forefeet as high as you can, keeping your heels on the ground. Then raise your heels as high as you can, keeping your toes on the ground.

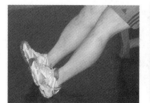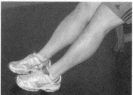

7. LEG LIFT

Hold on to a counter or chair for support. Step back with your leg while keeping your knee straight.

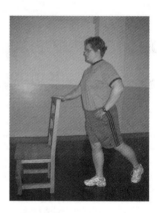

8. CALF STRETCH

Hold on to a chair or wall for support. Take a small step back with your right foot and place your foot flat on the floor. Gently lean forward until you feel a stretch in your calf. Relax and repeat with your left foot.

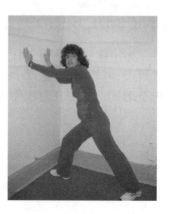

Lesson 4

Exercise Is Good

Objectives

Participants will

- Discuss the benefits of exercise on their health
- Identify reasons why they might want to exercise

HANDOUTS

also on CD-ROM

Participant Handout(s):
  Week 1 News
  Good Things About Exercise

MATERIALS

Blackboard and chalk

Pens or pencils

Camera to take photos of warm-ups and stretches

Personal Notebooks for handouts and pictures

Suggested Activities

INSTRUCTOR ACTIVITY	INSTRUCTOR SCRIPT/DIRECTIONS
DISTRIBUTE AND DISCUSS NEWSLETTER: Week 1 News	Give participants the **Week 1 News** handout. Discuss the newsletter.
REVIEW	*We have been talking about what being healthy means to each of us.* Review examples given by participants.
	We also talked about the benefits of physical activity, different types of exercises that we can do, and the types of clothes we should wear. Review examples from Lessons 2 and 3.
INTRODUCE LESSON	*Today, we are going to talk about what's good about exercise.*
	NOTE: Benefits of exercise is a theme that will be discussed throughout the program.
DISTRIBUTE AND DISCUSS PARTICIPANT HANDOUT: Good Things About Exercise	Distribute the **Good Things About Exercise** handout. Discuss the following six benefits of exercise: weight control, improved posture, strong bones and muscles, heart works better, more energy, and fun.
ASK	*Can anyone tell me why you might start an exercise program?*
RECORD RESPONSES	Write responses on the board.

INSTRUCTOR ACTIVITY	INSTRUCTOR SCRIPT/DIRECTIONS
DISCUSS	Discuss additional reasons why people would want to start an exercise program: • Lose or control weight • Get more energy to do what I want to do • Sleep better • Make my body feel better • Feel more confident • Like my body better • Decrease joint pain and stiffness • Meet new people • Feel happier • Feel less stressed (relieve tension) • Get in shape • Look better • Reduce my cholesterol level • Lower my blood pressure
SUMMARIZE	*There are many specific benefits to exercising regularly.* *Exercise can keep us healthy and helps us do the things we like to do.*

Evaluation

• Can participants describe the benefits of exercise on health?

• Can participants identify why they might start an exercise program?

Week 1 News

NEWSLETTER FOR THE EXERCISE AND NUTRITION HEALTH EDUCATION CLASS

Different Types of Exercises We Can Do

We have been learning about the benefits of different types of exercises.

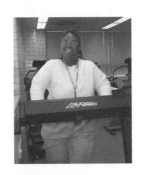

- **Warm-ups** help to "wake up" and "loosen up" our muscles, relieve stiffness, and prevent injuries.

- **Stretches** help to maintain or increase muscle strength.

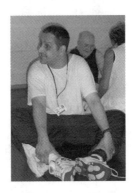

- **Aerobic** exercises help increase the health of our heart and improve our ability to do our usual daily activities.

- **Cool-down** exercises are done after we exercise to keep us from feeling dizzy.

We talked about what *being healthy* means to each of us. Being healthy means eating good foods, feeling happy, having good relationships, sleeping well, working, going to dances, keeping your room clean, keeping your body clean, not being sick, and having friends.

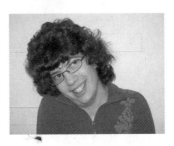

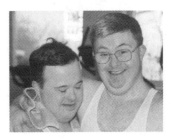

We Talked About the Benefits of Physical Activity and Exercise and How We Can Be More Flexible

We learned the benefits of physical activity and exercise, such as losing or controlling weight, getting more energy to do what we want to do, sleeping better, making our bodies feel better, feeling more confident, liking our bodies better, and decreasing joint pain and stiffness.

We also began learning some stretches and warm-ups that we should always do before we exercise.

Good Things About Exercise

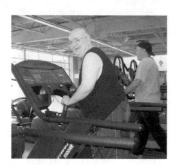

Weight control

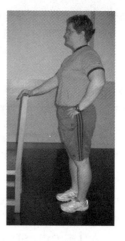

Good posture

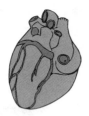

Heart works better

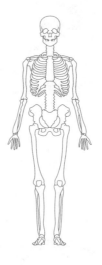

Healthy bones

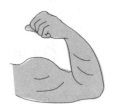

Healthy muscles

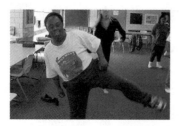

More energy

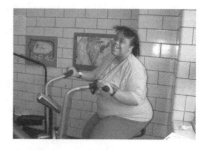

Fun

What Do Different Exercises Do for My Body?

also on
CD-ROM

Objectives

Participants will

- Identify different types of exercises
- Discuss the benefits of stretching/
  flexibility exercises, aerobic exercises,
  balance exercises, and strength/
  endurance
- Practice an aerobic exercise using an
  aerobic video

HANDOUTS

Instructor Reference(s):

    Aerobic Exercise Activities

Participant Handout(s):

    Tips: Warm-Ups *(see Lesson 3 for handout)*

    Tips: Stretching *(see Lesson 3 for handout)*

    Tips: Aerobic Exercises *(see Lesson 3 for
      handout)*

    Tips: Cool-Downs *(see Lesson 3 for handout)*

    Warm-Ups *(see Lesson 3 for handout)*

    Stretches *(see Lesson 3 for handout)*

    Balance Exercises: Anytime/Anywhere

MATERIALS

DVD player and TV

Aerobics video (e.g., Richard Simmons's aerobic
    video, National Association on Down
    Syndrome video, Tai Chi dancing tape)

Camera to take photos of participants doing the
    exercise video for their notebooks

Magazine pictures of different types of exercises
    (e.g., stretching, strength and endurance,
    aerobic)

Personal Notebooks for handouts and pictures

Suggested Activities

INSTRUCTOR ACTIVITY	INSTRUCTOR SCRIPT/DIRECTIONS
REVIEW	*In the last class, we talked about the benefits of regular exercise. What were some of the benefits of regular exercise that were important to you?*
INTRODUCE LESSON	*Today, we are going to talk about how different types of exercises can benefit us.*

INSTRUCTOR ACTIVITY	INSTRUCTOR SCRIPT/DIRECTIONS
REVIEW STRETCHING EXERCISES	*We have talked about warm-ups and stretches. Stretches can increase our **flexibility**. Can anyone tell us why it's good for us to be flexible (or to be able to move our arms, legs, and neck as much as we can)?*
RECORD RESPONSES	You may supplement participants' responses by saying: *Being flexible keeps your joints and muscles from becoming stiff. This can decrease pain in our joints. It can also decrease our risk of injury.*
REVIEW	Review **stretching** exercises to increase **flexibility**. You may do neck rolls, reaching and stretching, toe touching, and side bends for 5 minutes. Remind participants to avoid jerky or sudden movements or stretching to the point of pain.
ASK (BALANCE EXERCISES)	***Balance exercises*** *are another type of exercise that we can do to keep our bodies in shape. Can anyone tell us why balance exercises are good for us to do?*
SAY	*Balance exercises can help you do the things that you like to do as you age. They can also keep you from falling.*
DISTRIBUTE AND DISCUSS PARTICIPANT HANDOUT: Balance Exercises: Anytime/Anywhere	Refer to the **Balance Exercises: Anytime/Anywhere** handout. These types of exercises also improve your balance. You can do them almost anytime, anywhere, and as often as you like, as long as you have something sturdy nearby to hold onto if you become unsteady. Have participants practice the balance exercises.
ASK (AEROBIC EXERCISES)	*Another type of exercise is **aerobic exercise**. Can anyone tell us why aerobic exercises are good to do? When we do aerobic exercises, we keep our whole body moving fast enough to increase our heart rate and long enough so that our body has to use more oxygen. The goal of the exercise is to strengthen our cardiovascular system, or our heart, lungs, and blood vessels. How do we benefit from this?*
RECORD RESPONSES	*What types of things can you do for aerobic exercise?* Supplement responses with the following: running, fast walking, bike riding, skiing, swimming, and doing an aerobics video.
ASK (STRENGTH AND ENDURANCE EXERCISES)	*Other exercises include **strength and endurance** exercises. Can anyone tell us why strength and endurance exercises are good?*
SAY	*Strength and endurance exercises help our muscles push or carry something (e.g., pushing heavy furniture, carrying groceries up the stairs).*
COMPLETE STRENGTH EXERCISES	Ask participants to hold a book in one arm and then bend and straighten both arms for about 2 minutes. Participants will note which arm becomes tired sooner. Other strength exercises that can be practiced include sit-ups (abdominal muscles) and pushups (upper body).

INSTRUCTOR ACTIVITY	INSTRUCTOR SCRIPT
COMPLETE ENDURANCE EXERCISES	Sit-ups and pushups can be used as a test of participants' endurance.
MAGAZINE PICTURES	Have participants identify stretching exercises for flexibility, aerobic exercises, balance exercises, and strength and endurance exercises in the pictures.
ASK	*Does anyone have an aerobic video at home? How often do you exercise with this video? Does anyone go to an exercise class?*
DISCUSS INSTRUCTOR REFERENCE: Aerobic Exercise Activities	*Today, you are going to do an aerobic exercise with an aerobics video.* Instruct the group on how to do warm-ups and stretches before starting the aerobic video. Refer to the **Aerobic Exercise Activities** reference.
BEGIN VIDEO	Have participants participate with the aerobics video. Depending on the group, you may only want to do 10–15 minutes the first time.
ASK	*Did you enjoy the exercise video (state the name of the video)? Would you be able to do this at home or at work?*
SUMMARIZE	*There are four important groups of exercise that must be in your fitness program. These include flexibility/stretching, aerobics to increase our heart rate, balance exercises, and strength and endurance exercises.* *It is essential that all of our muscles (including the heart) receive exercise. This cannot be done by using only one type of exercise.* Review and summarize the benefits of aerobic exercise. Solicit responses from participants (e.g., health benefits, being with friends).

Evaluation

- Can participants identify different types of exercises?

- Did participants participate in the aerobics video?

- Are participants able to identify the benefits of the video?

Aerobic Exercise Activities

Aerobic exercise involves four distinct activities:

1. **Warm-ups**—Warm-ups and stretches prepare the body for exercise and should last for 5–10 minutes. Warm-ups will raise the body temperature, heart rate, and breathing rate for the same reason that we allow our cars to warm up on a cold January morning in Chicago. Our bodies will function better if they have warmed up before exercising.

2. **Stretches**—Ideally, stretching should be done before and after each aerobic exercise session. Unfortunately, stretching is often the most neglected part of an exercise program.

3. **Aerobic exercise**—The goal of aerobic exercise is to maintain our heart rate within a target heart rate zone for a minimum of 20 continuous minutes. If an individual cannot complete 20 continuous minutes, break the session into short multiple bouts.

   Begin the exercise with the warm-up. After the warm-up, begin to increase the intensity of the aerobic activity (e.g., bike, treadmill, stepper) to get the heart rate within the desired range through activities, such as

   • *Bike:* Resistance (or revolutions per minute), speed of pedaling

   • *Treadmill:* Speed or angle of elevation

   • *Stepper:* Rate of stepping or height of step

4. **Cool-downs**—Cool-downs follow the aerobic exercise and should last for 5–10 minutes. Cool-downs help the body transition from exercise to rest. The cool-down phase gives the body time to decrease its heart rate and blood pressure.

Balance Exercises: Anytime/Anywhere

Balance exercises can improve your balance. You can do them almost anytime, anywhere, and as often as you like. You just need to have something sturdy nearby to hold onto if you need to keep yourself steady.

Anytime/Anywhere Balance Exercises

One type of balance exercise is called Anytime/Anywhere. This is a great exercise that you can do almost anytime and anywhere you want to do it.

Three Different Anytime/Anywhere Balance Exercises:

1. Walk heel to toe. Position your heel just in front of the toes of your opposite foot each time you take a step. Your heel and toes should touch or almost touch.

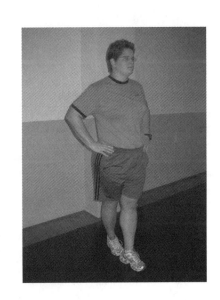

2. Stand on one foot (while waiting in line at the grocery store or at the bus stop, for example). Alternate feet every 10 seconds.

3. Stand up and sit down without using your hands in a slow, controlled movement.

Source: U.S. National Institutes of Health, National Institute on Aging. (2009). *Chapter 4: Sample exercises—balance.* Available online at http://www.nia.nih.gov/HealthInformation/Publications/ExerciseGuide/04d_balance.htm

---

Lesson 6

Good Nutrition

Objectives

Participants will

- Discuss the benefits of nutrition on their health
- Discuss the effect of nutrition on exercise and/or physical activity
- Discuss the effect of nutrition on physical and emotional well-being
- Understand the advantages of including different types of food in their diet

HANDOUTS

also on CD-ROM

Instructor Reference(s):

MyPlate

Getting Started with MyPlate Online Tools

The Food Groups

Making Your Own Nutrition Cards

MATERIALS

Blackboard and chalk

Pens or pencils

Nutrition cards (may create pictures that show different types of food)

Computer with Internet access

Personal Notebooks for handouts and pictures

💡 Idea

Field Trip: Visit a corner convenience store. Have participants plan to take money for the visit.

Suggested Activities

INSTRUCTOR ACTIVITY	INSTRUCTOR SCRIPT/DIRECTIONS
REVIEW	*In our last class, we talked about four different types of exercises that you should have in your fitness program. Can anyone tell me what these exercises are and why they are important? The exercises include flexibility/stretching, aerobics to increase our heart rate, balance exercises, and strength and endurance.*
	Discuss the types of exercises and the importance of doing them.
INTRODUCE NEW LESSON	*Today, we are going to talk about foods that are good for us to eat.*
	NOTE: The benefits of nutrition is a theme that will be discussed throughout the program.
ASK	*Can anyone tell me why you might want to eat healthy foods?*

Diet and lifestyle recommendations revision 2006: A scientific statement from the American Heart Association Nutrition Committee. (2006). *Circulation, 114,* 2–96. Available online at http://circ.ahajournals.org/cgi/reprint/CIRCULATIONAHA.106.176158

INSTRUCTOR ACTIVITY	INSTRUCTOR SCRIPT/DIRECTIONS
DISCUSS AND RECORD RESPONSES	Write responses on the board. *Eating many different types of food can keep us healthy and give us the energy we need to do the things we like to do.*
	We need to eat many different foods to give us strength to exercise.
	Eating good foods may also help us feel happy and less depressed.
ASK	*Can anyone give me some examples of "good" foods?*
DISCUSS INSTRUCTOR REFERENCES: MyPlate Getting Started with MyPlate Online Tools	*When you think about eating foods, it is helpful to think about **different types of foods**. For example, healthy foods can prevent three things that can cause you to have a heart attack: 1) high blood pressure, 2) high blood cholesterol, and 3) too much body weight.*
	Visit www.ChooseMyPlate.gov to identify the amount of each food group you need daily.
	Have participants identify foods that they like and discuss to which group each type of food belongs (e.g., an apple is a type of fruit).
DISCUSS	*It's important to identify foods that we like and how often we can eat these foods.* Review general guidelines to healthy eating.
	• Choose an overall balanced diet with foods from major food groups, emphasizing fruits, vegetables, and grains (American Heart Association Guidelines).
	• Eat different types of fruits, vegetables, and grain products.
	• Include fat-free and low-fat dairy products.
	• Eat lean meats, fish, and poultry.
	• Limit foods that are high in calories and/or low in nutritional quality, including those with a high amount of added sugar.
ASK	• *What types of **vegetables** do you like?*
	• *What types of **fruits** do you like?*
	• *What types of **breads** and cereal do you like?*
	• *What types of **meat** do you like?*
	• *What types of **dairy products** do you like?*
	• *What types of **candy** or other junk food do you like?*
RECORD RESPONSES	Write participants' responses on the board.
ASK AND RECORD RESPONSES	*How often do you eat **fruits and vegetables?*** Write participants' responses on the board. *In general, fruits and/or vegetables are good to eat at every meal and with your snacks.*

INSTRUCTOR ACTIVITY	INSTRUCTOR SCRIPT/DIRECTIONS
DISCUSS INSTRUCTOR REFERENCE: The Food Groups	*Why is it good to eat* **fruits and vegetables?** Record responses. Refer to **The Food Groups** reference. *Fruits and vegetables help to do the following: 1) heal cuts and bruises, 2) keep gums healthy, and 3) protect your body from illness.*
	How often do you eat **breads and grains?** Record responses and discuss the benefits of including breads and grains with each meal.
	Why is it good to eat **breads and grains?** Record responses. *Breads and grains give our bodies energy for work and play.*
	How often do you eat **meat and dairy** *products?* Record responses. *Milk, yogurt, and cheese are good for keeping your bones and teeth strong. Meats are good for growth and tissue repair.*
	How often do you eat **sweets, oils, and fats?** Record responses.
	Fats are high in calories. It's good to think about how much fat, oil, and sweets you eat every day.
	Because some of our favorite foods are candy, cookies, and other sweet foods, we want to eat them in moderation, (unless your health care provider has advised you to not eat certain foods because of a medical condition.)
NUTRITION CARDS ACTIVITY	Have participants take five cards with different foods on each card. Go around the circle and have each person identify whether his or her card is a fruit, vegetable, bread, grain, meat, dairy product, or fat.
	Ask each person whether he or she likes that particular item of food.
REVIEW INSTRUCTOR REFERENCE *(OPTIONAL)*: Making Your Own Nutrition Cards	Refer to the **Making Your Own Nutrition Cards** reference if you want to create your own cards.
TAKE A FIELD TRIP *(OPTIONAL)*	Visit a convenience store with participants. Have participants identify different types of foods in the food groups, such as fruits, breads, dairy, or junk foods.
	Discuss which foods might be best to eat as a snack after they exercise.
	Have participants select a food that they would like to eat as a healthy snack after they exercise.

INSTRUCTOR ACTIVITY	INSTRUCTOR SCRIPT/DIRECTIONS
SUMMARIZE	*There are many specific benefits of good nutrition.*
	We need to eat different types of foods to keep us healthy and feeling good about ourselves.
	It is important to find good foods that we like.
	Eating good foods also helps us do things we like to do. It will be easier to exercise and be active if we eat foods that are good for us.

Evaluation

- Can participants identify the benefits related to eating a variety of good foods?

- Can participants state foods that they like and dislike?

- Can participants state the differences bewteen fruits, vegetables, breads, grains, meats, dairy products, and fats?

- Can participants state reasons why they might want to eat more fruits and vegetables and fewer sweets and high-fat foods?

Helpful Hints

The field trips are designed to give participants opportunities to experience being physically active and making healthy choices in their community. Units that have field trip activities may be taught with or without the field trip.

Unit 1

Lesson 6

Good Nutrition

MyPlate

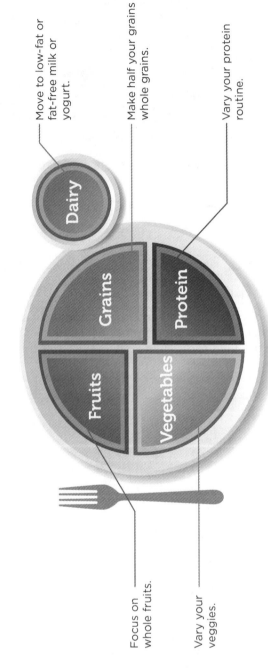

USDA
United States Department of Agriculture

MyPlate, MyWins: Make it yours

Find your healthy eating style. Everything you eat and drink over time matters and can help you be healthier now and in the future.

Move to low-fat or fat-free milk or yogurt.

Make half your grains whole grains.

Vary your protein routine.

Focus on whole fruits.

Vary your veggies.

ChooseMyPlate.gov

Limit the extras.
Drink and eat beverages and food with less sodium, saturated fat, and added sugars.

MyWins

Create 'MyWins' that fit your healthy eating style.
Start with small changes that you can enjoy, like having an extra piece of fruit today.

U.S. Department of Agriculture. ChooseMyPlate.gov Website. Washington, DC. Retrieved, June 15, 2016 from www.ChooseMyPlate.gov.

Getting Started with MyPlate Online Tools

ChooseMyPlate.gov website has great online tools. Here are some of them that you can use during your program.

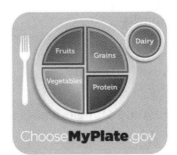

Step 1   Using a computer, go to www.ChooseMyPlate.gov.

Step 2   Click on "Online Tools".

Step 3   Familiarize yourself with the online tools.

SuperTracker   Can help you plan, analyze, and track your diet and physical activity.

What's Cooking? USDA Mixing Bowl   Is an interactive tool to help with healthy meal planning, cooking and grocery shopping.

MyPlate Daily Checklist   Shows your daily food group targets— what and how much to eat within your calorie allowance.

BMI Calculator   Enter your weight and height into BMI (Body Mass Index) calculator to find out your current weight status.

Portion Distortion   To see if you know how today's portions compare to the portions available 20 years ago, quiz yourself.

Quizzes   Test your knowledge about the MyPlate food groups and other nutrition-related information.

U.S. Department of Agriculture. ChooseMyPlate.gov Website. Washington, DC. Retrieved, June 15, 2016 from www.ChooseMyPlate.gov.

The Food Groups

Food Groups	Foods in a group have similar nutrients and have the same function in our bodies. For example, protein is found in both peanuts and meat.
Snacks	Foods we eat between breakfast, lunch, and dinner.
Nutritious	Feeding our bodies.
Less Nutritious	Non-nutritious foods that make us feel full but do **not** feed our bodies.
Feeding Our Bodies	Eating foods that have nutrients help our bodies feel strong, keep us from getting sick, or cause us to weigh too much or too little.
Nutritious Snacks	Nutritious snacks have ingredients that feed our bodies (e.g., fruits, raw vegetables, nuts, whole wheat bread).
	Non-nutritious snacks contain a lot of sugar, salt, and fat (e.g., doughnuts, soda pop, candy, potato chips).

1. **Milk group**—Milk or foods made from milk, such as yogurt, cheese, and ice cream. Butter comes from milk but it is mostly fat, so it goes in another group.

   Main function: Keeps bones and teeth strong

2. **Meat group**—Beef, pork, hamburgers, hot dogs, eggs, fish, and chicken. Also, beans, peas, and nuts because they contain protein.

   Main function: Growth and repair of tissue

3. **Fruit group**—Apples, oranges, bananas, and the juices from fruits.

   Main function: Helps heal cuts and bruises, keeps gums healthy, helps protect body from illness, makes skin softer and healthy looking

4. **Vegetable group**—Potatoes, carrots, cabbage, spinach, corn, and the juices from vegetables.

   Main function: Helps heal cuts and bruises, keeps gums healthy, helps protect body from illness, helps us see better at night.

5. **Bread and cereal group**—Bread, crackers, rice, and pasta, such as spaghetti and macaroni.

   Main function: Gives body energy for work and play

6. **Combination foods**—Many food groups are combined in one meal. For example, pizza may have foods from the milk group, meat group, vegetable group, and the bread and cereal group.

Making Your Own Nutrition Cards

If you want to create your own nutrition cards, you can make them yourself in a few easy steps.

1. **Include participants in the process of making the nutrition cards.**

2. **Collect old food magazines or advertisements from grocery stores.** Cut out foods from different food groups.

3. **Sort foods.** Put pictures of each of the foods in folders.

    Fats, oils, and sweets

    Milk group

    Meat group

    Fruit group

    Vegetable group

    Bread and cereal group

Lesson 7

How Much Energy Does It Take?

Objectives
Participants will • Discuss various energy needs for different activities

also on
CD-ROM

HANDOUTS
Participant Handout(s): Week 2 News Physical Activity Observation Sheet *(see Lesson 1 for handout)* What Activity Needs the Most Energy?

MATERIALS
Blackboard and chalk Pens or pencils Personal Notebooks for handouts and pictures

Suggested Activities

INSTRUCTOR ACTIVITY	INSTRUCTOR SCRIPT/DIRECTIONS
DISTRIBUTE AND DISCUSS NEWSLETTER: Week 2 News	Give participants the **Week 2 News** handout. Discuss the newsletter.
REVIEW	*We have been talking about the benefits of exercise and good nutrition. What are some examples of fruits, vegetables, breads, grains, meats, dairy products, and fats?* Review examples given by participants. *We have also talked about different types of exercises that we do and would like to do. What are some exercises that you would like to do or would like to try?* *We also did aerobic exercises to the _____ exercise video. Did you like that video? Would you be able to exercise with this video at home or work? Who would you like to ask to do it with you?*
INTRODUCE LESSON	*Today, we will talk about what it means to have "energy." This class will help you think about different kinds of activities and how much energy those activities need. Before we exercise, we need to think about how we feel.*

DISCUSS
PARTICIPANT HANDOUT:
   Physical Activity Observation
   Sheet

Using the **Physical Activity Observation Sheet** (Lesson 1), ask everyone how they feel. It is important for us to recognize when we might feel low on energy and need to change our diet or try to get more exercise so that we can feel better or more "energized."

*What does **energy** mean to you?* Participants may say being able to do different things during the day.

*What does it mean to have **lots of energy** or **high energy** to you?*

*What kinds of things can you do if you have **lots of energy** or **high energy?***

RECORD RESPONSES

Record participants' responses on the board.

ASK

Some activities use a lot of energy. What are some examples of these activities? Wait for response.

Some activities use less energy. What are some examples of these activities? Wait for response.

DISTRIBUTE
PARTICIPANT HANDOUT:
   What Activity Needs the
   Most Energy?

Distribute the **What Activity Needs the Most Energy?** handout.

Let us look at our handout. Tell me what activities need a lot of energy. Discuss different energy levels for different activities in the handout.

Supplement replies with examples from the handout.

SUMMARIZE

Some of our daily activities need more energy than others.

Review activities that people can do that need a lot of energy and activities that need little energy.

Evaluation

- Can participants identify different activities that require a lot of energy?

- Can participants identify different activities that require a little energy?

Week 2 News

NEWSLETTER FOR THE EXERCISE AND NUTRITION HEALTH EDUCATION CLASS

Good Things About Exercise

This week we talked about good things related to exercise.

- Weight control
- Improved posture
- Strong bones
- Strong muscles
- Heart works better
- More energy
- Fun
- Meet new people
- Sleep better
- Less pain in my body
- Feel better

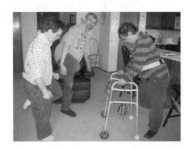

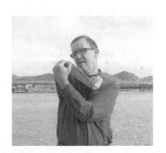

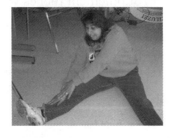

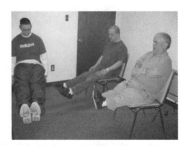

This week we learned that we can do different types of aerobic exercises such as dancing, walking, swimming, and Tae Bo. We did aerobic dancing to a video. In these pictures, we are warming up and stretching before we do aerobic exercise.

We Discussed Foods We Like to Eat and Foods that We Want to Try to Eat More of Every Day

People also said they liked to eat good foods, including bananas, peaches, apples, and apricots.

As for changes, we talked about eating better foods; for example, eating foods like salads, vegetables, and fruits. We also talked about having portions of fruits and vegetables. In addition, we talked about taking a walk with family and friends after eating a "heavy" meal.

Health Matters: The Exercise and Nutrition Health Education Curriculum for People with Developmental Disabilities
by Beth Marks, Jasmina Sisirak, and Tamar Heller

What Activity Needs the Most Energy?

Which of the following activities need a lot of energy?

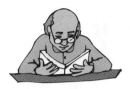

Reading

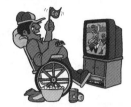

Watching television

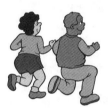

Jogging

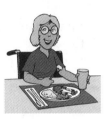

Eating

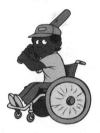

Playing ball

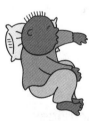

Sleeping

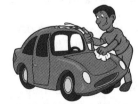

Washing the car

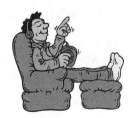

Relaxing

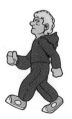

Walking

Healthy Choices/ Self-Advocacy

Objectives

Participants will

- Identify health practices that are healthy behaviors
- Discuss the importance of health behaviors to achieve and maintain their exercise and nutrition goals

HANDOUTS

also on **CD-ROM**

Instructor Reference(s):

   The Americans with Disabilities
      Act and Your Rights (*see Appendix A*)

Participant Handout(s):

   Good Health Habits

   Healthy Choices

MATERIALS

Blackboard and chalk

Video: *Self-Advocacy: Freedom, Equality, and Justice for All*

Reminder Envelope

Personal Notebooks for handouts and pictures

HOMEWORK

Have participants bring in their favorite picture of themselves.

Suggested Activities

INSTRUCTOR ACTIVITY	INSTRUCTOR SCRIPT/DIRECTIONS
REVIEW	*We have been talking about what it means to have "energy." Some of our daily activities need more energy than others. What are some activities that take a lot of energy? What are some activities that need a little energy?*
INTRODUCE LESSON	*Today, we are going to talk about things that we can do that will keep us healthy. We will also talk about how to make healthy choices.*
DISCUSS	*We do many things each day that can make us healthy and some that can make us sick.* Discuss the importance of making good choices for healthy behaviors. Note that participants have the right to make choices that affect their health.

INSTRUCTOR ACTIVITY	INSTRUCTOR SCRIPT/DIRECTIONS
DISTRIBUTE AND DISCUSS PARTICIPANT HANDOUT: Good Health Habits	Ask participants to name habits they have learned that will keep them healthy. Have them identify habits that will make them unhealthy (or sick).
	Distribute the **Good Health Habits** handout. Supplement participants' replies with examples from the handout.
RECORD RESPONSES	Record participants' responses on the board.
DISTRIBUTE AND DISCUSS PARTICIPANT HANDOUT: Healthy Choices	Work with participants individually on their **Healthy Choices** handout. *We can choose many different things for ourselves. This exercise will help us think about the choices that we can make and learn how these choices can affect our health. We will also learn how to communicate our choices.* Remind participants that there are no right or wrong answers, and this is not a test.
DISCUSS	Discuss the pictures of healthy behavior and behaviors that may not be healthy. Ask questions about participants' choices and preferences related to each picture. You might ask these questions:
	• *Did you decide what to eat this morning for breakfast?*
	• *What do you like to eat for breakfast?*
	• *Do you like to eat cake?*
	• *How much cake should you eat?*
	Discuss with participants that some—not all—behaviors may be healthy in moderation if they enjoy the activity.
DISCUSS	*With rights, you also have responsibilities. For example, you have a right to choose to have a job. If you decide to have a job, you have a responsibility to be at work on time. Just as you decide what type of job you like to have, you also have a right to decide the types of exercises you like to do and when you like to do them.*
	For example, some of us may like to use a treadmill to get our heart rate up, whereas some of us may like to run, do jumping jacks, or go speed walking for exercise. Also, some of us may decide at the end of this course that we like to exercise by ourselves in our home, while others may decide that we like to exercise with our friends at a gym or in an aerobics class.
	NOTE: A variety of examples can be given. The goal is to get participants to understand that they can make choices about different types of activities they may like to do and when they would like to do them.
DISCUSS	*We will continue talking about self-advocacy and making healthy choices during the next 10 weeks and when we have our Lifelong Learning classes.*

INSTRUCTOR ACTIVITY	INSTRUCTOR SCRIPT/DIRECTIONS
SHOW VIDEO	Show the video **Self-Advocacy: Freedom, Equality, and Justice for All**[2] to participants. You may need to discuss the video frame by frame depending on the types of questions being asked by group participants.
SUMMARIZE	*Some of our daily activities can help us stay healthy, and others can make us feel bad or result in injuries. We can help keep ourselves healthy by eating right, exercising, getting enough sleep, bathing our bodies, brushing our teeth, staying out of the sun, dressing for the weather, and preventing accidents.*
	Review the ways in which people can advocate for themselves to make individual choices.
GIVE OUT HOMEWORK	*For our next class, please bring in your favorite picture of yourself.* Send a note home with each participant in a **Reminder Envelope.**

Evaluation

- Can participants identify health behaviors that will help them stay healthy?

- Are participants able to make choices to do the things they enjoy?

Helpful Hints

When discussing healthy behaviors, stress that participants have a choice. Some choices may have negative consequences. For example, eating candy may cause you to gain weight. Having carrots might be a better alternative to candy if you are trying to lose weight. Encourage participants to advocate for themselves whenever possible. This is also a good time to bring in the concept of taking responsibility for your choices.

Also, depending on time and the conversation, you may want to refer to **The Americans with Disabilities Act and Your Rights** reference (see Appendix A) to discuss rights for individuals with disabilities.

Source: [2]Advocating Change Together (ACT). *Self-advocacy: Freedom, equality, and justice for all* [Video]. St. Paul, MN: Author. Available online at http://www.selfadvocacy.com

Good Health Habits

Nutrition

Starting with breakfast, eat at least 3 meals each day. Select different kinds of food, and avoid sweets and fats.

Exercise

Get some exercise every day.

Sleep

Get between 6–8 hours of sleep each night.

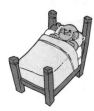

Prevent Illness

- Cover your mouth when you cough.
- Don't touch the blood of anyone with any part of your body.
- See your health care provider for checkups.

Taking Care of Your Body

- Take a bath or shower every day.
- Brush your teeth at least two times a day and floss.
- Stay out of the sun and choose clothes so that you will be comfortable when it's hot or cold.

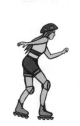

Safety

- Wear a seatbelt in the car.
- Wear a helmet when you ride a bike or rollerblade.

Getting Along

Be kind to others.

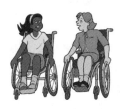

Source: McElmurry, B., Newcomb, B.J., Lowe, A., & Misner, S.M. (1995). *Primary Health Care Curriculum Grade K–8 for Urban School Children.* Chicago: University of Illinois at Chicago, College of Nursing, Global Halth Leadership Office.

Healthy Choices/Self-Advocacy

Healthy Choices

Circle pictures of healthy choices.

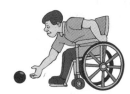
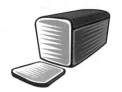
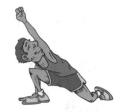

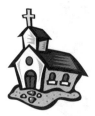
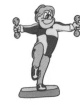
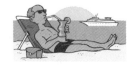

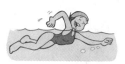
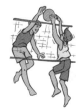

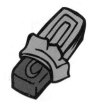

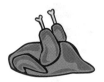

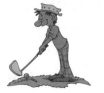

Health Matters: The Exercise and Nutrition Health Education Curriculum for People with Developmental Disabilities
by Beth Marks, Jasmina Sisirak, and Tamar Heller

Changing Lifestyle

What Are the Things We Do?

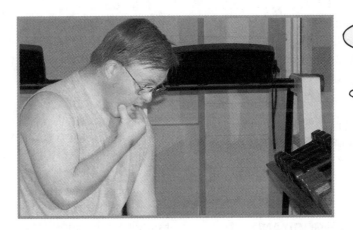

I'm thinking about it!

The contemplation stage is the second stage of behavior change. People in this stage become aware that they should change their behavior and are seriously thinking about making changes in their behaviors. However, people have not made a commitment to take action. At this time, it is helpful to work with participants to consider making lifestyle changes by assessing their exercise and nutrition behaviors.

Unit 2 Contents

Lesson 9

What Do I Think of Me?

Objectives

Participants will
- Identify good things about themselves and things they want to change
- Discuss things that make people unique
- State what their height and weight is

HANDOUTS

also on CD-ROM

Participant Handout(s):
  Good Things About Me

MATERIALS

Blackboard and chalk

Camera to take photos of each participant

Favorite pictures from participants

Height and weight scale

Video: *Disability Identity and Culture*

Personal Notebooks for handouts and pictures

💡 Idea

Field Trip: Take a field trip with participants to a local department store. Have participants identify which section of the department store has the most meaning to them.

Suggested Activities

INSTRUCTOR ACTIVITY	INSTRUCTOR SCRIPT/DIRECTIONS
REVIEW	*In our last class, we talked about ways that we can stay healthy during our daily activities. For example, we can stay healthy by eating right, exercising, and getting enough sleep. What are some other ways that you can stay healthy?*
INTRODUCE LESSON	*Today, we are going to talk about ourselves so that we can do the things that will keep us healthy and happy.*
REVIEW HOMEWORK: Favorite Picture	Ask participants to show their favorite pictures that they brought from home and say what they like about the picture.
ASK	*How would you describe yourself? What are good things about you?*
RECORD RESPONSES	List participants' contributions on the board. Examples of descriptions include hair, eyes, height, weight, skin color and type, race, physical features, talents, personality, and health status.

Source: McElmurry, B., Newcomb, B.J., Lowe, A., & Misner, S.M. (1995). *Primary Health Care Curriculum Grade K–8 for Urban School Children.* Chicago: University of Illinois at Chicago, College of Nursing, Global Halth Leadership Office.

INSTRUCTOR ACTIVITY	INSTRUCTOR SCRIPT/DIRECTIONS
DISTRIBUTE AND DISCUSS PARTICIPANT HANDOUT: Good Things About Me	Review examples of what other people have identified as good things about themselves.
ASK	*Can you identify at least four things that you think about yourself?* Try to have participants state two good things about themselves and two things that they would like to change. You may also have group members identify good things that they like about each other.
TAKE PICTURES	Take photos of each participant conveying something good about him- or herself.
COMPLETE HEIGHT AND WEIGHT SCALE EXERCISE	Have each participant measure his or her weight in a private space. Ask participants if they think their weight is too much, too little, or about right for their height.
WATCH A VIDEO *(OPTIONAL)*	Watch the video *Disability Identity and Culture*[3].
TAKE A FIELD TRIP *(OPTIONAL)*	Take a field trip with participants to a local department store. Have participants identify which section of the department store has the most meaning to them (i.e., that they can identify with or like). These sections may include the following: music, books, cosmetics, clothing, electronics, sports and recreation, gardening, home decorating, or hobbies. Participants can buy something from the section of the store they like the most.
	Note: Depending on your group, you may need to have additional staff on the field trip to help participants identify things that have meaning to them.
SUMMARIZE	*We all have things in common, but we are all different in how we feel, think, act, and look. Beginning today, we'll try to think more about what makes each of us unique so that we can help each other be comfortable with who we are.*
	We described things we liked about ourselves and talked about things we want to change. Sometimes it's easier to talk about our weak areas than our strengths. What we like about ourselves is often the same things others like about us, so it is important to be with those people we like and who like us.

EVALUATION

- Did participants describe unique characteristics about themselves?

- Did participants identify at least two good things and two things they would like to change?

---

[3]Advocating Change Together (ACT) (Producer). *Disability identity and culture* [Video]. St. Paul, MN: Author. (Available online at http://www.selfadvocacy.com)

HELPFUL HINTS

The field trips are designed to give participants opportunities to experience being physically active and making healthy food choices in their community. Units that have field trip activities may be taught with or without the field trip.

Participants may find it more difficult to identify their strong points or their weak points.

Help participants understand that the things we like about ourselves are usually the same things that other people like about us and that it is important to be with people who like us.

Examples of things people want to change include eating better, losing weight, and getting more exercise.

You may also consider showing the film *Disability Identity and Culture*. This is a 22-minute documentary that discusses what it's like to be a person with a disability in America.

Good Things About Me

A good thing about me
is that I like to have fun.

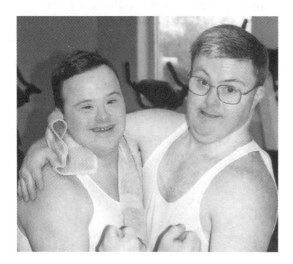

A good thing about me
is that I'm a good friend.

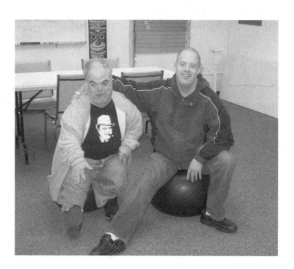

A good thing about me
is that I'm a good dancer.

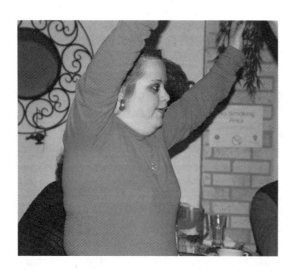

Good things about me include
being an attractive woman and
a nice person to others.

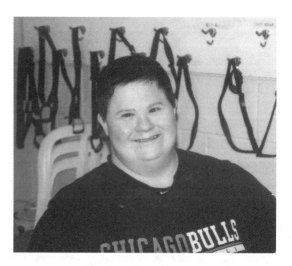

Health Matters: The Exercise and Nutrition Health Education Curriculum for People with Developmental Disabilities
by Beth Marks, Jasmina Sisirak, and Tamar Heller

Lesson 10

What Is My Heart Rate?

Objectives
Participants will • Discuss the meaning of heart rate (HR) • Identify things that affect heart rate • Describe reasons why it is important to monitor heart rate during physical activity or exercise

also on CD-ROM

HANDOUTS

Instructor Reference(s):
    Calculating Target Heart Rate Zone
Participant Handout(s):
    Week 3 News
    What Is Heart Rate?

MATERIALS
Blackboard and chalk Pens or pencils Heart rate monitor watch Wrist blood pressure monitor (see Appendix E for more information on heart rate watches and blood pressure monitors.) Personal Notebooks for handouts and pictures

Suggested Activities

INSTRUCTOR ACTIVITY	INSTRUCTOR SCRIPT/DIRECTIONS
DISTRIBUTE AND DISCUSS NEWSLETTER: Week 3 News	Give participants the **Week 3 News** handout. Discuss the newsletter.
REVIEW	*We have been talking about how much energy it takes to do different types of physical activity and exercises. We discussed keeping ourselves healthy by eating right, exercising, and getting enough sleep.* *We also talked about things that we like about ourselves and some things we would like to change.* Review examples from Lesson 9.
INTRODUCE LESSON	*Today, we will talk about the meaning of heart rate. Your heart is a muscle, and it is the most important muscle in your body.*
ASK	*What is heart rate?* Wait for responses.

INSTRUCTOR ACTIVITY	INSTRUCTOR SCRIPT/DIRECTIONS
ANSWER	*Heart rate is the number of times your heart beats in 1 minute.*
ASK	*What is a normal heart rate?* Wait for responses.
ANSWER	*Your heart rate should be between 60 and 100 beats per minute.*
DISTRIBUTE PARTICIPANT HANDOUT: What Is Heart Rate?	Work with participants individually on their **What Is Heart Rate?** handout.
PRACTICE USING BLOOD PRESSURE MONITOR TO GET HEART RATE	Have participants practice taking their blood pressure by using the Wrist Blood Pressure Monitor. Write down each participant's blood pressure in his or her Personal Notebook.
ASK	*What affects heart rate?*
RECORD RESPONSES	Selected responses could include the following: • Exercise, age, and hormones • Medications[4] (speed up or slow down your heart rate) • Caffeine and cigarettes speed up your heart rate • Stress • Body temperature (cool temperatures lower your heart rate; high temperatures increase your heart rate) • Dehydration increases your heart rate • Different illnesses, health conditions, general health status, and emotional state (e.g., excited, frightened, stressed)
ASK	*Why is heart rate important during exercise?*
RECORD RESPONSES	Selected responses could include the following: • Your heart rate increases when you do any physical activity or exercise. • How hard you exercise is reflected in your heart rate. The harder you exercise, the higher your heart rate. • Because hard work alone does not guarantee better results, it is important to exercise within your personal *Target Heart Rate (THR)* (see the **Calculating Target Heart Rate Zone** reference for more information). • Your heart beats at a certain rate when you're resting, but when you exercise you want to get your heart to a target rate that depends on your age and how in shape your heart is.

[4]Heller, T., Hsieh, K., & Rimmer, J. (2004). Attitudinal and psychological outcomes of a fitness and health education program on adults with Down syndrome. *American Journal on Mental Retardation, 109*(2), 175–188.

INSTRUCTOR ACTIVITY	INSTRUCTOR SCRIPT/DIRECTIONS
REFER TO INSTRUCTOR REFERENCE: Calculating Target Heart Rate Zone	Calculate participants' Target Heart Rate (THR) Zone. Most people will start at a beginner level.
COMPLETE POLAR HEART RATE MONITOR EXERCISE	After calculating participants' THR zone, work with them to put their Polar Heart Rate Monitors on their chests and watches on their wrists.
	Once participants have their Polar Heart Rate Monitor on, have them jog in place or hold their arms above their head while opening and closing their fingers. Complete either one of these exercises for about 5 minutes (or as long as they can do it).
	After exercising for 5 minutes, have participants look at their heart rate on their watch.
SUMMARIZE	*Several things can increase our heart rates. For example, exercise, medications, and caffeine can make our heart rates go up.*
	Review different types of activities that can increase heart rate.
	Running, playing basketball, and dancing are three things on the handout that can increase heart rate.

EVALUATION

- Can participants identify their heart rates?

- Can participants identify which activities increase their heart rates?

HELPFUL HINTS[5]

Some medications increase heart rate, whereas others decrease heart rate. The following is a list of medications that affect heart rate.

Increase Heart Rate	Decrease Heart Rate
Nitrates	Beta blockers
Calcium channel blockers	Propafenone
Vasodilators	
Antiarrhythmic agents like Quinidine and Disopyramide	
Thyroid medications	

[5]Heller, T., Hsieh, K., & Rimmer, J. (2004). Attitudinal and psychological outcomes of a fitness and health education program on adults with Down syndrome. *American Journal on Mental Retardation, 109*(2), 175–188.

Calculating Target Heart Rate Zone

Male	220 – age = maximum heart rate
Female	226 – age = maximum heart rate

Calculating Target Heart Rate for Exercise

Maximum heart rate X exercise level = Target Heart Rate Zone

Exercise Level

Beginner: 50%–60% of maximum heart rate

Intermediate: 61%–70% of maximum heart rate

Advanced: 71%–80% of maximum heart rate

Calculating Target Heart Rate Zone Example

Calculate the Target Heart Rate for 26-year-old Judy.

$$226 - 26 = 200 \text{ (maximum heart rate)}$$

Beginner Target Heart Rate:

$$200 \text{ X } .50 \text{ (50\%)} = 100$$
$$200 \text{ X } .60 \text{ (60\%)} = 120$$

Answer: Judy's heart rate should be between 100 and 120 beats per minute during exercise.

Source: American College of Sports Medicine. (2006). *ACSM's guidelines for exercise testing and prescriptions* (7th ed.). Indianapolis, IN: Author.

Week 3 News

NEWSLETTER FOR THE EXERCISE AND NUTRITION HEALTH EDUCATION CLASS

How to Stay Healthy

We have talked about things that we can do to stay healthy.

- Nutrition
- Exercise
- Prevent illness
- Sleep
- Care of your body
- Safety
- Getting along with others

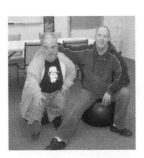

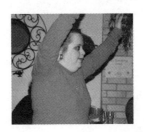

This week we continue practicing different types of stretches and warm-ups before class. We should always stretch and warm-up before we exercise.

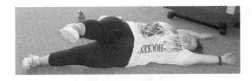

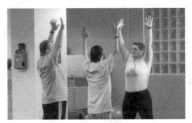

We Learned Some Things about Ourselves and Choices We Would Like to Make to Take More Responsibility for Our Health

Some people said they liked being with friends and family. In their free time, people enjoy doing things like walking and fishing with boyfriends and girlfriends. People like to dance, listen to music, and watch television shows. People also said that they liked to eat good foods, including bananas, peaches, and apricots.

We also started talking about being responsible for our health by exercising and eating good foods. We identified foods that we like to eat but that are not nutritious. For example, some of us like coffee, soda, and desserts. But, we should only eat these things in small amounts.

What Is Heart Rate?

Heart rate is the number of heart beats per minute

Normal heart rate: 60–100 beats per minute

Directions: Circle all of the activities that you think will increase your heart rate.

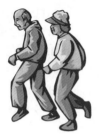

Running

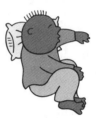

Sleeping

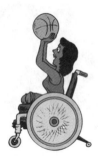

Playing basketball

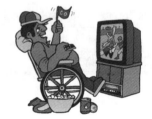

Watching television

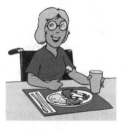

Eating

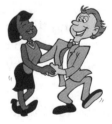

Dancing

Lesson 11

What Is My Blood Pressure?

Objectives

Participants will

- Discuss the meaning of blood pressure (BP)
- Identify things that affect blood pressure
- Describe reasons why it is important to monitor blood pressure during physical activity or exercise

HANDOUTS

also on CD-ROM

Instructor Reference(s):

    Blood Pressure and Exercise

Participant Handout(s):

    What Is Blood Pressure?

MATERIALS

Blackboard and chalk

Pens or pencils

Heart rate monitor watch

Wrist blood pressure monitor (See Appendix E for more information on the heart rate watches and blood pressure monitors.)

Personal Notebooks for handouts and pictures

Suggested Activities

INSTRUCTOR ACTIVITY	INSTRUCTOR SCRIPT/DIRECTIONS
REVIEW	*In our last class, we talked about some things that can increase our heart rates. What are different types of activities that can increase heart rate?* Wait for responses.
INTRODUCE LESSON	*Today, we will talk about blood pressure. This class will help you think about blood pressure while you exercise.*
ASK	*What is blood pressure?* Wait for responses.
ANSWER	*Blood pressure is blood flow through your heart. It is measured by reading two numbers. One is the beating of the heart (systolic) and the other is the heart relaxing (diastolic).*
ASK	*What is normal blood pressure?* Wait for responses.
ANSWER	*Normal blood pressure is below 120/80.*
ASK	*What is high blood pressure?* Wait for responses.
ANSWER	*High blood pressure, also known as hypertension, is 140/90 or higher.*
ASK	*Why is blood pressure important?* Wait for responses.

INSTRUCTOR ACTIVITY	INSTRUCTOR SCRIPT/DIRECTIONS
ANSWER	*Making sure that our blood pressure is within normal limits is very important. It prevents us from getting heart disease, kidney failure, eye complications, and other health problems. Untreated high blood pressure can result in having a stroke.*
ASK	*What affects our blood pressure?*
RECORD RESPONSES	• **Medications**[6] may increase or decrease blood pressure • Physical activity/exercise • Caffeine and cigarettes increase your blood pressure • Stress/anxiety • Sleep • Relaxation • Different illnesses and health conditions • Eating/drinking • Atmospheric pressure • Diet can have positive or negative effects on blood pressure • Hardening of arteries • Standing up too fast may decrease your blood pressure
ASK	*How does physical activity and exercise affect blood pressure?* Wait for responses.
ANSWER	*Any exercise will help lower your blood pressure.* **Endurance exercises,** *such as walking, jogging, swimming, stair climbing, and bike riding can help control blood pressure. Even weight lifting can be used to treat high blood pressure* **(hypertension).** *Practically any physical exercise you can think of can be used to lower your blood pressure.*
DISCUSS INSTRUCTOR REFERENCE: Bood Pressure and Exercise	Refer to the **Blood Pressure and Exercise** reference for more information about blood pressure and exercise.
DISCUSS	• It is normal for your blood pressure to increase during a hard physical activity. • Blood pressure will go back to normal soon after you stop exercising. (See following activity.) • . If you have high blood pressure, it is important to monitor it during physical activity.

---

[6]Heller, T., Hsieh, K., & Rimmer, J. (2004). Attitudinal and psychological outcomes of a fitness and health education program on adults with Down syndrome. *American Journal on Mental Retardation, 109*(2), 175–188.

INSTRUCTOR ACTIVITY	INSTRUCTOR SCRIPT/DIRECTIONS
COMPLETE ACTIVITY	Participants will measure their blood pressure while resting and after they do jumping jacks.

1. Measure resting blood pressure and record that number on the **What Is Blood Pressure?** handout.

2. Do jumping jacks for 1 minute.

3. Measure blood pressure right after completing the jumping jacks.

4. *Is there a difference in blood pressure?* (It should be slightly higher after jumping jacks.)

REVIEW PARTICIPANT HANDOUT: What Is Blood Pressure?	Review the **What Is Blood Pressure?** handout with participants.
SUMMARIZE	*Several things can increase our blood pressure. For example, exercise, medications, and caffeine can make our blood pressure go up.*

Review different types of activities that can increase blood pressure.

Running, bike riding, and weight lifting are three things that can increase blood pressure.

EVALUATION

- Can participants state their blood pressure?

- Can participants identify which activities increase or decrease their blood pressure?

HELPFUL HINTS

Some medications[7] increase or interfere with blood pressure. The following is a list of classes of medications that affect blood pressure:

- Oral contraceptives
- Steroids
- Nonsteroidal anti-inflammatory agents (Aleve, Codeine, Ibuprofen, Motrin)
- Nasal decongestants and other cold remedies
- Appetite suppressants
- Antidepressants

For more information, you may want to talk with a health care provider.

---

[7]Heller, T., Hsieh, K., & Rimmer, J. (2004). Attitudinal and psychological outcomes of a fitness and health education program on adults with Down syndrome. *American Journal on Mental Retardation, 109*(2), 175–188.

Blood Pressure and Exercise

Normal values: 120/80 mm Hg (SBP/DBP)

	SBP		
DBP	< 120	120–139	> 140
< 80	Optimal	Prehypertension	High
80–89	Prehypertension	Prehypertension	High
> 90	High	High	High

Sources: American College of Sports Medicine. (2006). *ACSM's guidelines for exercise testing and prescriptions* (7th ed.). Indianapolis, IN: Author; American Heart Association (2003).

SBP (Systolic Blood Pressure):

maximum pressure exerted when heart contracts

DBP (Diastolic Blood Pressure):

pressure in arteries when the heart is at rest

mm Hg: millimeters of mercury

Hypertension: high blood pressure

DO NOT EXERCISE IF

SBP is > 200 mm Hg   **DBP is >100 mm Hg**

What Is Blood Pressure?

Blood Pressure (BP)

- Blood flow through your heart

- Changes depending on activity, temperature, diet, how you feel, posture, physical state, and medication use

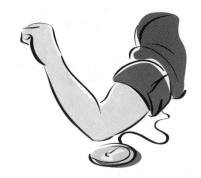

Normal BP: below 120/80 mm Hg

Blood Pressure Cuff

- Soft

- Wraps around your arm or your wrist to see how fast and heavy your blood is flowing

- Is used to find out how well your heart is sending blood through your body

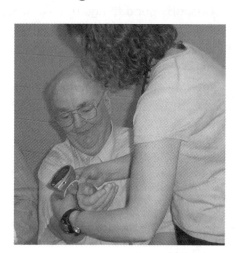

How to prevent high blood pressure:

- Maintain healthy weight

- Do not smoke

- Do regular physical activity

- Eat less salt, and eat as many fruits and vegetables as you can

- Avoid drinking too much alcohol

- Relax

My BP (resting) _____   My BP (after activity) _____

Lesson 12

What Exercises Do I Like in My Community?

Objectives

Participants will

- Describe good things related to regular exercise
- Discuss things that make it hard to exercise
- Identify exercises they are doing now

HANDOUTS

also on **CD-ROM**

Participant Handout(s):

Exercises and Activities I Like

MATERIALS

Blackboard and chalk

Pens or pencils

Magazines (select a variety of sports, recreation, and leisure magazines)

Scissors

Personal Notebooks for handouts and pictures

💡 Idea

Field Trip: Visit a community park with participants.

Suggested Activities

INSTRUCTOR ACTIVITY	INSTRUCTOR SCRIPT/DIRECTIONS
REVIEW	*In our last class, we talked about several things that can increase our blood pressure. For example, exercise, medications, and caffeine can make our blood pressure go up.* *Different types of activities can increase the heart rate. Running, bike riding, and weight lifting are three things that can increase blood pressure.*
INTRODUCE LESSON	*Today, we are going to talk about exercises that we have done and what we like to do.*
DISCUSS	Review and discuss positive and negative aspects of regular exercise. *Let's list some of the ways that exercise helps us look, feel, and remain healthy. Some of these things may make us feel good or bad.*
RECORD RESPONSES	Have participants identify positive and negative things related to exercising. You may want to provide examples of the positive aspects of exercise first and then solicit responses. Then, review examples of some negative aspects of exercise, and ask participants for additional responses.

	Record additional responses from participants on the board.
COMPLETE EXAMPLES OF GOOD AND BAD THINGS RELATED TO EXERCISE	Some good things related to exercise are similar to the reasons that people want to start an exercise program as discussed in Lesson 4. You may want to add the following good things related to exercise to the discussion:

- Helps our bodies become more flexible
- Increases our heart rate and blood circulation and strengthens our heart muscle, which makes it easier for nutrients and oxygen to reach our body's cells
- Helps our bodies last longer
- Helps us to be more alert
- We may get along better with our friends and family because we are happier with ourselves

Bad things related to exercise may include the following:

- May make us too tired to do usual work or activities
- May not be safe, and we may get hurt
- May not have anyone to exercise with us
- Can cost too much money

COMPLETE PARTICIPANT HANDOUT: Exercises and Activities I Like	Distribute the **Exercises and Activities I Like** handout. Have participants circle the exercises and activities they like to do.
COMPLETE MAGAZINE ACTIVITY	Using magazines with pictures of different exercises and recreational activities is another way of having participants identify exercises that they may be doing. Give each participant a magazine. Have them identify and cut out pictures of exercises that they are doing or would enjoy doing.
	You may also ask about activities they might be doing in Special Olympics or with their family and friends.
	Have participants show their pictures to the class and discuss the pros and cons of the exercises that they selected.
ASK	Ask participants to tell the group about any exercises they do or have done. Ask them to demonstrate the activity if it is appropriate.
TAKE A FIELD TRIP *(OPTIONAL)*	Visit a community park with participants. Take a tour of the park and discuss different activities (physical activities and other activities available). Also, try to identify parks in your community that may have fitness stations along the trails. Have participants try these stations.

INSTRUCTOR ACTIVITY	INSTRUCTOR SCRIPT/DIRECTIONS
SUMMARIZE	Summarize good and bad things related to exercising.
	Review the types of exercise that people like to do or would like to try.

EVALUATION

- Did participants discuss positive and negative aspects of regular exercise?

- Did participants identify the types of exercises that they are doing now and what they might like to do?

HELPFUL HINTS

The field trips are designed to give participants opportunities to experience being physically active and making healthy choices in their community. Units that have field trip activities may be taught with or without the field trip.

Exercises and Activities I Like

Directions: Circle the exercises or activities that you like to do.

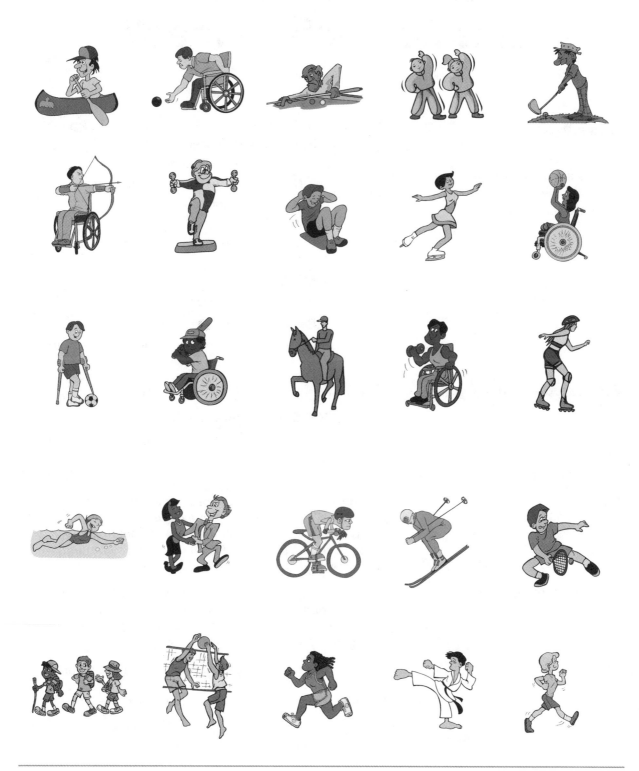

Lesson 13

What Are Good and Bad Influences?

Objectives
Participants will
• Identify influences that may affect their ability/choices to engage in exercise or physical activity

also on CD-ROM

HANDOUTS
Instructor Reference(s):
Positive Things Related to Exercise
Negative Things Related to Exercise
Participant Handout(s):
Week 4 News
Influences on My Exercise and Nutrition Plan

MATERIALS
Blackboard and chalk
Pens or pencils
Personal Notebooks for handouts and pictures

Suggested Activities	
INSTRUCTOR ACTIVITY	**INSTRUCTOR SCRIPT/DIRECTIONS**
DISTRIBUTE AND DISCUSS NEWSLETTER: Week 4 News	Give participants the **Week 4 News** handout. Discuss the newsletter.
REVIEW	*This past week, we talked about our heart rates and blood pressure. We also talked about exercises that we are doing and what we would like to learn how to do. In addition, we talked about activities we like to do in our community. What are some things that you like to do?*
INTRODUCE LESSON	*Today, we are going to talk about why people exercise and why they don't exercise. We are also going to talk about things inside of us and things around us that affect our ability to exercise.*
DISCUSS	Write the word "influence" on the board and then draw two columns. One column is for **internal influences,** and the other column is for **external influences.**
ASK	*What are some things that influence why we do or do not exercise?* Wait for responses.

INSTRUCTOR ACTIVITY	INSTRUCTOR SCRIPT/DIRECTIONS
SAY	***Influences from ourselves*** *are things that we are born with or learn—thoughts, feelings, values, skills, and self-esteem.*
	Influences that are outside of us *may be the people we know and who are close to us, or they may be people we know at work. Not all influences have the same effect on all of us. Also, influences can be good or bad. We may not always be able to control all of the things that affect us, but we can try very hard to make the choices that will be good for us.*
ASK	Ask participants to identify additional influences that may affect their opportunity or choices in being able to exercise.
DIVIDE INTO SMALL GROUPS	Suggest that participants discuss positive and negative influences that have an effect on their life.

DISTRIBUTE AND DISCUSS PARTICIPANT HANDOUT:
  Influences on My
    Exercise and Nutrition Plan
	Distribute the **Influences on My Exercise and Nutrition Plan** handout. Work with the participants to complete the handout.

ASK	• *What's important to you and your family (e.g., job, church, pets)?* • *Which people are important to you?* • *What kinds of activities do you like to do?* • *What do you like about yourself?*

REFER TO
INSTRUCTOR REFERENCES:
  Positive Things Related to Exercise
  Negative Things Related to Exercise
	Use the **Positive Things Related to Exercise** and **Negative Things Related to Exercise** references to guide discussion on positive influences and barriers to regular exercise.

RETURN TO LARGE GROUP	Ask participants to review their answers with the group. Discuss how their answers influence their behaviors.
SUMMARIZE	*Our thoughts, feelings, and actions affect our health and happiness. Information, people, and events in our environment also affect our health and happiness.* *Also, many things affect our choices to be physically active, such as being too tired or not having anyone to exercise with us. We may also decide to exercise if we feel that it will help us feel better or meet new people.*

EVALUATION

• Can participants identify influences that affect their health and ability/choices to exercise?

Positive Things Related to Exercise

- More energy for family and friends

- Relieve tension

- Feel more confident

- Sleep better

- Feel good about myself

- Like my body better

- Would be easier to do usual activities (improve my endurance)

- Feel less stressed

- More comfortable with my body

- More positive outlook on life

- Look better

- Feel happier

- Lose or control my weight

- Be in a better mood

- Make my body feel better (lower blood pressure)

- Decrease joint pain and stiffness

- Meet new people

Negative Things Related to Exercise

- Too tired to do my usual work or activities

- Difficult to find exercises that are not affected by bad weather

- Heart would beat too fast

- Would get out of breath

- Takes too much time

- Less time to spend with family or friends

- Would be too tired at the end of the day

- Costs too much money

- Don't have a way of getting to an exercise program

- Don't like to exercise

- Exercise is boring

- Exercising is too hard

- Exercise will not make me healthier

- Don't know where to exercise

- Exercising is too painful

- Don't have anyone to exercise with me

- Don't know how to exercise

Week 4 News

NEWSLETTER FOR THE EXERCISE AND NUTRITION HEALTH EDUCATION CLASS

Heart Rate and Blood Pressure

We talked about things that affect our heart rate and blood pressure.

- Physical activity

- Exercise

- Medications

- Caffeine and cigarettes

- Stress

- Different illnesses and health conditions

- Dehydration can increase heart rate

- Diet can have a positive or negative effect on blood pressure (BP)

- Sleep can affect BP

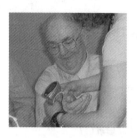

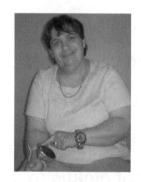

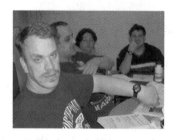

How to Prevent High Blood Pressure

Maintain healthy weight

Don't smoke

Do regular exercise

Eat less salt and eat as many fruits and vegetables as you can

Avoid drinking too much alcohol

Relax

We Discussed Exercises We Like To Do in Our Community

This week, we also talked about exercises that we like to do. We visited a park in our community and talked about different types of activities that we could do in our local park.

Influences on My Exercise and Nutrition Plan

Directions: Use this handout to write down all of the people, events, or things that influenced your exercise and nutrition plan.

Internal influences	External influences
Example: My thoughts about how I look and act, my feelings, my values, my skills, and my self-image	*Example:* My friend(s), mom, dad, or another support person

Exercise and nutrition goal(s): _____

_____

Is this goal a priority?   YES   NO

Resources needed   Who is responsible?

_____

_____

	Barriers	Ways around barriers	Who is responsible
1.			
2.			
3.			

I plan to accomplish this goal by: _____

Lesson 14

Am I Drinking Enough Water?

Objectives

Participants will

- Discuss the importance of drinking water
- State the amount of water to drink each day
- Identify signs of dehydration

HANDOUTS

also on
CD-ROM

Instructor Reference(s):

How Much Water Should I Drink?

Participant Handout(s):

Am I Drinking Enough Water Every Day?

Bottled or Tap Water?

Participant Game: Am I Drinking Enough Water Every Day?

MATERIALS

Blackboard and chalk

Pens or pencils

Personal Notebooks for handouts and pictures

Suggested Activities

INSTRUCTOR ACTIVITY	INSTRUCTOR SCRIPT/DIRECTIONS
REVIEW	*In our last class, we talked about why people exercise and why they don't exercise. We also talked about things inside of us and things around us that affect our ability to exercise.*
ASK	*What are some things that help you exercise? What are some reasons why you might not want to exercise?*
INTRODUCE LESSON	*Today, we will talk about the importance of drinking water. We need to make sure that we drink plenty of water every day. We cannot live without water.*
ASK	*Why is water important?*
RECORD RESPONSES	<ul><li>Carries nutrients and oxygen to cells</li><li>Aids digestion and absorption of food</li><li>Decreases our appetite</li><li>Lubricates joints</li><li>Prevents bloating</li><li>Helps convert food into energy</li><li>Helps fat metabolism</li><li>Protects organs</li><li>Regulates body temperature and blood circulation</li><li>Removes toxins and waste</li></ul>

INSTRUCTOR ACTIVITY	INSTRUCTOR SCRIPT/DIRECTIONS
REFER TO INSTRUCTOR REFERENCE: How Much Water Should I Drink?	Use the **How Much Water Should I Drink?** reference to guide discussion on how much water you should drink every day and the common causes of dehydration.
DISCUSS PARTICIPANT HANDOUTS: Am I Drinking Enough Water Every Day? Bottled or Tap Water?	Distribute the **Am I Drinking Enough Water Every Day?** and **Bottled or Tap Water?** handouts. Discuss the handouts with participants. You may ask the following questions: • *What happens to you if you don't drink enough water?* • *What are some things that you can do to make sure that you drink enough water?*
COMPLETE PARTICIPANT GAME: Am I Drinking Enough Water?	Work with participants on the water game. Answer their questions.
SUMMARIZE	*Several things can make us lose water in our bodies. For example, vomiting, sweating, and fevers can cause dehydration or loss of water in our bodies.* *When we need to drink more water, we may notice that our mouths, skin, or lips are dry.*

EVALUATION

- Can participants state the importance of drinking water?
- Can participants state how much water they should drink every day?
- Can participants report the signs of dehydration?

HELPFUL HINTS

Individual differences:
- Some people (e.g., athletes, construction workers) may require more water.
- People with certain health conditions (e.g., renal disease, congestive heart failure) may require less water.
- Certain medications may dehydrate the body and necessitate drinking more water.

Tips:
- Go to the bathroom before exercising.
- Eating fruits and vegetables that are juicy, such as watermelons, oranges, cucumbers, and tomatoes will help you reach your daily water intake.

How Much Water Should I Drink?

How much water should I drink?

Although fluid needs can be very different between individuals, a general rule of thumb is:

Drink six to eight 8-ounce glasses of water each day

What causes dehydration (loss of water in our body)?

- Vomiting or spitting up

- Having diarrhea

- Sweating

- Drinking alcohol

- Breathing fast or panting

- Having a high fever

- Drinking caffeinated beverages (soda, coffee, tea)

Source: Mayo Clinic. (2008). *Water: How much should you drink every day?* Available online at http://www.mayoclinic.com/health/water/NU00283

Health Matters: The Exercise and Nutrition Health Education Curriculum for People with Developmental Disabilities
by Beth Marks, Jasmina Sisirak, and Tamar Heller

Am I Drinking Enough Water Every Day?

What happens if I don't drink enough water? (What are the signs of dehydration?)

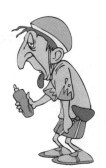

- Increased thirst

- Dry, itchy, and/or saggy skin

- Headache, weakness, or lightheadedness

- Dry mouth

- Dark urine

- Constipation

- Trouble staying cool or keeping warm

How can I make sure I am getting enough water during the day?

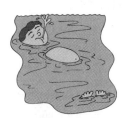

- Start and end your day with a glass of water.

- Do not substitute coffee, tea, or soda for water— they contain caffeine that causes dehydration.

- Drink water before and during meals.

- Carry a water bottle wherever you go.

- While exercising, drink water every 15 minutes.

- Freeze a bottle overnight so you will have cold water all day.

- Get some of your water supply from such foods as watermelon, cantaloupe, grapes, oranges, cucumbers, lettuce, and celery.

Bottled or Tap Water?

Which one should I drink: bottled or tap water?

Choosing one type of water over another is a personal choice.

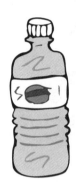

Bottled water

- Bottled water is not necessarily cleaner or safer than most tap water

- Quality regulated by the U.S. Food and Drug Administration

- Sometimes tastes better than tap water

- More expensive than tap water

- Do not reuse bottled water containers—they cannot hold up to repeated use and washings; even the heat from the dishwasher will start damaging such containers.

- Does not contain fluoride, which promotes strong teeth and prevents tooth decay.

Tap water

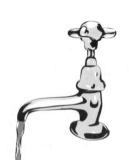

- Water coming from a tap is safe for human and animal consumption unless labeled as nonpotable.

- Quality is regulated by the Environmental Protection Agency (EPA).

- Contains fluoride, which promotes strong teeth and prevents tooth decay.

- If you do not mind drinking tap water and want to use the same water container multiple times, sports bottles made of heavier plastic with wider mouths can be cleaned and reused.

Source: Bullers, A.C. (2002, July-August). Bottled water: Better than the tap? *FDA Consumer Magazine,* 36(4), 14–18.

Participant Game: Am I Drinking Enough Water Every Day?

1. Can alcohol cause dehydration?   Yes   No

2. How many 8-ounce glasses of water should you drink each day?

   A. 1–2 glasses   B. 3–4 glasses   C. 5–7 glasses   D. 6–8 glasses

3. Circle the drink that does not have caffeine.

   A. Coffee   B. Orange juice   C. Tea   D. Soda/cola

4. From the following choices, what is the best beverage to satisfy your water needs?

   A. Tea   B. Diet soda   C. Beer   D. Water

5. How often should you drink water during exercise?
   A. Only after exercise
   B. Every hour
   C. Every 15 minutes
   D. Every 30 minutes

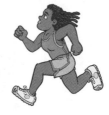

6. I can get dehydrated by:
   A. Vomiting or spitting up   B. Having a high fever
   C. Sweating   D. Having diarrhea
   E. Breathing fast or panting   F. All of the above

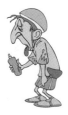

Answers:
1. Yes   2. D   3. B   4. D   5. C   6. F

Lesson 15

What Foods Do I Like to Eat?

Objectives

Participants will

- Review benefits of good nutrition on their health
- Identify favorite foods
- Discuss their eating habits

HANDOUTS

also on
CD-ROM

Instructor Reference(s):
  Soft Foods

Participant Handout(s):
  Foods and Beverages I Like to Eat and Drink
  Putting Foods I Like to Eat on the MyPlate

MATERIALS

Blackboard and chalk

Pens or pencils

Magazines with pictures or food stickers of different types of foods and meals

Scissors

Personal Notebooks for handouts and pictures

Idea

Field Trip: Take a field trip to the local grocery store.

Suggested Activities

INSTRUCTOR ACTIVITY	INSTRUCTOR SCRIPT/DIRECTIONS
REVIEW	*In our last class, we talked about some things that can make us lose water in our bodies. For example, vomiting, sweating, and fevers can cause dehydration or loss of water in our bodies.*
	When we need to drink more water, we may notice that our mouths, skin, or lips are dry. What are some ways that we can make sure that we drink enough water during the day?
INTRODUCE LESSON	*Today, we are going to talk about foods we like to eat. We are also going to discuss our eating habits: what kinds of foods we eat during the day, how often we eat, how much we eat, and the people who eat with us.*
ASK	*How does a person look who eats a balanced diet?*
RECORD RESPONSES	Responses may include the following: • Hair is shiny • Eyes are clear and bright • Weight is normal for height, age, and body build

- Good appetite
- Digests food easily
- Gets rid of waste without difficulty
- Has energy during the day and sleeps well at night

ASK

If I asked why people eat food, many of you would probably say they are hungry or like the taste of some foods.

But let's think back to times when we ate food even though we weren't hungry. Why do you suppose we did that?

Solicit responses. Supplement responses. *People may eat foods that are not nutritious (healthy) because they value the company of friends more than food.*

DISCUSS

Certain foods make us think of holidays and happy periods in our lives. We may eat because we are bored, frustrated, want attention, or are happy.

CONTINUE

In choosing what we eat, we should make sure that we select different kinds of foods so we get the nutrients we need. A balanced diet allows the body to produce energy, grow and repair body tissues, and work properly. A well-nourished person looks and feels healthy.

ASK

Ask if anyone has trouble chewing and/or swallowing any foods or if they are allergic to any types of foods.

DISCUSS

Some foods may be difficult for us to eat or we may be allergic to some foods.

REFER TO INSTRUCTOR REFERENCE:
  Soft Foods

We need to choose foods that are easy for us to chew or swallow and will not cause us to have an allergic reaction or choke. There are different ways of substituting meats, fruits, vegetables, and grains with foods that are easier to chew and swallow.

For example, foods with skins or seeds, raisins, nuts, whole leaves of lettuce, or foods that can easily break apart in the mouth (e.g., dry crackers, scrambled eggs, dry cereals) may be difficult for people who have problems chewing or swallowing.

Refer to the **Soft Foods** reference for more information.

DISCUSS PARTICIPANT HANDOUTS:
  Foods and Beverages I Like to Eat and Drink
  Putting Foods I Like to Eat on the MyPlate

Now, let's talk about the foods you like to eat. Distribute handouts to participants. Have them circle the foods that they like to eat. They may like sweets and other less nutritious foods. Explain that it's okay to like less nutritious foods, but these foods need to be eaten in small amounts.

Next, have participants look through magazines and cut out pictures of food. Participants can use these food pictures to place their food choices on the MyPlate.

INSTRUCTOR ACTIVITY	INSTRUCTOR SCRIPT/DIRECTIONS
CONTINUE	Have participants show their pictures to the class and discuss the pros and the cons of the foods they selected.
	Have them identify such food choices as a fruit, vegetable, bread, grain, meat, dairy product, fat, or oil.
	Talk about the importance of limiting how much they eat or substituting the food item with low-fat alternatives or soft foods that are easier to chew and swallow.
TAKE A FIELD TRIP *(OPTIONAL)*	Before going to the grocery store, discuss an upcoming holiday or a season that you are in. Look up fruits and vegetables that are in season at http://www.fieldtoplate.com, and then go to a grocery store and find the fruits and vegetables that are in season. How do they look (e.g., fresh, juicy)? Look at the fruits and vegetables that are not in season. How do they look (e.g., green, hard, not even on the shelves)? For example, you may not be able to find strawberries in every season.
	If you choose to do a holiday, discuss what foods are typically eaten for that holiday. Discuss healthier alternatives to a holiday meal. Participants will then go to the grocery store. Identify holiday foods and find healthier alternatives for these foods.
SUMMARIZE	Summarize the importance of nutrition on exercise/ physical activity, physical and emotional well-being, stress, and long-term exercise/physical activity.
	It's important to pick foods that we like so that we can eat a balanced diet every day.

EVALUATION

- Can participants state the benefits of good nutrition on their health?
- Did participants identify their favorite foods?
- Did participants discuss their eating habits?
- Did participants identify healthy foods and unhealthy foods?

HELPFUL HINTS

The field trips are designed to give participants opportunities to experience being physically active and making healthy choices in their community. Units that have field trip activities may be taught with or without the field trip.

When participants identify foods high in fats or oils, stress that the goals is not necessarily to not eat these foods but to reduce the amount and frequency.

Present alternatives to the foods high in fat that they can have in small quantities every day.

Read the nutrition facts on food labels to choose foods that have less than 3 grams of fat and more than 2 grams of fiber per serving to lower your fat intake and increase your fiber.

Soft Foods

Dairy foods:

- Low-fat or no-fat cottage cheese
- Nonfat, sugar-free yogurt
- Frozen or regular sugar-free or fat-free pudding
- Sugar-free or fat-free ice cream
- Low-fat frozen yogurt or ice cream

Fruits and vegetables:

- Unsweetened applesauce
- Canned peaches and pears in their own juice
- Soft fruits—watermelon, honeydew, cantaloupe, bananas, strawberries, or ripe peaches (chewed thoroughly)
- Any vegetables (EXCLUDING CORN), including potatoes cooked soft and mashed with a fork
- Soups—it may be necessary to blend slightly to break up large chunks—split pea soup, bean soups
- Fat-free refried beans

Breads and grains:

- Unsweetened oatmeal
- Cream of Wheat and grits
- Cornmeal

Meat, fish, poultry, and eggs:

- Baked/poached fish fillets or crabmeat—cooked very soft and moist
- Tuna salad, chicken salad
- Eggs—scrambled, soft-boiled, and in the form of egg salad. (Because eggs are high in fat and cholesterol, they should only be eaten every once in a while.)
- Peanut butter is very high in fat, but it is also a good source of protein, so use sparingly.

Source: American Cancer Society. (2008). *Trouble swallowing.* Available online at http://www.cancer.org/docroot/MBC/content/ MBC_6_2X_Difficulty_with_swallowing.asp

Unit 2

Lesson 15

What Foods Do I Like to Eat?

Foods and Beverages I Like to Eat and Drink

Directions: Circle the foods that you like to eat.

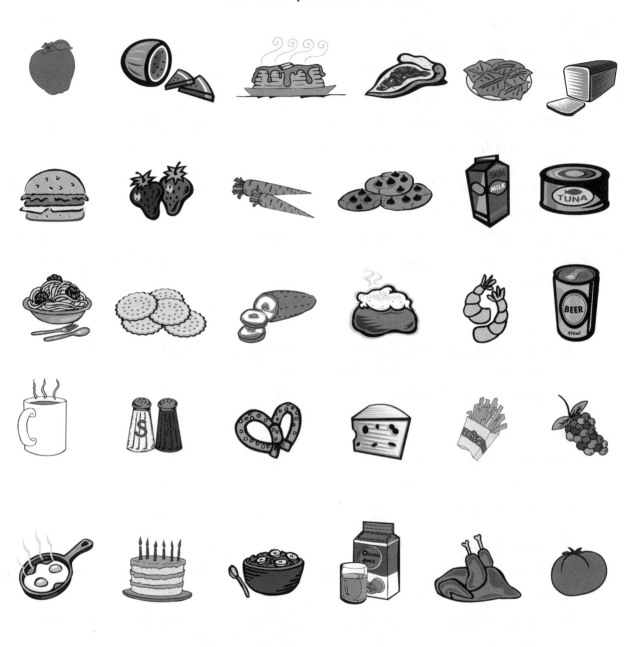

Health Matters: The Exercise and Nutrition Health Education Curriculum for People with Developmental Disabilities
by Beth Marks, Jasmina Sisirak, and Tamar Heller

Putting Foods I Like to Eat on the MyPlate

Directions: Place pictures of food items on the MyPlate in each corresponding category.

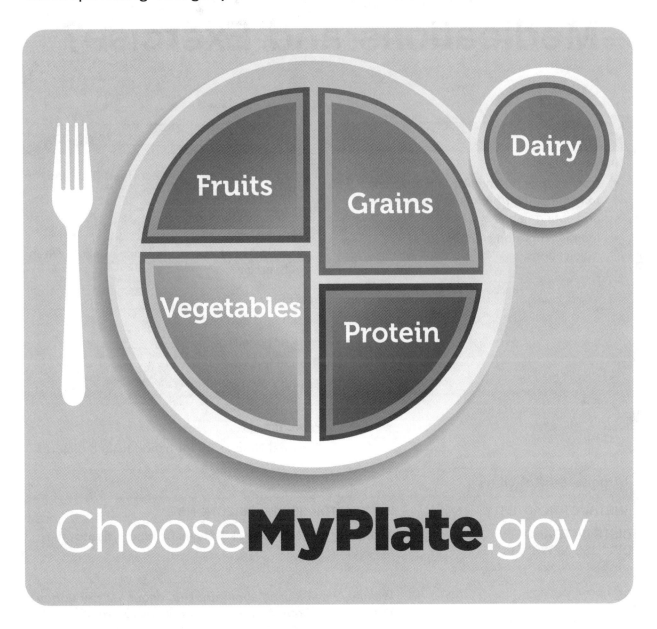

How About My Medications and Exercise?

also on
CD-ROM

Objectives

Participants will

- Discuss how the medications they take may affect their body, physical activity, and eating habits
- Identify common side effects of medications

HANDOUTS

Instructor Reference(s):

How Do Medications Affect Heart Rate and Blood Pressure?

Participant Handout(s):

Week 5 News

How Do My Medications Make Me Feel When I Exercise?

MATERIALS

Blackboard and chalk

Pens or pencils

Orange juice

Strong flavored mints

Small paper cups

Paper towels

Personal Notebooks for handouts and pictures

Suggested Activities

INSTRUCTOR ACTIVITY	INSTRUCTOR SCRIPT/DIRECTIONS
DISTRIBUTE AND DISCUSS NEWSLETTER: Week 5 News	Give participants the **Week 5 News** handout. Discuss the newsletter.
REVIEW	*We have been talking about drinking enough water during the day and about the things that help us to exercise and things that make it hard for us to exercise.*
	We have also been talking about the importance of nutrition on exercise/physical activity, physical and emotional well-being, stress, and long-term exercise/ physical activity.
	It's important to pick foods that we like so that we can eat a balanced diet every day.

Source: Pronsky, Z.M. (2008). *Food–medication interactions* (15th ed.). Birchrunville, PA: Food Medication Interactions.

INSTRUCTOR ACTIVITY	INSTRUCTOR SCRIPT/DIRECTIONS
INTRODUCE LESSON	*Today, we will talk about how medications affect our bodies. Medications may make our bodies feel better. Some medications may make one part of our body feel better but also do something to another part of the body that is not expected. This is called a medication side effect.*
ASK AND DISCUSS	*Does anyone want to share if they have taken any medications? You don't have to tell us what medication you were taking, but just think about how that medication made you feel.* *Did this medication make you feel a certain way?*
DISCUSS	**Medications may make us:** • More hungry—we may gain weight • Less hungry—we may lose weight • More thirsty—we may get dehydrated • Tired or sleepy—we cannot pay attention or stay awake • Dizzy—we may have a hard time walking or keeping our balance • Shaky—we may have a hard time doing certain tasks, like stitching, writing, or holding something firmly • Bloated and/or constipated—our stomachs may feel full, or we may not be able to go to the bathroom • Nauseated—we may feel uncomfortable or sick
DISCUSS	**Medications may change sense of smell, taste, and perception of texture. Medications may give us:** • Cotton or dry mouth • Metallic taste • Things may smell differently or you may lose your sense of smell
ASK	*Has anyone felt any of these changes?*
DISCUSS	**You may experience the following when you take medications:** • Vomiting • Diarrhea • Constipation • Dehydration *All of these things are called medication side effects. Side effects impact how we feel, which may affect our physical activity.*
REFER TO INSTRUCTOR REFERENCE: How Do Medications Affect Heart Rate and Blood Pressure?	Use the **How Do Medications Affect Heart Rate and Blood Pressure?** reference to guide discussion on how our medications may change our heart rate and blood pressure.

INSTRUCTOR ACTIVITY	INSTRUCTOR SCRIPT/DIRECTIONS
COMPLETE PARTICIPANT ACTIVITY: The Taste, Smell, and Flavor Experiment	1. Take a sip of orange juice. Discuss the taste, smell, and flavor. 2. Take a mint and let it melt in your mouth. 3. Take another sip of orange juice. Discuss the taste, smell, and flavor.
ASK	*Has the taste, smell, or flavor of orange juice changed? Why?* *This is called a medication side effect. The mint changes how we taste the orange juice.*
DISTRIBUTE AND DISCUSS PARTICIPANT HANDOUT: How Do My Medications Make Me Feel When I Exercise?	Distribute the **How Do My Medications Make Me Feel When I Exercise?** handout. Discuss the handout with participants.
ASK	*How do medications change our senses of smell, taste, and flavor?*
SUMMARIZE	*Medications that we take can affect our bodies. Although medications make our bodies feel better, some medications may make one part of our bodies feel better but also do something to another part of our bodies that is not expected. Does anyone remember what this is called?* *This is called a medication side effect.*

EVALUATION

- Can participants state how medications can alter taste, smell, and flavor of foods?
- Can participants state common side effects from taking medications?

How Do Medications Affect Heart Rate and Blood Pressure?

ANTIDEPRESSANTS

Mechanism of action:
- Block the uptake of norepinephrine (hormone) into the central nervous system synapses

Commonly used to treat:
- Depression

Effect at rest:
- Increase HR, may cause hypotension (abnormally low BP)

Effects during exercise:
- Increase HR, decrease or maintain BP, and increase the risk for arrhythmias (irregular heart beats)

Caution:
- Careful with cardiac rehabilitation

Examples:
- Prozac
- Norpramin
- Elavil

BETA BLOCKERS

Mechanism of action:
- Blocks beta-receptors of the sympatheic nervous system. Some agents act primarily on beta-receptors in the heart. These are called *cardioselective.* Beta-blockers decrease HR, BP, and contractility of the heart, thus reducing the demand for oxygen by the heart.

Commonly used to treat:
- Angina pectoris, hypertension (high blood pressure), previous myocardial infarction (heart attack), arrhythmias (irregular heartbeats), migraine headaches

Effect at rest:
- Decreased HR, decreased BP, decreased arrhythmias (irregular heatbeats)

Effect during exercise:
- Increased exercise ability in patients with angina (chest pain), exercise ability decreased in patients without angina (chest pain), decreased exercise ischemia (not enough blood getting to a place, causing lack of oxygen), decreased HR, decreased BP

Examples:
- Inderal
- Lopressor

BRONCHODIALATORS/ANTIHISTAMINES

Mechanism of action:
- Inhibit bronchial smooth muscle constriction in patients with asthma or Chronic Obstructive Pulmonary Disease (COPD)

Sources:
Pronsky, Z.M. (2008). *Food–medication interactions* (15th ed.). Birchrunville, PA: Food Medication Interactions.
Durstine, K.L., & Moore, G.E. (2003). *ACSM's exercise management for persons with chronic diseases and disabilities* (2nd ed.). Champaign, IL: Human Kinetics.

How About My Medications and Exercise?

How Do Medications Affect Heart Rate and Blood Pressure?

BRONCHODIALATORS/ANTIHISTAMINES *(continued)*

Commonly used to treat:
- Asthma, COPD

Effect at rest:
- May produce arrhythmia (irregular heart beat), bronchodialtors may increase HR or BP

Effect during exercise:
- May produce Premature Ventricular Contractions (PVCs) and dysrhythmias (abnormal heart rhythm), bronchodialtors may increase HR or BP

Examples:
- Theo-Dur
- Theophylline

Note: The decongestant pseudoephedrine (sometimes combined with certain antihistamines) can increase HR and BP. This effect may lessen after continued use.

CALCIUM CHANNEL BLOCKERS

Mechanism of action:
- Causes a vasodilation (widening of blood vessels) and a lower resting BP

Commonly used to treat:
- Angina pectoris (chest pain), coronary artery spasm, arrhythmias (irregular heart beats), hypertension (high blood pressure)

Effect at rest:
- *Nifedipine (Procardia)*—increased HR and BP
- *Other calcium channel blockers*—decreased HR, decreased BP, decreased ischemia (not enough blood pressure getting to a place, causing lack of oxygen). Check individual medication!

Effect during exercise:
- Same as rest, may increase exercise ability

Examples:
- Cardizem
- Procardia

DIGITALIS

Mechanism of action:
- Improves myocardial (heart) contraction by altering the calcium utilization of the myocardial cell.

Commonly used to treat:
- Congestive heart failure (CHF), atrial fibrillation (complex irregular hear beat), atrial flutter (irregular beat)

How Do Medications Affect Heart Rate and Blood Pressure?

DIGITALIS *(continued)*

Effect at rest:
- May decrease HR

Effect during exercise:
- May decrease HR, will improve exercise ability only in people with atrial fibrillation or CHF

Examples:
- Lanoxin
- Digitalis

DIURETICS

Mechanism of action:
- Most diuretics alter renal (kidney) function, causing an increase in the excretion of fluid.
- CAUTION: Sodium and potassium levels may be depleted. Calcium supplement may also be necessary.

Commonly used to treat:
- Hypertension (high blood pressure), edema (swelling)

Effect at rest:
- Decreased BP

Effect during exercise:
- May decrease BP, may affect congestive heart failure (CHF) patients, may cause arrhythmias (irregular heart beat)

Examples:
- Lasix
- Dyazide
- Hydro-Diuril

THYROID MEDICATION (ONLY LEVOTHYROXINE)

Mechanism of action:
- Hormonal regulation

Commonly used to treat:
- To correct abnormal and irregular release of hormones due to thyroid dysfunction

Effect at rest:
- Increase HR and BP, may increase ischemia (not enough blood getting to a place, causing lack of oxygen)

Effect during exercise:
- Same effects as rest may be exaggerated

Examples:
- Syntrox

Week 5 News

NEWSLETTER FOR THE EXERCISE AND NUTRITION HEALTH EDUCATION CLASS

How Can We Make Sure that We Drink Enough Water Every Day?

- Start and end your day with a glass of water.

- Do not substitute coffee, tea, or soda for water. They contain caffeine that causes dehydration.

- Drink water before and during meals.

- Carry a water bottle wherever you go.

- While exercising, drink water every 15 minutes.

- Freeze a bottle of water so you have cold water all day.

- Get some of your water supply from foods such as watermelon, cantaloupe, grapes, oranges, cucumbers, lettuce, and celery.

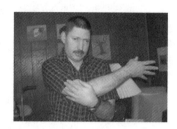
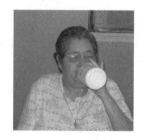
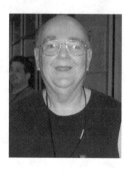
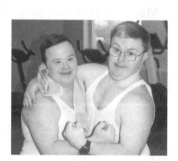

We talked about the importance of nutrition on exercise/physical activity, physical and emotional well-being, stress, and long-term exercise/physical activity.

Good and Bad Influences

We talked about things that help us exercise and things that make it hard for us to exercise regularly. We also talked about having our friends or family encourage us to exercise or to exercise with us.

How Do My Medications Make Me Feel When I Exercise?

Medications may make us:

More hungry—
weight gain

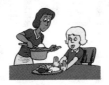

Less hungry—
weight loss

More thirsty

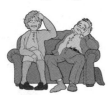

Tired/sleepy

Dizzy

Shaky

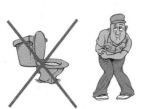

Bloated/
constipated

Nauseated

Medications may change sense of smell, taste, and texture (how things feel):

- Cotton or dry mouth
- Metallic taste
- Things may smell differently or you may lose your sense of smell.

You may experience the following:

- Diarrhea
- Constipation
- Dehydration
- Vomiting

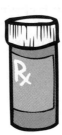

Unit 3

Making Lifestyle Changes

Setting Goals

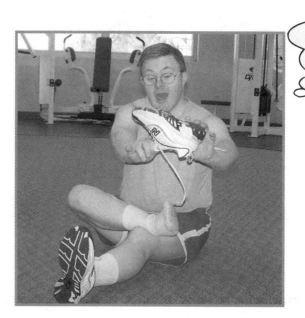

I'm making plans!

During the third stage, preparation, people are ready to take action and change a specific behavior. You should structure your classes on setting goals and examining barriers and influences that may affect participants' abilities to exercise or eat a more nutritious diet.

Unit 3 Contents

Lesson 17

Things to Remember When Exercising

Objectives	HANDOUTS
Participants will	Participant Handout(s):
• Describe the things they need to do in order to exercise	Things to Remember When Starting an Exercise Plan
• Discuss types of clothing to wear when they exercise	**MATERIALS**
	Blackboard and chalk
	Pens or pencils
	Personal Notebooks for handouts and pictures

Suggested Activities

INSTRUCTOR ACTIVITY	INSTRUCTOR SCRIPT/DIRECTIONS
REVIEW	*In our last class, we talked about how medications that we take can affect our bodies. Although medications can make our bodies feel better, some medications may make one part of our body feel better but also do something to another part of the body that is not expected.*
ASK	*Does anyone want to share with the class how some of your medications make you feel?*
INTRODUCE LESSON	*Today, we are going to talk about things that we need to do before we start an exercise program.*
DISTRIBUTE PARTICIPANT HANDOUT: Things to Remember When Starting an Exercise Plan	Distribute the **Things to Remember When Starting an Exercise Plan** handout.
ASK AND REVIEW PARTICIPANT HANDOUT	Ask participants questions about the types of things they need to have and do before they exercise. Review the handout. Add additional responses from participants.
TAKE PICTURES	Take pictures of participants demonstrating things that they should do before starting their exercise program as appropriate for their Personal Notebooks.
SUMMARIZE	Review participants' responses and the handout.

EVALUATION

• Are participants able to describe the things they need to do before they exercise?

Things to Remember When Starting an Exercise Plan

GET AN OK

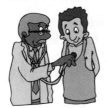

FROM YOUR DOCTOR
OR HEALTH CARE PROVIDER

CHOOSE A GOOD TIME

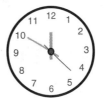

TO EXERCISE

WEAR THE RIGHT CLOTHES

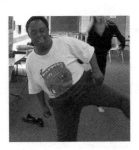

- Sweat pants
- T-shirt
- Tennis shoes

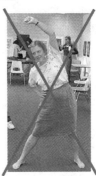

STRETCH FIRST...

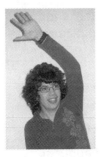

with trunk side bends

...THEN WARM UP

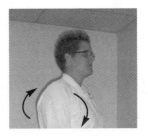

beginning with shoulder rolls

START SLOWLY

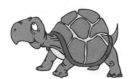

EXERCISE REGULARLY

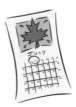

Use a calendar to mark the days
and times that you want to exercise

Community Fitness Center Visit

Using Exercise Machines Safely

Objectives

Participants will

- Discuss how to stay safe during physical activity
- Review when to slow down or stop exercising

HANDOUTS

also on CD-ROM

Instructor Reference(s):

  Warm-Ups, Stretches, and Cool-Downs Safety Tips

Participant Handout(s):

  Staying Safe During Physical Activity

MATERIALS

Blackboard and chalk

Pens or pencils

Heart rate monitors

Personal Notebooks for handouts and pictures

Idea

Field Trip: Visit to a local community fitness center.

Suggested Activities

INSTRUCTOR ACTIVITY	INSTRUCTOR SCRIPT/DIRECTIONS
REVIEW	*In our last class, we talked about some things we need to do before we exercise. Can anyone tell us what some of those things were?*
	It's important to make sure that we feel okay to exercise. We should make sure that we have eaten and have taken our medications (if we are taking medications). We should also make sure that we are wearing loose fitting and comfortable clothes.
INTRODUCE LESSON	*Today, we will talk about how to stay safe during physical activity and exercise. In this class, we will talk about the importance of* **warm-ups** *and* **stretching** *and exercising at a slow and steady pace without overdoing it.*

INSTRUCTOR ACTIVITY	INSTRUCTOR SCRIPT/DIRECTIONS
REFER TO INSTRUCTOR REFERENCE: Warm-Ups, Stretches, and Cool-Downs Safety Tips	Review the **Warm-Ups, Stretches, and Cool-Downs Safety Tips** reference.
ASK AND DISCUSS	*What should we do before we start exercising?*
	Always start with 5–10 minutes of warm-up exercises. These are low-intensity exercises, such as brisk walking, jumping jacks, or easy jogging to get your muscles going. After warming up, you should stretch for another 5–10 minutes. Let's do some warm-ups. Let's do some stretches.
	Warm-ups and stretches are a must!
ASK AND WAIT FOR RESPONSES	*Should you start exercising as fast as you can or should you start slowly and build up?*
	Your workout should not be so intense that you feel pain, fatigued, unwell, or gasping for air.
	Exercise at a slow and steady pace!
ASK AND WAIT FOR RESPONSES	*How hard (or fast) should you exercise?*
	For your heart (cardiovascular activity), exercise so you feel that your heart is working harder but you do not feel short of breath. You should be able to have a normal conversation while exercising.
	Don't take your breath away!
ASK AND WAIT FOR RESPONSES	*What about heart rate monitors?*
	Use your heart rate monitors to see how hard you are exercising. (Medication for your heart or blood pressure may affect your heart rate, so please check with your health care provider.)
	Don't take your breath away!
ASK AND WAIT FOR RESPONSES	*How fast should your heart beat?*
	For beginners, aim for 50% to 60% of your maximum heart rate. Your maximum heart rate can be estimated using the following formula:
	Men—[220 minus (your age)]
	Women—[226 minus (your age)]
	Review Heart Rate Session (Lesson 10)
	Your heart is your guide!
ASK AND WAIT FOR RESPONSES	*What should you do at the end of your exercise session?*
	End your exercise sessions with slow, cool-down exercises and stretches.
	Don't forget cool-downs!

INSTRUCTOR ACTIVITY	INSTRUCTOR SCRIPT/DIRECTIONS
ASK AND WAIT FOR RESPONSES	*What if you get too hot?* • *End exercise sessions with slow cool-down exercises.* • *In general, take sips of water every 15 minutes while exercising.* • *Plain water is the best for activities that take less than an hour.* • *Wear loose fitting clothes that allow your skin to breathe.* **Don't get too hot!**
ASK AND WAIT WAIT FOR RESPONSES	*When should you get help from your staff or nurse?* *Tell your staff or nurse if you are feeling:* • *Moderate to severe pain* • *Pain that interferes with daily activity or sleep* • *Swelling of the injured area* • *An inability to perform normal activities* **Keep yourself safe!**
ACTIVITY	Show some examples of warm-ups and stretches. Pick some of the warm-ups and stretches (from Lesson 3) and do them with participants.
DISTRIBUTE AND DISCUSS PARTICIPANT HANDOUT: Staying Safe During Physical Activity	Distribute and review the **Staying Safe During Physical Activity** handout. Write down individual target heart rates.
TAKE A FIELD TRIP *(OPTIONAL)*	Prearrange a visit to a local community fitness center. Have fitness center personnel give participants a tour of the fitness center. Talk to participants about different exercise equipment that is available. Have a fitness center employee show you how to use equipment safely. Give participants an opportunity to explore different equipment after they do their warm-ups and stretches. Explore other options and physical activities at the center.
SUMMARIZE	*It's important to stay safe during physical activity and exercise. Today, we talked about the importance of doing warm-ups, stretches, and cool-downs and exercising at a slow and steady pace without overdoing ourselves.*

EVALUATION

• Did participants talk about ways to stay safe when exercising?

• Did participants explain when they should slow down or stop exercising?

HELPFUL HINTS

The field trips are designed to give participants opportunities to experience being physically active and making healthy choices in their community. Units that have field trip activities may be taught with or without the field trip.

Refer to the participant handouts in Lesson 3 to review tips related to warm-ups, stretches, and cool-downs.

Refer to the **Recharging Through an Exercise Program** and **Common Exercise Techniques** references in Lesson 3.

Unit 3

Lesson 18

Community Fitness Center Visit

Warm-Ups, Stretches, and Cool-Downs Safety Tips

WARM-UPS

Warm-ups should raise the heart rate and warm the particular muscle groups that will be used during physical activity. Some examples include the following:

- Doing jumping jacks

- Lightly jogging in place

- Briskly walking around the block or around a large room

- Cycling at a slow, leisurely pace and gradually increasing the speed

- Walking at a brisk pace and as your heart rate and breathing increase, pick up the speed to a jog

- Doing arm circles

- Swimming slow and easy laps

STRETCHING

Stretching should be part of both your warm-up and cool down. Some tips to remember while stretching include:

- Only stretch a muscle to the point of mild discomfort. If it hurts, you are pushing too hard—ease off.

- Do not bounce. Instead, hold the stretch for between 10 and 30 seconds.

- Stretch opposing muscle groups one after the other. For example, stretch your quadriceps (muscles on the front of the thigh) then stretch your hamstrings (muscles on the back of the thigh).

- Remember to keep breathing normally as you stretch.

- See the **Tips: Stretching** handout (Lesson 3).

Source: State of Victoria, Australia. (2008). *Exercise-injury prevention.* Available online at http://www.betterhealth.vic.gov.au/bhcv2/bhcarticles.nsf/pages/Exercise_injury_prevention?open

Warm-Ups, Stretches, and Cool-Downs Safety Tips

COOL-DOWNS

Some of the many health benefits of cooling down after physical activity include:

- Helps to gently return heart rate, breathing, and blood pressure to normal

- Improves flexibility

- Reduces the risk of injury

- Removes waste products from muscle tissue (e.g., lactic acid) and helps to reduce the risk of soreness

It is important to cool down after exercising to further reduce the risk of injury. Some tips to remember while cooling down include:

- Cool down for several minutes

- Taper off your activity. For example, if you have been running, cool down by slowing down to a jog then a brisk walk for a few minutes.

- Finish your cool-down routine with 10 minutes of gentle stretches.

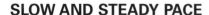

Community Fitness Center Visit

Staying Safe During Physical Activity

WARM-UPS AND STRETCHES ARE A MUST!

- Start with 5–10 minutes of warm-up exercises, such as **brisk walking, jumping jacks, or easy jogging** to get your muscles going.

- Follow your warm-up with **gentle stretching**.

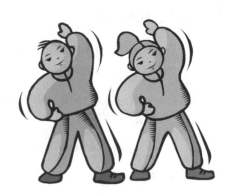

SLOW AND STEADY PACE

Start slowly to give your body time to adjust.

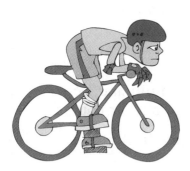

DON'T TAKE YOUR BREATH AWAY!

- You should not feel pain, tired, unwell, or gasping for air during physical activity.

- For your heart, exercise so you feel that your heart is working harder but you do not feel short of breath.

- You should be able to have a normal conversation while exercising.

YOUR HEART IS YOUR GUIDE

Check your heart rate monitor to see how hard you are working your body.

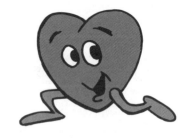

HOW FAST SHOULD YOUR HEART BEAT?

Your trainer will tell you how fast your heart should beat.

My target heart rate range is _____ beats/minute.

Source: American College of Sports Medicine. (2006). *ACSM's guidelines for exercise testing and prescriptions* (7th ed.). Indianapolis, IN: Author.

Health Matters: The Exercise and Nutrition Health Education Curriculum for People with Developmental Disabilities by Beth Marks, Jasmina Sisirak, and Tamar Heller

Staying Safe During Physical Activity

DON'T FORGET YOUR COOL-DOWNS!

End your exercise session with low intensity cool-down exercises and stretches.

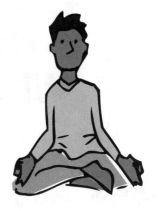

IT'S TOO HOT!

- Drink water before, during, and after physical activity.

- Take sips of water every 15 minutes while you exercise.

- **Plain water** is the best for activities of less than an hour.

- Wear loose fitting clothes that allow your skin to breathe.

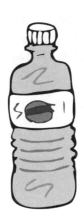

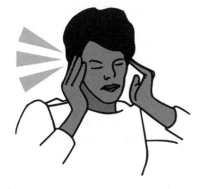

TELL YOUR STAFF OR NURSE IF YOU ARE FEELING:

- Moderate to severe pain

- Pain that interferes with daily activity or sleep

- Swelling of the injured area

- An inability to perform normal activities

Lesson 19

How to Breathe When We Exercise

also on
CD-ROM

Objectives

Participants will

- Identify the importance of correct breathing
- Discuss breathing techniques
- Practice proper breathing techniques during physical activity

HANDOUTS

Instructor Reference(s):

Breathing Techniques During Exercise

Participant Handout(s):

Week 6 News

Breathing Techniques During Exercise

How I Breathe When I Exercise

MATERIALS

Blackboard and chalk

Pens or pencils

Carpeted, quiet, low-traffic room where all participants can lie down comfortably (you may bring blankets or mats)

Stopwatch

Personal Notebooks for handouts and pictures

Suggested Activities

INSTRUCTOR ACTIVITY	INSTRUCTOR SCRIPT/DIRECTIONS
DISTRIBUTE AND DISCUSS NEWSLETTER: Week 6 News	Give participants the **Week 6 News** handout. Discuss the newsletter.
REVIEW	*We have talked about how our medications affect our bodies and how we feel when we exercise. We have also talked about staying safe when we exercise.* *We also discussed things that we should remember when we exercise. Can anyone tell me what some of those things are?*
INTRODUCE LESSON	*Today, we will talk about breathing. This class will help you think about your breathing. Our lungs breathe automatically. When we are sitting down, our breathing is usually slow. When we engage in a physical activity, such as running, fast walking, or riding a bike, our breathing becomes faster and we may run out of breath. This is normal. Your body runs on oxygen, just as a car runs on gas. When you start to exercise, whether running, walking, or doing any other*

physical activity, your muscles need more oxygen. The body meets this need by supplying oxygen-rich blood to the muscles. The lungs work harder to absorb this oxygen out of the air.

ASK

Why is proper breathing important?

DISCUSS RESPONSES

Examples of responses include the following:

- Provides the only way your body and organs can get oxygen that is vital for your survival
- Gets rid of waste products and toxins from your body
- Relieves stress quickly and easily
- Increases digestion of food
- Improves the health of your brain, spinal cord, and nerves
- Maintains the strength and health of your lungs
- Reduces the workload for your heart

ASK AND WAIT
FOR RESPONSES

When I'm lifting a weight, should I inhale when I'm picking up the weight or as I release? And, does it really make a difference?

It does make a difference. Imagine how hard it would be to do a crunch while inhaling instead of exhaling.

REFER TO
INSTRUCTOR REFERENCE:
    Breathing Techniques
      During Exercise

Refer to the **Breathing Techniques During Exercise** reference.

DISTRIBUTE AND DISCUSS
PARTICIPANT HANDOUT:
    Breathing Techniques
      During Exercise

Distribute the **Breathing Techniques During Exercise** handout.

Why is proper breathing important?

- Discuss BREATHING TECHNIQUES.
- Practice SIMPLE BREATHING TECHNIQUES.
- DO BREATHING AND PHYSICAL ACTIVITY.
- Do any other breathing technique and try it—or try all of them.

COMPLETE
PARTICIPANT HANDOUT:
    How I Breathe When I Exercise

Distribute the **How I Breathe When I Exercise** handout. Review the worksheet together.

SUMMARIZE

Review and summarize the benefits of correct breathing. Demonstrate how to do proper breathing techniques.

EVALUATION

- Are participants able to identify benefits of correct breathing?
- Can participants demonstrate proper breathing techniques?

Breathing Techniques During Exercise

Exhale (on exertion) when your muscles contract (when lifting), and inhale when they lengthen as they return to the starting position (when releasing). It is understandable why this is so confusing because your muscles move your limbs in so many planes and directions. THIS TAKES PRACTICE.

1. **Pressing or extending motions** (moving the weight away from your body):

   Exhale when you push and **inhale** when you return to the starting position. These movements include leg extensions, press machines, overhead shoulder presses, back and lateral shoulder flies, and tricep presses or extensions.

2. **Moving the weight toward your body:**

   Exhale when you pull and inhale when the muscle is lengthening. These movements include **hamstring** curls, rowing motions (seated or bent over), **lateral pull-downs, chest flies,** and **bicep curls.** Much of our confusion over when to breathe out comes from not knowing which phase (contraction or lengthening) we are in when we start an exercise.

It is very important to keep breathing while you exercise. You should not hold your breath when lifting weights. **Even breathing in reverse is much better than not breathing at all.** Make sure you breathe throughout each repetition. If you are not doing that, your face may turn red and you will be out of breath by the end of the set.

Source: California Air Resources Board. (n.d.). *Breathing and exercise.* Available online at http://www.arb.ca.gov/knowzone/teachers/lessons/k-6/exercise.htm

Week 6 News

NEWSLETTER FOR THE EXERCISE AND NUTRITION HEALTH EDUCATION CLASS

Staying Healthy with Exercise

We have been talking about ways to stay safe with exercise.

- Warm-ups and stretches are a must!

- Keep a slow and steady pace!

- Don't take your breath away!

- Remember to do cool downs at the end!

- Avoid getting too hot!

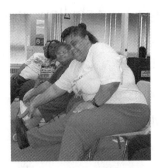

This week we talked about going to the grocery store and the foods we like to eat.

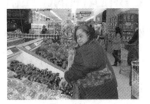

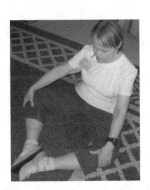

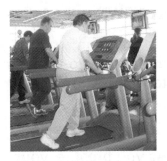

We Talked About Things to Remember When We Exercise

It is important to make sure that we feel okay to exercise.

We should make sure that we have eaten and have taken our medications (if we are taking medications).

We should also make sure that we are wearing loose fitting and comfortable clothes.

Breathing Techniques During Exercise

TECHNIQUES FOR CORRECT BREATHING

- We should breathe through the nose. Take a breath through the nose.

- Our noses have little hairs that prevent dust, tiny insects, and other particles from reaching and possibly injuring the lungs. Use a mirror to look at the hairs in your nose.

- Our noses warm up the cool air before it reaches the lungs.

- Long deep breaths are better than shallow breaths.

SIMPLE BREATHING TECHNIQUE

1. Take a deep breath slowly through your nose.

2. Hold the breath for a couple of seconds.

3. Exhale smoothly through your mouth.

4. Repeat several times.

LYING DOWN BREATHING TECHNIQUE

1. Lie down on a rug or blanket on the floor with your legs straight and slightly apart, your toes pointed comfortably outwards, arms at your sides not touching your body, your palms up, and your eyes closed (relaxed body position).

2. Take a deep breath slowly through your nose.

3. As you breathe, your chest and stomach should move together. If only your chest seems to rise and fall, your breathing is shallow and you are not using the lower part of your lungs.

4. As you inhale, you should feel your stomach rising as if your stomach is filling with air.

5. As you exhale, your stomach comes back in, like a balloon releasing all of its air.

6. This inhale and exhale process should continue comfortably and smoothly.

7. Your chest and abdomen should rise as you inhale and fall as you exhale.

8. Repeat several times.

Source: California Air Resources Board. (n.d.). *Breathing and exercise.* Available online at
http://www.arb.ca.gov/knowzone/teachers/lessons/k-6/exercise.htm

Breathing Techniques During Exercise

THE RELAXING SIGH TECHNIQUE

Sighing and yawning during the day are signs that you are not getting enough oxygen. A relaxing sigh releases a bit of tension.

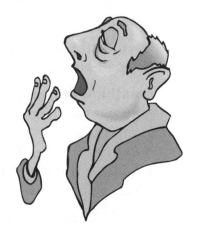

1. Sit or stand up straight.

2. Sigh deeply, letting out a sound of deep relief as the air rushes out of your lungs.

3. Let new air come in naturally.

4. Repeat this procedure 8–12 times whenever you feel the need for it, and experience the feeling of relaxation.

DEEP, RELAXED BREATHING TECHNIQUE

Although this exercise can be practiced in a variety of poses, the following is recommended for beginners:

1. Lie down on a blanket or rug on the floor. Bend your knees and move your feet about eight inches apart, with your toes turned outward slightly. Make sure your spine is straight.

2. Place one hand on your abdomen and one hand on your chest.

3. Inhale slowly and deeply (counting to 10) through your nose into your abdomen to push up your hand as much as feels comfortable. Your chest should move only a little and only with your abdomen.

4. Continue Step 3 until it becomes rhythmic and comfortable. Now smile slightly, inhale through your nose and exhale (counting to 10) through your mouth, making a quiet, breezy sound as you gently blow out. Your mouth, tongue, and jaw will be relaxed. Take long, slow, deep breaths raising and lowering your abdomen. Hear the sound and feel your breathing as you become more and more relaxed.

5. When you first begin this technique, do it for 5 minutes. When you become more comfortable with it, you may extend it up to 20 minutes.

6. Upon ending a session, stay still for a few minutes and try to keep your entire body relaxed.

7. The purpose of this technique is to develop a good, relaxing breathing method. It may be practiced anytime, especially during stressful situations.

How I Breathe When I Exercise

BREATHING AND PHYSICAL ACTIVITY

What to do:

1. Have a stopwatch this worksheet ready. You should have one worksheet per participant.

2. **Breathing at rest.** The participant is sitting down. The timer/recorder will give the participant the following instructions: "When I say start, begin counting your breaths. Breathe normally." Have another person count breaths with you. The timer tells the particpant when to start. After 1 minute, the timer asks the participant how many breaths he or she has taken. Record the number on the worksheet.

3. Breathing during physical activity. The timer/recorder tells the participant, "When I say start, begin jumping jacks. After 15 seconds, I will say stop. Stop jumping and immediately start counting your breaths." The timer tells the participant to start. After 15 seconds, the timer tells the participant to stop jumping. After an additional 15 seconds, the timer asks the participant for a breath count. The recorder writes the number of breaths on the worksheet and multiplies it by 4. The timer asks the participant, "Were your breaths deeper while you exercised?" The recorder writes down the answer. Breathing is usually shallow and faster after physical activity.

4. Repeat Steps 2 and 3 until each participant has had a turn.

5. **Comparing results.** Discuss the variety of results. What other things could cause widely varying results (physical condition, respiratory illness such as asthma).

"Does a person breathe more or less during exercise such as jumping jacks?"

How much more or less? _____

Breaths in one minute at rest: _____

Breaths after 15 minutes of exercise _____ x 4 = _____

Is the breathing deeper after jumping? _____

_____

Source: California Air Resources Board. (n.d.). *Breathing and exercise.* Available online at http://www.arb.ca.gov/knowzone/teachers/lessons/k-6/exercise.htm

Lesson 20

Why Do We Clean Equipment?

Objectives
Participants will • Identify influences that may affect their ability/choices to engage in exercise activities

HANDOUTS
Participant Handout(s):   Why Do We Clean Equipment?

also on CD-ROM

MATERIALS
Blackboard and chalk
Pens or pencils
Rags
Spray bottle
Cleaning solution: Check with the manufacturer of the equipment to see what they recommend for a cleaning solution. Usually diluted 409 can be used for cleaning.
Personal Notebooks for handouts and pictures

Suggested Activities

INSTRUCTOR ACTIVITY	INSTRUCTOR SCRIPT/DIRECTIONS
REVIEW	*In our last class, we talked about your breathing. Our lungs breathe automatically. When we are sitting down, our breathing is usually slow. When we do physical activity, such as running, fast walking, or riding a bike, our breathing becomes faster and we may run out of breath. This is normal.*
ASK AND WAIT FOR RESPONSE	*Can anyone show us how to breathe when you are exercising?*
INTRODUCE LESSON	*Today, we are going to talk about the importance of cleaning exercise equipment after we use it. We will also talk about how to clean the equipment.*
ASK AND WAIT FOR RESPONSE	*Why is it important to clean equipment?* • Prevents us from getting sick • Kills off any bacteria and germs that we may have on our hands and body • Keeps us from spreading our germs to others • Makes equipment last longer
ASK AND WAIT FOR RESPONSE	*How often should you clean equipment?* • After every use.

INSTRUCTOR ACTIVITY	INSTRUCTOR SCRIPT/DIRECTIONS
ASK AND WAIT FOR RESPONSE	*What should you clean?* • Areas where your hands and body touch, such as handles and seats (where you can leave sweaty marks) • Top surface of seat, computer console, and frame (when cleaning console, spray cloth first) • Dust in hard-to-reach areas
ASK AND WAIT FOR RESPONSE	*What supplies do you need to clean equipment daily?* • Rag • Spray bottle • Cleaning solution: Check with the manufacturer of the equipment to see what they recommend for a cleaning solution. • Usually diluted 409 can be used for cleaning.
DISTRIBUTE AND DISCUSS PARTICIPANT HANDOUT: Why Do We Clean Equipment?	Distribute and discuss the **Why Do We Clean Equipment?** handout Ask the following questions: • *What equipment needs to be cleaned?* • *What parts of the equipment do you clean?*
COMPLETE PARTICIPANT ACTIVITIES	Using **Why Do We Clean Equipment?** as a guide, complete the following activities with participants: • Make a list of your exercise equipment. (You may even take pictures of your equipment.) • Post a list of your equipment in a visible place. • Identify the areas that should be cleaned. • Clean equipment after each use.
SUMMARIZE	Summarize the importance of cleaning equipment. Have participants demonstrate how to clean the equipment and identify equipment that they will clean.

EVALUATION

• Can participants identify the importance of cleaning equipment?

• Can participants demonstrate how to clean equipment?

Why Do We Clean Equipment?

List of Our Exercise Equipment

Equipment   Areas to be cleaned

1. _____

2. _____

3. _____

4. _____

5. _____

6. _____

7. _____

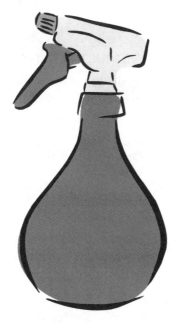

Lesson 21

Nutrients We Need

Objectives

Participants will

- Learn about the functions of carbohydrates, proteins, and fat
- Discuss the reasons people need carbohydrates, proteins, and fat
- Identify good sources of carbohydrates, proteins, and fat

HANDOUTS

also on CD-ROM

Instructor Reference(s):
  Types of Nutrients We Need
  Blood Sugar and Exercise
  Nutrient Game Answers
Participant Handout(s):
  What Nutrients Do We Need for Physical Activity?
  Participant Game: What Nutrients Do We Need?

MATERIALS

Blackboard and chalk
Pens or pencils
Unsalted crackers (carbohydrates)
Can of water-packed tuna (protein)
Cooking oil (fat)
Preparation bowls
Spoons and napkins
Personal Notebook for handouts and pictures

Idea

Field Trip: Participants will go to a restaurant of their choice for a meal. Participants should plan to bring money.

Suggested Activities

INSTRUCTOR ACTIVITY	INSTRUCTOR SCRIPT/DIRECTIONS
REVIEW	*In our last class, we talked about the importance of cleaning exercise equipment. Who can tell us what equipment we need to clean? How do we clean the equipment?*
INTRODUCE LESSON	*Today, we are going to talk about nutrients that we need for physical activity, such as **carbohydrates, proteins, and fats**.*
ASK	*What do you remember seeing in the grocery store the last time you went there?*
RECORD RESPONSES	Thousands of food packages with these words on them: • Low fat • Protein enriched • Fat free • Good source of complex carbohydrates • Low carb

INSTRUCTOR ACTIVITY	INSTRUCTOR SCRIPT/DIRECTIONS
ASK	*What do these words mean?*
REFER TO INSTRUCTOR REFERENCES: Types of Nutrients We Need Blood Sugar and Exercise	*What are carbohydrates, proteins, and fats? We need them for our bodies, but how do we get them?* Use the **Types of Nutrients We Need** reference to guide the discussion. You may also use the **Blood Sugar and Exercise** reference as a resource to guide your discussion. *Note:* This is especially important if any participants have diabetes.
ASK AND WAIT FOR RESPONSE	*Have you ever felt hungry and found it kind of hard to think?*
ANSWER	*That's because you were running out of glucose or energy and your brain needed more fuel.*
COMPLETE ACTIVITY: Taste Test: Why Are Some Carbohydrates Salty and Others Sweet?	*Why are some carbohydrates salty and others sweet?* Have everyone wash their hands. Have each participant taste three items: crackers, packed tuna, and cooking oil. Tell participants to put the crackers in their mouths and leave them there until the crackers start dissolving.
ASK AND WAIT FOR RESPONSES	***What do you taste?*** *Does the taste turn from salty to sweet? Why?*
DISCUSS	*Our taste buds cannot taste the sugar until complex carbohydrates start breaking down to simple sugars. The digestive enzymes in our mouths start this process, and if you keep a starchy food in your mouth long enough, it will start to taste sweet!*
ASK AND WAIT FOR RESPONSES	***What about tuna?*** *What is the texture of tuna? Proteins are used to build up tissues like our muscles. It's important to eat protein when we are exercising.* ***What about oil?*** *How does it feel in your mouth?*
DISCUSS	*Even though our bodies needs **some** fat to work properly, our bodies don't need as much as most people eat. It's a good idea to avoid eating a lot of fat because it can contribute to **obesity** (when a person weighs much too much for his or her height) and other health conditions that can occur when we get older, like heart disease or adult-onset diabetes.* *Foods with a lot of fat in them taste good—like cookies, chocolate, hamburgers, and french fries. It is okay to eat them once in a while.*

INSTRUCTOR ACTIVITY	INSTRUCTOR SCRIPT/DIRECTIONS
DISTRIBUTE AND DISCUSS PARTICIPANT HANDOUT: What Nutrients Do We Need for Physical Activity?	Distribute and review the **What Nutrients Do We Need for Physical Activity?** handout.
COMPLETE PARTICIPANT GAME: What Nutrients Do We Need?	Have participants complete the **Participant Game: What Nutrients Do We Need?** handout. Read the question out loud and answer the questions together. Good discussion points: some foods are made up of different nutrients. For example, an egg is a good source of protein and fat. *What are other foods that have more than one nutrient in them?*
REFER TO INSTRUCTOR REFERENCE: Nutrient Game Answers	Use the **Nutrient Game Answers** reference to guide your discussion.
TAKE A FIELD TRIP (OPTIONAL)	Participants will go to a restaurant of their choice for a meal (brunch, lunch, dinner). As a group, look at the menu and discuss different nutrients on the menu. Encourage participants to find healthy options and options that are not as healthy. When the food is ordered and everyone is eating their meal, ask them to identify different types of nutrients by taste (e.g., fat is greasy, bread tastes sweet if you leave it in your mouth).
SUMMARIZE	*Let's summarize what we learned today. We discussed three types of nutrients, including* **carbohydrates, proteins, and fats.** *Which nutrient is a major source of energy? Carbohydrates can give our bodies fuel. Which nutrient can build up and repair muscles? Protein's biggest job is to replace and build tissue in our bodies. Which nutrient stores energy in your body? Fat insulates our bodies from the cold and cushions our organs.*

EVALUATION

- Can participants state the functions of carbohydrates, proteins, and fats?
- Can participants identify the reasons they need carbohydrates, proteins, and fats?
- Can participants identify good sources of carbohydrates, proteins, and fats?

HELPFUL HINTS

The field trips are designed to give participants opportunities to experience being physically active and making healthy choices in their community. Units that have field trip activities may be taught with or without the field trip.

Types of Nutrients We Need

CARBOHYDRATES

Major source of energy

Why do we need carbohydrates?

- Gives all the cells in your body the energy they need.

- They let you run, jump, think, blink, breathe, and more.

What are sources of carbohydrates?

- Two different types: sugars and starches.

- Sugars are called **simple carbohydrates.** This is because your body digests them quickly and easily. Simple carbohydrates are usually sweet tasting, like cookies, candy, soda, and other sugary foods. Some come from nature—apples, bananas, grapes, and raisins; fruit cocktail, oranges, and pears; ice cream and frozen yogurt—both are good ways to get simple carbohydrates.

- Starchy carbohydrates have their own name, too: **complex carbohydrates.** These carbohydrates take longer to be digested than simple carbohydrates do. Complex carbohydrates are found in foods like bread, noodles, cereals, and rice, and in lots of tasty vegetables, such as corn, potatoes, and sweet potatoes.

PROTEINS

Build up, keep up, and replace the tissues, such as muscles

Why do you need proteins?

- Protein's biggest job is to build up, keep up, and replace the tissues in your body.

- Your muscles, your organs, and even some of your hormones are made up mostly of protein.

- Making a big muscle? Taking a deep breath with your big lungs? Running down the street on your strong feet? You have got the power of protein!

What are sources of protein?

- Meat, chicken, fish, eggs, cheese, yogurt, milk, beans (lentils and peas), and nuts. Some proteins are leaner than others.

- Choose lean protein such as chicken breast, fish, and skim milk.

Types of Nutrients We Need

FATS

Fats store energy

Our bodies can make fat.

Fat insulates our bodies from the cold and provides some cushioning for our organs.

Fat sounds like it is always a bad thing that people avoid eating, but actually our bodies need some fat to work correctly.

Why do we need fat?

- Fat is the body's major form of energy storage. Our bodies can make fat.

- Fat gives our bodies energy.

- Some fats help make up important hormones that we need to keep our bodies at the right temperature or keep our blood pressure at the right level.

- Fat helps us have healthy skin and hair.

- Fat is our bodies' very own storage and moving service: it helps vitamins A, D, E, and K hang out **and** get transported through the bloodstream when our bodies need them!

What are sources of fat?

- Oils, butter, fried foods

- Fats come from many sources, but not all fats are created equal! **Saturated fat** is the main dietary cause of high blood cholesterol. It is found in foods from animals, such as beef, pork, bacon, butter, cream, cheese, and milk, and some foods from plants such as coconut, cocoa butter, and palm and canola oils.

- **Hydrogenated fat** is found in processed foods that undergo a chemical process called hydrogenation. The common foods with hydrogenated fats are margerine and shortening. This type of fat also raises blood choleseterol. *Trans*-fatty acids are also formed during this process of hydrogenation, and they may raise cholesterol levels even more than saturated fats.

- **Unsaturated (polyunsaturated and monounsaturated) fats** are found mainly in fish (salmon, trout, herring), nuts (walnuts, hazelnuts, pecans, peanuts), seeds, oils from plants (olive, canola, sunflower, soybean), avocados, and olives. Unsaturated fats may help lower your blood cholesterol level.

Blood Sugar and Exercise

Before starting any new physical activity program, get your health care provider's OK to exercise.

Exercise can help you improve your blood sugar control.

Remember to check your blood sugar BEFORE, DURING, and AFTER exercise. This will help you track how your body responds to exercise and help you prevent rapid blood sugar changes.

Check your blood sugar BEFORE physical activity

Think about these general guidelines:

- **Lower than 100 milligrams per deciliter (mg/dL).** Your blood sugar is too low to exercise. Eat a small snack containing carbohydrates, such as fruit or crackers, before starting your exercise.

- **100 to 250 mg/dL.** For most people, this is a safe blood sugar range. You may start your exercise!

- **250 mg/dL or higher.** Caution zone! Test your urine for ketones (compound made when your body breaks down fat for energy). Too many ketones indicate that your body doesn't have enough insulin to control blood sugar. Exercising with high levels of ketones may lead to a serious health complication, ketoacidosis, that needs immediate treatment. Wait for the levels of ketones to come down before exercise.

- **300 mg/dL or higher.** Do not exercise! Your blood sugar may be too high and is putting you at risk for ketoacidosis. Wait for the levels of ketones to come down before exercise.

Watch for symptoms of low blood sugar DURING physical activity

Your blood sugar may change during exercise. If you are feeling shaky, dizzy, faint, or confused or have changes in coordination or vision, stop exercising and eat or drink something to raise your blood sugar level. Check your blood sugar and recheck it again 15 minutes later after your snack.

Check your blood sugar AFTER physical activity

After exercise, check your blood sugar immediately. Exercise uses up reserve sugar stored in your liver and muscles. Your body will rebuild these stores by taking sugar from your blood. The longer you exercise, the longer your blood sugar will be affected.

Source: Mayo Clinic. (2009). *Diabetes and exercise: When to monitor your blood sugar.* Available online at http://www.mayoclinic.com/health/diabetes-and-exercise/DA00105

Nutrient Game Answers

Foods that are **high in fat** are in **bold**:

Skim milk	**Chicken***
Tomato	Cereal
Hamburger	**Whole milk**
Eggs	**French fries**
Peanut butter	Apple

*Chicken breast is low in fat, but chicken with skin on and dark meat such as legs and wings are high in fat.

Foods that are **high in protein** are in **bold**:

Chicken	**Cheese** (also high in fat)
Green beans	Pasta
Tuna	Orange juice
Skim milk	Crackers
Cucumber	**Eggs**

Foods that are **high in carbohydrates** are in **bold**:

Orange juice	Cheese
Cereal	**Crackers**
Eggs	Chicken
Spinach	**Skim milk**
Pasta	**Rice**

What Nutrients Do We Need for Physical Activity?

CARBOHYDRATES

Major source of energy

Eat more of these: apples, bananas, grapes, raisins, fruit cocktail, oranges, and pears.

Eat these only once in a while: ice cream, frozen yogurt, candy, and cookies

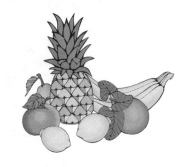

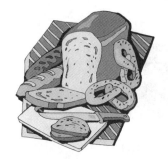

Sources: bread, noodles, cereals, rice, and all veggies, such as corn, potatoes, and sweet potatoes

PROTEINS

Build up, keep up, and replace such tissues as muscles

Lean protein: chicken breast, fish, low-fat yogurt and milk, beans (lentils and peas), and nuts.

High-fat protein: red meat, eggs, and cheese.

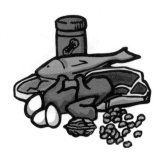

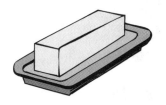

FATS

Energy storage.

Our bodies can make fat.

Fat insulates our bodies from the cold and provides some cushioning for our organs

Fat helps us have healthy skin and hair.

Sources: cookies, chocolate, eggs, cheese, fast food, hamburgers, and french fries.

Participant Game: What Nutrients Do We Need?

Directions: Circle the foods that are high in fat.

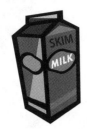

Skim milk

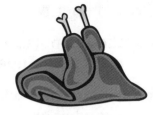

Chicken

Tomato

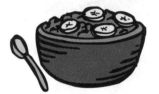

Cereal

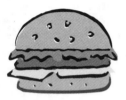

Hamburger

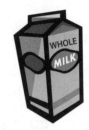

Whole milk

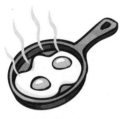

Eggs

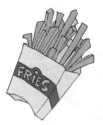

French fries

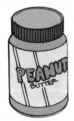

Peanut butter

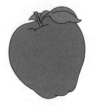

Apple

Participant Game: What Nutrients Do We Need?

Directions: Circle the foods that are high in protein.

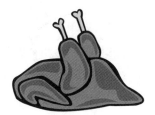

Chicken

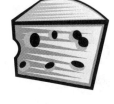

Cheese

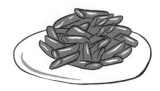

Green beans

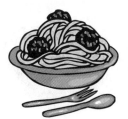

Pasta

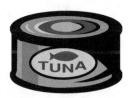

Tuna

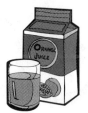

Orange juice

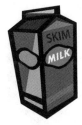

Skim milk

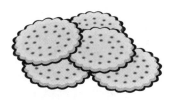

Crackers

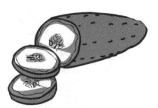

Cucumber

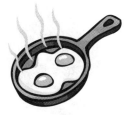

Eggs

Nutrients We Need

Participant Game: What Nutrients Do We Need?

Directions: Circle the foods that are high in carbohydrates.

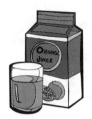

Orange juice

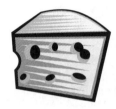

Cheese

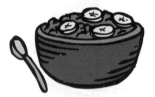

Cereal

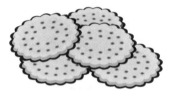

Crackers

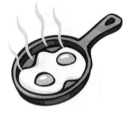

Eggs

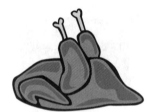

Chicken

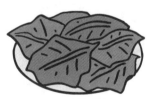

Spinach

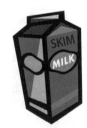

Skim milk

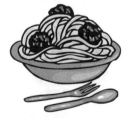

Pasta

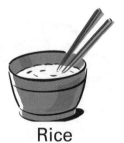

Rice

 Health Matters: The Exercise and Nutrition Health Education Curriculum for People with Developmental Disabilities
by Beth Marks, Jasmina Sisirak, and Tamar Heller

Exercise Plans

Becoming More Active

Objectives	HANDOUTS
Participants will	Participant Handout(s):
• Discuss the effects of lifestyle on their health	Week 7 News
• Identify one or two exercises they would like to do	Exercise Plan
• State where they would like to do their exercises (e.g., home, work, community center)	**also on CD-ROM**
• Write down their exercise goals	

HANDOUTS

Participant Handout(s):

Week 7 News

Exercise Plan

MATERIALS

Blackboard and chalk

Pens or pencils

Pictures of different types of exercises

Reminder Envelope

Personal Notebooks for handouts and pictures

Suggested Activities

INSTRUCTOR ACTIVITY	INSTRUCTOR SCRIPT/DIRECTIONS
DISTRIBUTE AND DISCUSS NEWSLETTER: Week 7 News	Give participants the **Week 7 News** handout. Discuss the newsletter.
REVIEW	*We have talked about using proper breathing techniques when we exercise. We also discussed the need to clean exercise equipment after we use it and how to clean the equipment.*
	In our last class, we talked about three types of nutrients, including carbohydrates, proteins, and fats. Which nutrient is a major source of energy? Which nutrient can build up and repair muscles? Which nutrient stores energy in our bodies?
INTRODUCE LESSON	*Today, we are going to talk about things that we can change and things that we cannot change. We are also going to discuss our goals for doing exercises.*
DISCUSS	*We have been talking about our own preferences for exercising and the foods we like. Things that we like to do and eat make us unique people. We also are different in how we look.*

INSTRUCTOR ACTIVITY	INSTRUCTOR SCRIPT/DIRECTIONS
ASK	*What are some differences in how we look?*
WAIT FOR RESPONSES	Supplement responses by adding hair texture and color, having a disability, body structure and shape, and eye color.
ASK	*Can any of these things be changed?*
CONTINUE	*Some people use plastic surgery to change their looks they don't like (most often their nose and ears). Dentists can change the way your teeth look in your mouth. However, for the most part, there is little that we can do about the things that we were born with, so we must learn to accept them.*
	What we look like is affected by what we are born with, our environment, and what we do every day—our lifestyle, how we live, what we eat, and the activities that we do.
ASK	*What are some activities that we can do that influence the way we look and how we feel?*
RECORD RESPONSES	Examples may include the following: • Exercise • Get enough sleep at night • Do things to relax (e.g., watching television) • Watch what we eat (regular meals, junk food versus fruits and vegetables) • Have fun with friends and family • Do preventive health activities (e.g., taking care of your teeth by visiting the dentist) • Pay attention to our appearance, posture, personal hygiene, selection and care of clothes, and so forth • Do things we like to do (work, hobbies)
DISCUSS	*Our lifestyle or what we do every day affects our health. For example, we can reduce our risk of getting heart disease if we reduce stress in our life, eat a variety of low-fat foods, exercise at least three times a week, and avoid drugs and alcohol.* *Let's talk about some exercises that you would like to do to stay healthy.*
DISTRIBUTE AND COMPLETE PARTICIPANT HANDOUT: Exercise Plan	Work with participants in small groups or individually on their **Exercise Plan** handout. You may show participants pictures of each type of exercise from the **Exercises and Activities I Like** handout (Lesson 12). Review the types of exercises they like and don't like to do.
ASK	Ask participants to discuss their exercise plans with the class.

INSTRUCTOR ACTIVITY	INSTRUCTOR SCRIPT/DIRECTIONS
SUMMARIZE	*Our health is affected by our bodies, things that we were born with, our lifestyles, or the way we live, where we live, and the people who live with us. All of these things combined make us different from each other.*
	Review some of the exercise plans and goals. Also, summarize where, when, and with whom people can exercise (e.g., home, community center, with a group, at work during their breaks).
DISTRIBUTE EXERCISE PLAN AND LETTER TO SUPPORT PERSON	Give participants a copy of their exercise plan and a letter to their support persons regarding their exercise plan.
	Have participants take the letter and a copy of their exercise plan home to their support person in their **Reminder Envelope** or include their plan with their newsletter.

EVALUATION

- Did participants discuss how their lifestyle affects their health?

- Did participants complete their exercise plan and identify exercises that they would like to do and where they want to do them?

Week 7 News

NEWSLETTER FOR THE EXERCISE AND NUTRITION HEALTH EDUCATION CLASS

Nutrients We Need to Exercise

This week, we talked about nutrients we need for exercising.

- Carbohydrates are a major source of energy for our bodies.

- Proteins help build up, keep up, and replace tissues like muscle.

- Fat is important for storage of energy and insulating our bodies from the cold.

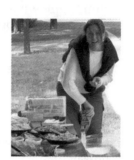

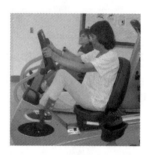

This week, we did aerobic exercises to a video tape. We also went to a restaurant and talked about different types of nutrients in our foods.

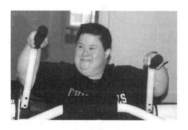

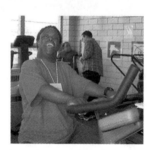

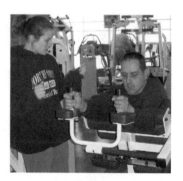

We Learned About Proper Breathing Techniques

Proper breathing is important for living. Breathing gets rid of waste products and toxins from the body, gives a quick and easy stress reliever, maintains the strength and health of the lungs, reduces the workload for the heart, increases food digestion, and improves the health of the brain, spinal cord, and nerves.

Exercise Plan

I have decided that I will spend _____ minutes per day exercising.

I would like to do exercises on the following days: (circle days)

Monday   Tuesday   Wednesday   Thursday

Friday   Saturday   Sunday

The exercise(s) I would like to do (or try) are:

_____ Exercises like we have been doing in the gym (lifting weights, biking, using rowing machines)

_____ Exercises like we have been doing in class (yoga, Tae Bo, aerobics, dancing)

_____ Other: _____

_____

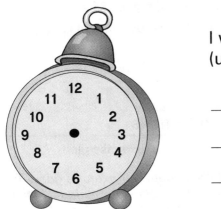

I want to do my exercises in the:
(use the clock to draw in the hands for the time)

_____ Morning

_____ Afternoon

_____ Evening

I want to do my exercises at:

_____ Home

_____ Work

_____ Other: _____

_____

Nutrition Plans

Making a Menu

Objectives

Participants will

- Review the MyPlate
- Identify food groups and the location on the levels of the MyPlate
- Identify foods that they would like to increase and decrease in their diet
- Create a menu plan (may be used for snacks or meals for the class or for home)
- Write down their nutrition goals

HANDOUTS

Instructor Reference(s):

   Shopping for Groceries

   Eating Fruits and Vegetables

   MyPlate *(see Lesson 6 for handout)*

Participant Handout(s):

   Nutrition Plan

   Meal Plan for a Day

MATERIALS

Blackboard and chalk

Pens or pencils

Pictures of different types of foods

Personal Notebooks for handouts and pictures

Suggested Activities

INSTRUCTOR ACTIVITY	INSTRUCTOR SCRIPT/DIRECTIONS
REVIEW	Review and discuss participants' exercise plans.
INTRODUCE LESSON	*In our last class, we talked about our exercise goals. Today, we are going to talk about our plans for eating a balanced diet, and we are going to create a menu plan.*
DISTRIBUTE AND COMPLETE PARTICIPANT HANDOUT: Nutrition Plan	Work with participants in small groups or individually on their **Nutrition Plan** handout. You may show participants pictures of different types of foods. Have them talk about foods they like and do not like.
ASK	Ask participants to identify foods that they would like to reduce in their diets and foods they would like to increase. Ask why they should add these foods to their diet.

INSTRUCTOR ACTIVITY	**INSTRUCTOR SCRIPT/DIRECTIONS**
ASK	Ask participants to identify foods that they eat for breakfast, lunch, and dinner. Discuss the importance of eating breakfast every day.
	Who do you usually eat with for breakfast, lunch, and dinner? Who prepares your meals? Do you make your own meals or do you help out with the cooking?
ASK	Ask participants to review their nutrition plans with the class.
DISTRIBUTE AND COMPLETE PARTICIPANT HANDOUT: Meal Plan for a Day	*Next, we are going to create a menu.* Depending on the availability of cooking appliances, you may create menus that people can take home or menus that can be made with the group during class.
	Work in small groups or with the entire group to create a menu. You can use the **Meal Plan for a Day** handout for the menu.
REFER TO INSTRUCTOR REFERENCES: Shopping for Groceries Eating Fruits and Vegetables MyPlate	Instruct participants to include foods from four groups to have a balanced diet, along with ways to increase fruits and vegetables in their diet. Refer to the **Shopping for Groceries** and **Eating Fruits and Vegetables** references.
	Show participants pictures of different types of foods.
	Have participants choose whether they want to make a menu for a specific meal or a series of different snacks. For example, participants may decide to have a menu of snacks that they can have after each class.
	Work on menus that include all of the food groups. You may use the **MyPlate** reference as a resource guide or go to the MyPlate web site at www.ChooseMyPlate.gov.
RECORD	Write down the menu plans on the board. Encourage consensus among group members.
SUMMARIZE	Review nutrition plans and goals. Summarize the types of food groups that should be included in a menu plan.

EVALUATION

- Did participants discuss the effect of their diet on their health?

- Did participants complete their nutrition plan and identify foods they would like to reduce and foods they would like to increase in their diet?

- Did participants develop a menu plan?

Shopping for Groceries

GETTING READY TO SHOP

- Plan your meals before heading to the store. Make a shopping list to reduce impulse purchases and to save money and time.

- Avoid shopping if you are hungry.

- Consider using store brands. They are usually less expensive than name brands, and the quality is generally comparable.

AT THE STORE: HEALTHY SHOPPING TIPS

- Read the Nutrition Facts on the food label.

Produce

- Eat fresh fruits and vegetables to increase your daily intake of vitamins, minerals, and fiber.

- You need 2–4 servings of fruit daily and 3–5 servings of vegetables daily.

Meat

- Buy the leanest cuts of meat (extra lean, loin, and round) and trim off any visible fat before cooking.

- Select chicken without the skin.

- Use extra lean ground beef (90%–95% lean), sirloin steak, round steak, lean pork, and boneless, skinless chicken breasts, thighs, or chicken fingers.

Seafood

- Eat fish at least once a week.

- It is best to bake, boil, or broil your fish.

- Flavor your fish with a twist of fresh lemon or lime.

Shopping for Groceries

Dairy

- Choose low-fat or skim milk, reduced-fat cheeses, and low-fat or nonfat yogurts.

- You need 2–4 servings of dairy products daily.

- Look for soy milk and soy-based alternatives for heart health.

Spices and Seasonings

- Get creative. Use seasonings like fresh or dried herbs, spices, and low-fat condiments that do not add fat or sodium to your foods.

- Use salsa, Dijon mustard, or spices like garlic, basil, thyme, or oregano to marinate your meats.

Salad Dressing

- Look for nonfat or light salad dressings to keep your total fat intake low.

- Dressings made with olive oil and canola oil offer the benefits of monounsaturated fats.

- Balsamic vinegar adds flavor to tossed greens and vegetables without the fat.

Canned Goods

- Avoid buying canned fruits and vegetables that you can buy fresh or frozen. Canned fruits and vegetables have more added sugar or sodium. The process of canning may destroy vitamins and minerals.

- Stock up on canned beans and chickpeas.

Eating Fruits and Vegetables

BREAKFAST

- Drink a glass of juice.
- Add a banana or strawberries to your cereal.
- Have a bowl of fruit like melon or peaches.
- Top your pancakes with fruit instead of syrup.

LUNCH

- Eat a salad or have vegetable soup.
- Add a carrot or celery to your lunch.
- Eat a piece of fruit (e.g., apple, plum) or have unsweetened applesauce.
- Add lettuce and tomatoes to your sandwich.

SNACK

- Snack on grapes or raisins.
- Have a glass of juice.
- Eat raw vegetables like carrots.

DINNER

- Add vegetables to your main dish.
- Use fruits as a garnish with your main dish.
- Add steamed vegetables as a side dish.

DESSERT

- Add fresh fruit to a dessert.
- Top frozen yogurt with pineapple or papaya.
- Add chopped fruit or berries to cakes or cookies.
- Have a piece of fruit for dessert.

Nutrition Plan

1. I have decided that I will eat more of the following foods:

   _____

   _____

   _____

2. I have decided that I will eat less of the following foods:

   _____

   _____

   _____

3. My favorite snacks (junk food) are:

   _____

   _____

   _____

4. I will eat the following snacks (junk foods) (note how much per day or week):

   _____

   _____

   _____

   _____ Morning   _____ Home

   _____ Afternoon   _____ Work

   _____ Evening   _____ Other _____

Meal Plan for a Day

Think of all of the foods you like to and should eat, and make up a menu for one day's meal. Be sure to include foods from each group on the MyPlate.

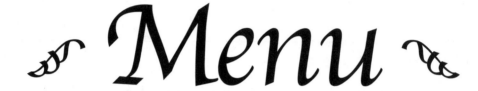

Breakfast

Lunch

Dinner

Snacks

Health Matters: The Exercise and Nutrition Health Education Curriculum for People with Developmental Disabilities
by Beth Marks, Jasmina Sisirak, and Tamar Heller

Lifestyle Changes

Doing My Program

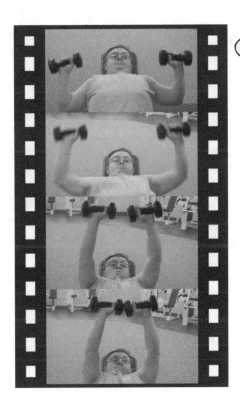

I'm doing it!

The fourth stage is when people are taking action and have changed their behavior(s). Participants are exercising and trying to include healthy foods in their diets. Classes should focus on reinforcing new behaviors to maintain their exercise and nutrition goals.

Unit 4 Contents

Lesson 24

Wants and Needs

Doing Different Exercises in My Community

Objectives
Participants will
• Identify the difference between wants and needs
• Describe general needs that must be met to achieve and maintain health
• Discuss needs that all human beings have in common

HANDOUTS

also on
CD-ROM

Instructor Reference(s):

What Do We Need?

MATERIALS

Blackboard and chalk

Pens or pencils

Personal Notebooks for handouts and pictures

💡**Idea**

Field Trip: Visit a miniature golf course (Putt-Putt Golf).

Suggested Activities	
INSTRUCTOR ACTIVITY	**INSTRUCTOR SCRIPT/DIRECTIONS**
REVIEW	*In our last class, we talked about our plans for eating a balanced diet, and we created a menu plan.* Have participants review their menu plans.
INTRODUCE LESSON	*Today, we will be talking about things that we need versus things that we want. We will also talk about how we can get the things that we need and want by asserting ourselves.*
ASK	*What are some things that you **need** to have?*
RECORD RESPONSES	Solicit responses (e.g., something a person must have to live, such as clothing, food, water, shelter). Record responses on the board.
ASK	*What are some things that you **want** to have?*
RECORD RESPONSES	Solicit responses (e.g., something a person desires to have but is not necessary to life or health, such as expensive clothes, junk food). Record responses on the board.

Source: McElmurry, B., Newcomb, B.J., Lowe, A., & Misner, S.M. (1995). *Primary Health Care Curriculum Grade K–8 for Urban School Children.* Chicago: University of Illinois at Chicago, College of Nursing, Global Halth Leadership Office.

INSTRUCTOR ACTIVITY	INSTRUCTOR SCRIPT/DIRECTIONS
REVIEW INSTRUCTOR REFERENCE: What Do We Need?	Review the **What Do We Need?** reference with participants. Discuss ways in which people can advocate for themselves to get their needs met.
WORK IN SMALL GROUPS	Divide participants into groups of two or three and (using **What Do We Need?**) ask them to select needs that are especially important in their lives. Regroup participants to discuss their ideas. Examples of needs for people include the following: • **Physical needs:** optimal nutrition, sleep, and rest • **Loving and belonging:** love and support of family and friends • **Safety and security:** security from harm and space to explore and understand who they are • **Esteem needs:** self-esteem is important at all ages • **Spirituality, religion, worship:** people of all ages may want the guidance of religion
TAKE A FIELD TRIP *(OPTIONAL)*	As a group, participants can go to a miniature (Putt-Putt) golf course. This is an opportunity to discuss our basic needs and wants to belong and be a part of a group. Playing golf can be a fun activity that can be an alternative to one's daily exercise routine. If it is winter and snow is on the ground, you can play golf online or you can find an indoor miniature (Putt-Putt) golf course in your area.
SUMMARIZE	*We all have many of the same basic needs, but they may change depending on how old we are, whether we are men or women, where we live, and where we work.* *Needs can change as we age. For example, nutrition needs, sleep needs, and exercise needs may change as we age.*

EVALUATION

• Can participants distinguish between wants and needs?

• Can participants describe general needs that must be met to achieve and maintain health?

• Do participants recognize that all human beings have the same basic needs?

HELPFUL HINTS

The field trips are designed to give participants opportunities to experience being physically active and making healthy choices in their community. Units that have field trip activities may be taught with or without the field trip.

What Do We Need?

WHAT ARE BASIC NEEDS?

Needs are essential as we grow.

There are three different types of needs. **Physical (body) needs** come first, followed by **psychosocial needs,** then **spiritual needs**.

WHAT ARE BODILY NEEDS?

Bodily needs are essential for our bodies and must be satisfied before any others are met. Examples of these needs are oxygen, water, food, elimination (e.g., urination), rest, sleep, exercise, sex, and not having pain.

For example: When a person is starving or thirsty, he or she spends time trying to find food or water and may have little energy or time for other needs. If a person cannot get oxygen, immediate action must be taken or that person will die.

WHAT ARE PSYCHOSOCIAL NEEDS?

- **Safety and Security Needs**

  We need a place to live to protect us from the outside. We like to feel secure from dangers by being in places we know, where we are used to doing the same things with people we can trust. We feel unsafe when we don't have this.

- **Loving and Belonging**

  We need to love and to be loved and to feel that we belong to a group. We feel unhappy when we are separated from our friends and family.

- **Esteem and Recognition**

  We have the need for self-esteem, the need to respect oneself and others, and the need to experience success in what we do.

WHAT ARE SPIRITUAL NEEDS?

We often need to have spirituality, religion, or worship in our lives. We need to believe in something beyond ourselves. We consider our relationship with a higher power. We wonder about the meaning of life.

Source: McElmurry, B., Newcomb, B.J., Lowe, A., & Misner, S.M. (1995). *Primary Health Care Curriculum Grade K–8 for Urban School Children.* Chicago: University of Illinois at Chicago, College of Nursing, Global Halth Leadership Office.

Lesson 25

What Is Good Pain and Bad Pain?

<table>
<tr><td colspan="2">

Objectives

Participants will

- Discuss and identify different types of pain
- Describe good pain and bad pain

</td></tr>
</table>

HANDOUTS

also on
CD-ROM

Instructor Reference(s):

How to Prevent Injury

Participant Handout(s):

Week 8 News

What Is Good Pain, and What Is Bad Pain?

MATERIALS

Blackboard and chalk

Pens or pencils

Personal Notebooks for handouts and pictures

Suggested Activities

INSTRUCTOR ACTIVITY	INSTRUCTOR SCRIPT/DIRECTIONS
DISTRIBUTE AND DISCUSS NEWSLETTER: Week 8 News	Give participants the **Week 8 News** handout. Discuss the newsletter.
REVIEW	*We have been talking about exercise and nutrition plans and goals. Does anyone want to discuss your plans for being more physically active and choosing healthy foods to eat? We also talked about things that we need versus things that we want. How can we get the things that we need and want by asserting ourselves?*
INTRODUCE LESSON	*Today, we will talk about what pain means to you. We will also learn about different kinds of pain and the difference between good pain and bad pain.*
ASK	*What does pain mean to you?*
RECORD RESPONSES	Listen to different responses. You may say to participants that pain is when someone feels physical or emotional hurt.
ASK, WAIT FOR RESPONSES, AND DISCUSS	*How do you describe different types of pain?* *Different conditions can cause different kinds of pain that are very different from each other. Pain can range from*

mild to severe. It may be steady or throbbing, stabbing or aching, pinching or burning. It can range from a little bit unpleasant to totally unbearable. Some kinds of pain only last a short while. Other types of pain can last for months, or even longer.

Give me some examples of pain. Wait for responses.

Let's talk about pain and physical activity.

Can any pain be good?

Actually, yes. Certain muscle aches are a sign of exertion— a sign that you are conditioning, rather than injuring, your body.

The burning sensation that you feel while trying to complete those last three repetitions, or the muscle soreness you experience a day or two after a workout or any physical activity are a sign that your muscles are building up. This pain goes away shortly after you stop doing the exercise. It is triggered by a buildup of **lactic acid,** *and you may experience it if you increase the weight or number of repetitions for a certain physical activity.*

Pain caused by injury is a different matter. Pain caused by injury can be **acute** *(short lasting), as with the sudden twisting of an ankle. Or it may be* **chronic** *(long lasting), as with a stress fracture or tendonitis that has worsened over time.*

As we get older, we may get pain from such chronic conditions as arthritis, rheumatic disease, back pain, and hip pain.

DISTRIBUTE AND DISCUSS PARTICIPANT HANDOUT:
  What Is Good Pain and What Is Bad Pain?

Distribute and review the **What Is Good Pain and What Is Bad Pain?** handout with participants. Discuss different types of pain and the difference between good and bad pain.

REFER TO INSTRUCTOR REFERENCE:
  How to Prevent Injury

Review the **How to Prevent Injury** reference with participants. Discuss ways in which people can prevent injuries.

SUMMARIZE

We learned about different kinds of pain today. We also learned the difference between good pain and bad pain. With good pain, you may feel a "mild burn," but bad pain may last for a long time.

EVALUATION

- Can participants state different types of pain?

- Can participants distinguish between good pain and bad pain?

- Can participants demonstrate ways to avoid injury?

HELPFUL HINTS

It is important to figure out the difference between **good pain**—the type that is part of the muscle strengthening process—and **bad pain**—the kind that may be caused by an injury.

Good Pain	Bad Pain
(Part of the muscle strengthening process)	(May be an injury)
"Mild" burn when you exercise	Lasts for a long time
Little soreness	Constant or does not go away
Goes away fast	Affects your walking

How to Prevent Injury

PREVENTING INJURIES

- **Warm-ups are a must! Stretch, stretch, stretch.** Working muscles shorten, which leads to injury unless you do something to maintain your flexibility. Always perform stretching exercises for all of the major muscles (and any others that you use during your workout) between 10 and 20 minutes before and after your workout.

- **Always start slow.** Your *cardiovascular system* usually shapes up faster than your *musculoskeletal system.* In other words, your lungs may be ready to run an extra 10 miles during the week, but your bones and tendons probably are not.

- **Do a variety of physical activities.** This spreads the workload around and challenges muscles you may not be using in your primary fitness activity.

- **Drink water before, during, and after physical activity.** Drink water every 15 minutes when you are exercising.

SAFETY TIPS FOR STRENGTH TRAINING

1. Demonstrate the proper technique for each exercise. If necessary, break the exercise into basic components.

2. Lift weights in a slow and controlled manner lasting about 2 seconds.

3. Lower the weights in a slow and controlled manner lasting about 2 seconds.

4. Exhale every time the weight is lifted.

5. Inhale every time the weight is lowered.

6. Encourage participants not to squeeze handles or free weights.

7. Check participants' form constantly during the early stages of the program.

   - Make sure feet are placed flat on the ground.

   - Make sure the entire back is touching the seat back.

   - Count each repetition with participants to complete the desired number of repetitions.

   - Stop the set if the participant does not use proper form.

Source: American College of Sports Medicine. (2006). *ACSM's guidelines for exercise testing and prescriptions* (7th ed.). Indianapolis, IN: Author.

How to Prevent Injury

SAFETY TIPS FOR TREADMILL USE

1. Explain and demonstrate how to properly use the treadmill before allowing participants to step on to the treadmill.

    *   Stand up tall.

    *   Take long strides.

    *   Look straight ahead, not down.

    *   Hold onto the handles for balance, not for support.

2. Participants must understand that they need to keep walking. They cannot stop while the belt is moving.

3. Do not allow participants to read or listen to headphones while on the treadmill.

4. Begin at a slow speed with participants holding onto handrails.

5. Stand next to participants in case they need assistance when stepping off the treadmill after a workout. It is not uncommon for them to feel slightly disoriented after using a treadmill the first couple times.

Week 8 News

NEWSLETTER FOR THE EXERCISE AND NUTRITION HEALTH EDUCATION CLASS

Needs or Wants

This week, we talked about things we need to have and things we want to have.

- Needs can change as we age. For example, nutrition needs, sleep needs, and exercise needs may change as we age.

- Wants are things we can live without (e.g., something a person would like to have but is not necessary to life or health, such as expensive clothes or junk food).

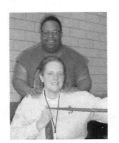

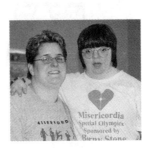

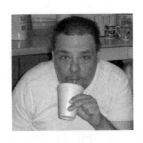

We have been making goals and plans for exercising, being more physically active, and making healthy food choices.

We also identified people who can help us meet our goals.

In exercise class, we talked about how to avoid injury.

Warm-ups are a must.

Always start slow.

Do a variety of physical activities.

Drink water before, during, and after physical activity.

We Talked About Important Needs in Our Lives

Physical needs: We all need to get enough healthy foods, sleep, exercise, and rest.

Loving and belonging: People need the love and support of family and friends.

Safety and security: People also need security from harm. At the same time, people need space to explore and understand who they are.

Esteem needs: Self-esteem is important at all ages.

Spirituality, religion, and worship: People may want the guidance of spirituality or worship.

PARTICIPANT HANDOUT

What Is Good Pain, and What Is Bad Pain?

What are different types of pain that you've had? Circle each answer.

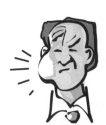
Toothache

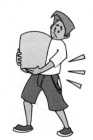
Back pain

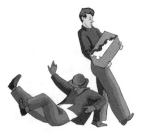
Falling down

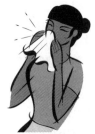
Fever/flu/cold

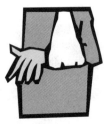
Sprain

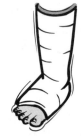
Broken bone

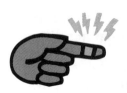
Cut

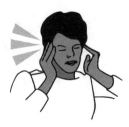
Headache

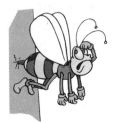
Bee sting

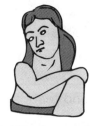
Stiff shoulder

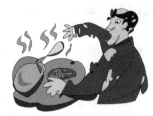
Burn

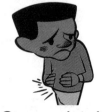
Stomachache

Good Pain	**Bad Pain**
Mild burn when you exercise	Lasts for a long time
Little soreness	Constant or does not go away
Goes away fast	Affects your walking

How Does Sleep Affect Physical Activity?

Objectives

Participants will
- Identify the importance of sleep
- State how much sleep they need at night
- Discuss the importance of physical activity on sleep

HANDOUTS

Instructor Reference(s):
   Helpful Hints for Good Sleep
Participant Handout(s):
   Exercise Helps You Sleep

also on CD-ROM

MATERIALS

Blackboard and chalk

Pens or pencils

Personal Notebooks for handouts and pictures

Suggested Activities

INSTRUCTOR ACTIVITY	INSTRUCTOR SCRIPT/DIRECTIONS
REVIEW	*In our last class, we learned about different kinds of pain and how to tell the difference between good pain and bad pain. Can anyone tell us the difference between good pain and bad pain?*
INTRODUCE LESSON	*Today, we will talk about sleep. Sleep is a very important part of your life. Not getting enough sleep can make you tired, nervous, and irritable. Being physically active will help you sleep better. This class will help you think about your sleeping habits.*
ASK	*Why is sleep so important?*
RECORD RESPONSES	• Keeps you in good health • Prevents injury and illness • Keeps your body functioning in top form physically, mentally, and spiritually • Helps you focus and think well
ASK	*How much sleep do you need?*
ANSWER	• 7–9 hours a night. • You might need more sleep if you are under a lot of stress or if you are sick.

INSTRUCTOR ACTIVITY	INSTRUCTOR SCRIPT/DIRECTIONS
REFER TO INSTRUCTOR REFERENCE: Helpful Hints for Good Sleep	Use the **Helpful Hints for Good Sleep** reference to guide your discussion.
ASK	*What kind of things can keep you up at night?*
ANSWER	• Drinking too much coffee, soda, tea, or any other drink with caffeine • Eating a big meal at the end of the day • Thinking or worrying about something
ASK	*Does exercise help you get a good night's sleep?*
ANSWER	• Makes you sleep better • Reduces depression and anxiety.
DISTRIBUTE AND DISCUSS PARTICIPANT HANDOUT: Exercise Helps You Sleep	Distribute and discuss the **Exercise Helps You Sleep** handout.
SUMMARIZE LESSON	*Today we talked about the importance of getting enough sleep and some things that keep us up at night. We also talked about exercise helping us sleep better.*

EVALUATION

- Can participants identify the importance of sleep?
- Can participants state how much sleep they need at night?
- Can participants discuss the importance of physical activity on their sleep?

Helpful Hints for Good Sleep

If people are having trouble sleeping, this is a list of some helpful hints to improve sleep habits:

- Reduce stimulants (e.g., tea, coffee, chocolate, cigarettes) that interfere with the quality of deep sleep.

- Reduce factors that might arouse you from sleep including external noise, having an uncomfortable bed, or experiencing extremes of temperature. Ear plugs are okay to use.

- Try to exercise (ideally at a level that causes you to sweat) at least 4–6 hours before going to bed.

- Get plenty of morning sunlight. Morning sunlight can help regulate your sleep–wake cycle.

- Make sure that medical problems that can interfere with sleep, such as asthma, heartburn, angina, arthritis, pain, or breathlessness are under control.

- Take a hot shower or bath before bed. Because your body temperature peaks during the daytime and falls during sleep, we tend to fall asleep as our body temperature begins to fall.

- Get out of bed at the same time each day.

- Avoid eating a large meal before going to bed. A drink high in carbohydrates with milk (which contains tryptophan) may help induce sleep, whereas high-protein foods may induce wakefulness.

- Avoid napping during the daytime.

Exercise Helps You Sleep

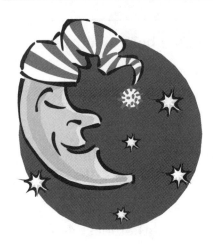

Exercise helps you sleep well.

Thirty minutes of daily physical activity can improve your sleep and give you more energy.

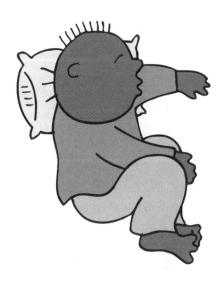

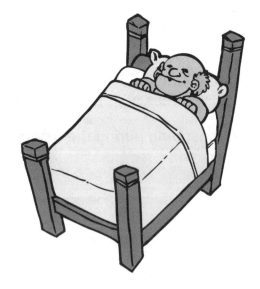

Negotiation and Compromise

Objectives

Participants will

- Discuss the process of negotiation
- Examine its role in helping to resolve conflicts
- State the steps involved in negotiating a fair solution to a conflict
- Practice skills of negotiation in order to reach a compromise
- Identify effective communication strategies that may be used to resolve conflicts with friends, family, and/or a support person

HANDOUTS

also on
CD-ROM

Instructor Reference(s):
   Negotiation Skills
   Vignettes for Negotiation

MATERIALS

Blackboard and chalk
Pens or pencils
Personal Notebooks for handouts and pictures

💡Idea

Field Trip: Participants are encouraged to go outside and participate in a community activity of choice.

Suggested Activities

INSTRUCTOR ACTIVITY	INSTRUCTOR SCRIPT/DIRECTIONS
REVIEW	*In our last class, we talked about sleep. How much sleep did everyone get last night?*
	Sleep is a very important part of our life. What happens to us if we don't get enough sleep? Not getting enough sleep may make us tired, nervous, and irritable.
	Does exercise help us sleep better?
	Being physically active will help you sleep better.
INTRODUCE LESSON	*Today we are going to talk about solving conflicts through **negotiation.***
	Introduce negotiation to participants by asking them to remember two situations when they really wanted something. In one instance they were successful, but in the other they lost out because they were not sure what to do. Explain that today they will learn a positive strategy for getting more of what they want and need from other people. This strategy is negotiation.

Source: McElmurry, B., Newcomb, B.J., Lowe, A., & Misner, S.M. (1995). *Primary Health Care Curriculum Grade K–8 for Urban School Children.* Chicago: University of Illinois at Chicago, College of Nursing, Global Halth Leadership Office.

INSTRUCTOR ACTIVITY	INSTRUCTOR SCRIPT/DIRECTIONS
CONTINUE	*Negotiation is deciding what you're willing to give up for something that you need or want. You also want to be fair and consider the needs of others. Negotiation is used in many different situations in life and is an important skill for you to develop.* *Negotiation is a process we use when we want to reach a fair agreement with someone to get something we need. Negotiation takes time. Sometimes we can resolve the issue ourselves, but other times we may need other people to give us advice.* Encourage participants to discuss their feelings about the conflict resolution strategies they have tried. If they have been practicing these strategies, they may be experiencing varying degrees of success in their efforts.
DISCUSS	*Let's think of some situations in which negotiations are used.* Provide examples of the kinds of things that people may negotiate. Focus on conflict resolution using **compromise**. *When we compromise, each person gives up something they want, and they each get something they want.*
ASK	*Has anyone tried to solve a conflict through compromise? What did you think of the activity? Did you feel that both people won? Why or why not? How much help do you get at home or at work when you are trying to solve a problem (or compromise)?* *Who do you talk to if you have a problem at work or at home? What do you do if someone is bothering you?* You may prompt with giving such examples as walking away or telling staff members, family members, or friends.
REFER TO INSTRUCTOR REFERENCE: Negotiation Skills	Refer to the **Negotiation Skills** reference. Discuss the reference by relating it to a situation that may be familiar to participants. Provide examples and discuss the steps in resolving conflicts through negotiation.
REFER TO INSTRUCTOR REFERENCE: Vignettes for Negotiation	Present vignettes/stories from the **Vignettes for Negotiation** reference to the group. Have group members provide solutions. You may want to role-play.
TAKE A FIELD TRIP *(OPTIONAL)*	Today's field trip is designed to incorporate physical activity (similar to Lesson 24 with the miniature (Putt-Putt) golf outing). Give participants a list of options (e.g., bowling, a community 5K walk/run event, a community bike ride event, an evening out at a dance club) and encourage them to negotiate as a group to decide which event they want to do. This field trip may be done on a different day depending on the activity that is selected.

INSTRUCTOR ACTIVITY	INSTRUCTOR SCRIPT/DIRECTIONS
SUMMARIZE	*Some problems are best resolved by using negotiation skills to reach a compromise (each person feels good about the outcome). This process isn't easy, and it requires a genuine desire on the part of both people to resolve the problem. It is important that we have people who can support us so that we can solve our problems.*

EVALUATION

- Did participants discuss the process of negotiation?

- Did participants practice skills of negotiation in order to reach a compromise?

- Were participants able to examine their role in helping to resolve conflicts?

- Did participants state effective communication strategies they can use to resolve conflicts with friends, family, and/or a support person?

HELPFUL HINTS

The field trips are designed to give participants opportunities to experience being physically active and making healthy choices in their community. Units that have field trip activities may be taught with or without the field trip.

Negotiation Skills

WHAT IS NEGOTIATION?

Negotiation is the process of deciding what you are willing to give up for something that you need or want. You want to make a fair trade and consider the needs of others as well as your own.

STEPS FOR SOLVING CONFLICTS THROUGH NEGOTIATION

1. First, decide **what problem** is **creating the conflict**.

2. Next, think of what **you want the most** from the situation. **What will you settle for** if you cannot have your first wish, and **what are you willing to give up** in return? Decide what **is not negotiable** under any circumstance. This step is easier if you really know yourself.

3. Find out what the other **person wants most** or **will settle for** in the situation.

4. Discuss your **first proposal** with the **other person.** If your proposal is fair, the other person will probably trust you and will likely suggest an equally fair proposal to you.

5. Be prepared for the possibility that your **first proposal may not be accepted.** You may need to have several discussions before an agreement is worked out. Be diplomatic.

6. Agree to a **compromise** if the details suit both of you.

How can you make sure that the other person will follow through with the trade?

Sometimes negotiations are finished by stating a promise or shaking hands, whereas at other times they must be put in writing. When the deal involves the approval of other people, you or the one you have traded with may have to talk about it again.

Source: McElmurry, B., Newcomb, B.J., Lowe, A., & Misner, S.M. (1995). *Primary Health Care Curriculum Grade K–8 for Urban School Children.* Chicago: University of Illinois at Chicago, College of Nursing, Global Halth Leadership Office.

Health Matters: The Exercise and Nutrition Health Education Curriculum for People with Developmental Disabilities
by Beth Marks, Jasmina Sisirak, and Tamar Heller

Vignettes for Negotiation

Note: Have group members participate in providing solutions.

SAMPLE SITUATIONS

- You would like to exercise at your local YMCA. You have no transportation or money. What can you do? How would you go about advocating for yourself?

- You would like to have healthy snacks while you are at work. However, the vending machines only have junk foods. What can you do? Who can you talk to so that you can have healthier options?

- You would like to watch a particular television show. Your roommate would like to watch another show. What do you do? How would you negotiate or resolve this conflict?

- You would like to have snacks in the evening when you are watching television. However, your house manager has decided not to have junk foods in your home. You know that these are foods that are high in fat, but you would like to have them sometimes. What do you do? How would you negotiate or resolve this conflict?

- You would like to move out of your mom's house into your own apartment. Your mom says no. How would you negotiate or resolve this conflict?

- You would like to marry your boyfriend/girlfriend and live together. How would you negotiate this? How would you go about advocating for yourself?

- Someone is bothering you on the bus. How would you negotiate or resolve this conflict?

Because we are unique individuals, it is inevitable that we will disagree with other people. Most disagreements occur among family, friends, and acquaintances. There are many strategies to resolve conflicts. Negotiation is just one way.

Can I Exercise if I Feel Sick?

Objectives
Participants will • Identify symptoms of illness • State how they feel

also on CD-ROM

HANDOUTS
Participant Handout(s): Week 9 News Can I Exercise if I Have Been Sick?

MATERIALS
Blackboard and chalk Pens or pencils Personal Notebooks for handouts and pictures

Suggested Activities

INSTRUCTOR ACTIVITY	INSTRUCTOR SCRIPT/DIRECTIONS
DISTRIBUTE AND DISCUSS NEWSLETTER: Week 9 News	Give participants the **Week 9 News** handout. Discuss the newsletter.
REVIEW	*We have been talking about how physical activity will help you sleep better. We also talked about solving problems by using negotiation skills to reach a compromise (each person feels good about what they received). Has anyone practiced negotiation in order to reach a compromise?*
INTRODUCE LESSON	*Today, we will talk about how we feel when we get sick. This class will help you think about how you feel. How you feel affects your physical activity.*
ASK AND WAIT FOR RESPONSES	*How does everyone feel today?* Wait for responses.
ASK	*How did you feel when you were sick?*
RECORD RESPONSES	• Not able to concentrate • Head was stuffed up • Runny nose • Body was aching • Felt sleepy, dizzy, or just tired • Throat was hurting • Did not have an appetite

INSTRUCTOR ACTIVITY	INSTRUCTOR SCRIPT/DIRECTIONS
ASK	*Should you exercise when you are sick?*
ANSWER	• If you are ill, stay away from exercise. Your lack of concentration can put you at risk of injury. • It's better to wait until you feel better, so you can exercise safely.
ASK	*When can you start exercising again?*
ANSWER	• Continue light exercise only 4–5 days after complete recovery in cases of a mild cold, muscle ache, or fever. • For more severe infections with these symptoms, allow 2–4 weeks of recovery before returning to intensive training.
DISTRIBUTE AND DISCUSS PARTICIPANT HANDOUT: Can I Exercise if I Have Been Sick?	Distribute and discuss the **Can I Exercise if I Have Been Sick?** handout with participants. Discuss different types of feelings.
SUMMARIZE	*We talked about how we feel when we get sick and how we can tell if we should not exercise. We also learned that if we have been sick, we should start exercising slowly. Exercise can also help keep us from getting sick.*

EVALUATION

• Can participants identify symptoms of illness?

• Can participants state how they feel?

HELPFUL HINTS

Physical activity and exercise build your immune system, so you will not get sick.

Week 9 News

NEWSLETTER FOR THE EXERCISE AND NUTRITION HEALTH EDUCATION CLASS

Sleep and Exercise

We have talked about the importance of sleep.

- Sleep can keep you in good health.

- Sleep can prevent injury and illness.

- Sleep can keep your body functioning.

- We need about 7–9 hours of sleep a night to help us think clearly.

- We may need more sleep if we are sick or stressed.

Exercise can help us sleep better at night!

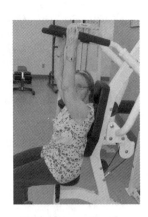

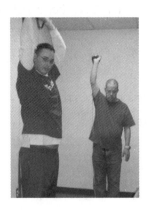

We are still doing our exercise program. This week we tried a new exercise video.

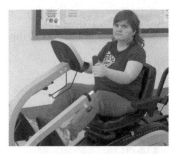

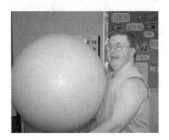

Steps for Solving Problems

Some problems are best resolved by using negotiation skills to reach a compromise (each person feels good about the outcome).

First, it is helpful to talk about your problem. Next, think of what you want to change.

What will you settle for if you cannot have your first wish, and what are you willing to give up in return? Decide what you are not willing to change.

This step is easier when you really know yourself.

Find out what the other person wants most or will settle for in the situation, then reach an agreement with the other person that makes you both feel okay.

Can I Exercise if I Have Been Sick?

Not feeling too well?

If you...

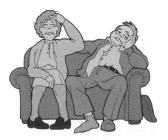

Feel tired, sleepy,
or dizzy

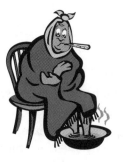

Feel cold, and
you are shivering

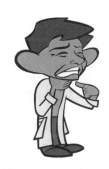

Have a sore throat

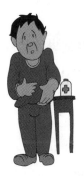

Have an aching body

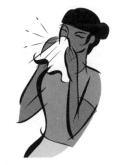

Have a runny nose

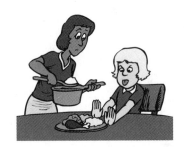

Have no appetite

Stay away from physical activity (exercise).

- Continue light exercise only 4–5 days after you feel better.

- If you are sick for a long time, wait 2–4 weeks before you start exercising again.

Lesson 29

Am I Meeting My Goals?

Objectives

Participants will

- Discuss the importance of setting exercise goals
- Identify skills or characteristics that will help them say "yes" to things that engage them in physical activities and other healthy behaviors

HANDOUTS

also on
CD-ROM

Participant Handout(s):

My Plan to Stay Physically Active

MATERIALS

Blackboard and chalk

Pens or pencils

Reminder Envelope

Personal Notebooks for handouts and pictures

Suggested Activities

INSTRUCTOR ACTIVITY	INSTRUCTOR SCRIPT/DIRECTIONS
REVIEW	*In our last class, we talked about how we feel when we get sick and how we can tell if we should not exercise. We also learned that if we have been sick, we should start exercising slowly. Exercise can also keep us from getting sick.*
INTRODUCE LESSON	*Today, we are going to talk about our individual plans for keeping our exercise goals. Goals are important in helping us direct our lives. When we set goals, we are able to deal with hard things and plan ways to either avoid or deal with them if they occur.*
CONTINUE	*People who want to have healthy lifestyles often feel good about themselves. When we feel good about ourselves, we are more likely to try new things, such as exercising and eating good foods.* *People who are willing to try new things often have the following characteristics:* • *High self-esteem—feel good about themselves* • *Clear goals* • *Behavior that is based on choice* • *Responsibility for the consequences of their actions*
DISTRIBUTE AND DISCUSS PARTICIPANT HANDOUT: My Plan to Stay Physically Active	Divide into small groups. Work with participants on the **My Plan to Stay Physically Active** handout. This should build on the **Exercise Plan** that they completed in Week 5.

CONTINUE	*This is your goal sheet. Remember, when you make a choice about something you want to do, you are making a goal for yourself. Think about the exercises we have done this week and think about the healthy foods we talked about. Doing these exercises or eating these foods are healthy choices you can make for yourself.*
	Have participants make any changes to their previous goals in the Exercise Plan or add additional goals. *Think about what you will have to do to make it happen. Write that down on your goal sheet.*
	If participants select an OUTDOOR activity, ask them to identify an INDOOR activity as well, in case of bad weather. Have them take the form home in their **Reminder Envelope** to their support person and request that they share their goals with their support person.
SUMMARIZE	Have participants summarize their exercise goals and how they plan on meeting their goals.
	It takes certain kinds of people to stand up for their rights and responsibilities and choose to do a certain activity that will help them stay healthy.
	Ask participants to identify how they can have a healthy lifestyle. Prompt them by saying that people who do this usually have chosen clear goals and can find people that will support their actions.

EVALUATION

- Did participants set exercise goals?

- Can participants identify characteristics that will help them engage in physical activities and other healthy behaviors?

My Plan to Stay Physically Active

GOAL(S):

1. _____

2. _____

3. _____

What are some steps I could take to reach these goals?

_____

COMMITMENT PLAN:

I will exercise _____ times a week for about _____ minutes each time.

What types of activity will you do?

_____

Will you exercise alone or with another person or group?

_____

Where will you exercise?

_____

What will you do on the days you don't feel like exercising?

_____

Lesson 30

Rewarding Myself

Objectives
Participants will
• Discuss the use of rewards as a motivator to exercise regularly
• Identify rewards for themselves when they engage in physical activity

HANDOUTS
None

MATERIALS
Blackboard and chalk
Pens or pencils
Personal Notebooks for handouts and pictures

♀Idea

Field Trip: Decide on an activity that participants can do as a group as a reward for making lifestyle changes.

Suggested Activities	
INSTRUCTOR ACTIVITY	**INSTRUCTOR SCRIPT/DIRECTIONS**
REVIEW	*In our last class, we talked about our plans for meeting our exercise goals.*
	Ask participants to talk about the ways in which they are keeping a healthy lifestyle. Also ask participants to name people in their lives who are supporting them to exercise and make healthy food choices.
INTRODUCE LESSON	*Today, we will talk about fun things that we can do for ourselves as a reward for achieving our exercise goals.*
DISCUSS	Discuss rewards for engaging in exercises, such as doing something nice for yourself for making an effort to exercise more, congratulating yourself after exercising, having more energy, or being in a better mood.
	Ask participants to identify their own ways in which they can reward themselves for exercising regularly. You may discuss some of the following rewards for exercising:
	• I am in a better mood and have less stress.
	• I do something nice for myself when I exercise.
	• I congratulate myself after I exercise.
	• I treat myself to something I like (new exercise outfit, exercise shoes, new exercise equipment, such as a stationary bike, aerobic video, rowing machine, treadmill).
	• I will get to see my friends if I attend an exercise program.
	• I keep a log that shows my progress.

INSTRUCTOR ACTIVITY	INSTRUCTOR SCRIPT/DIRECTIONS
TAKE A FIELD TRIP *(OPTIONAL)*	The goal for today's field trip is to have participants decide on an activity that they can do as a group as a reward for making lifestyle changes by making healthy choices. Some options that can be discussed include the following: a high school, college, or professional sports game or a museum such as a planetarium (if one is available) to see the stars at night. Encourage participants to make choices and negotiate with each other.
SUMMARIZE	Have participants summarize the ways in which they will reward themselves for exercising.

EVALUATION

- Did participants discuss the use of rewards to motivate themselves for exercising regularly?

- Did participants identify their own rewards to motivate themselves for exercising regulary?

HELPFUL HINTS

The field trips are designed to give participants opportunities to experience being physically active and making healthy choices in their community. Units that have field trip activities may be taught with or without the field trip.

New Lifestyle

Keeping My Program Going

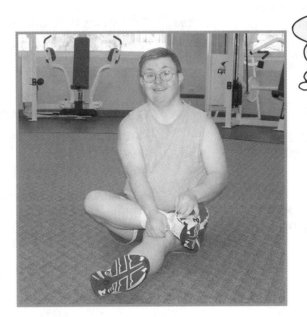

I'm still doing it!

The fifth stage is the maintenance stage. People in this stage are considering ways to prevent relapse. Activities should focus on reviewing what they have learned and different ways to help people continue with their health promotion program.

Unit 5 Contents

Lesson 31

Restructuring My Environment

Objectives
Participants will • Identify strategies for restructuring their environment to support exercising/physical activity • Discuss ways to increase support for physical activity

HANDOUTS	also on CD-ROM

Instructor Reference(s):
  Getting Past Barriers
Participant Handout(s):
  Week 10 News
  How Am I Doing?	

MATERIALS
Blackboard and chalk Pens or pencils Personal Notebooks for handouts and pictures

Suggested Activities

INSTRUCTOR ACTIVITY	INSTRUCTOR SCRIPT/DIRECTIONS
DISTRIBUTE AND DISCUSS NEWSLETTER: Week 10 News	Give participants the **Week 10 News** handout. Discuss the newsletter.
REVIEW	*We have been talking about things that help us stick with our exercise program and eat healthy foods. We can reward ourselves for exercising and eating a healthy, balanced diet. Meeting our goals can help us feel good about ourselves and keep us motivated to stick with our program.*
INTRODUCE LESSON	*Today, we are going to talk about how we can change our environment so that we can reach our exercise goals.*
DISCUSS	Discuss strategies for restructuring their environment to support exercising/physical activity. *To stay interested in exercising, we can* • *Keep things at work that remind us to exercise.* • *Keep a set of exercise clothes conveniently located so we can exercise whenever we have time.* • *Wear gym shoes to work so we can walk at lunch time.* • *Use a calendar to schedule exercise. Put the calendar in a place where it will remind us to exercise (e.g., kitchen).* • *Have our exercise partner call us to remind us to exercise.*

INSTRUCTOR ACTIVITY	INSTRUCTOR SCRIPT/DIRECTIONS
REFER TO INSTRUCTOR REFERENCE: Getting Past Barriers	Review the **Getting Past Barriers** reference with participants.
	Identify ways to increase support for physical activity, such as **social support** (e.g., family, staff), **access** (e.g., health clubs), **resources** (e.g., safe place for walking or jogging), and **programs** (e.g., affordable aerobics classes). Record participant responses.
DISTRIBUTE AND DISCUSS PARTICIPANT HANDOUT: How Am I Doing?	Divide participants into small groups and complete the **How Am I Doing?** handout
SUMMARIZE	Have participants summarize different ways that they can arrange their environment to support their efforts to exercise regularly.
	Identify key support people to help them negotiate the support they want to be able to exercise regularly.

EVALUATION

- Did participants identify ways to change the environment to meet exercise goals?

- Did participants discuss how support people can help structure their environment for success?

Getting Past Barriers

We all have days when we don't feel like doing the things we like to do. Sometimes we might be sick and it is important to rest. Other times, we may not be in the mood or have other things to do that wear us out. Here are some things to remember on the days when exercising seems like a burden:

- The **One-Minute Rule.** If you don't feel like exercising, put your shoes on and exercise for at least 1 minute. You'll probably stay out for 30 minutes and feel great.

- If the **weather** keeps you inside, do **stretching and strengthening exercises or use an aerobics tape.** This will keep you in the habit of exercising and help maintain the benefits to your health that you have already gained through exercising regularly.

- If you are **feeling down,** exercising often gives you more energy and lifts your spirits. Following the **routine from the exercise class** may help improve your mood. Starting a **walking group** at work may brighten your day by being in a social setting.

- **Keep exercise fun.** Do something you enjoy—walk with a family member or friend, ride an exercise bike while watching television, or try something new. **Vary your activities** if you find yourself becoming bored with the same old routine.

- **Set goals that you can reach** so you can see the progress you are making. Long-term goals are important so that you have something to work toward, but short-term goals help us feel a sense of accomplishment and provide motivation to keep on going.

- If you develop a **medical condition,** ask your doctor what kind of exercise is safe for you.

- **Keep a log** of how much you exercise so you can see the great work that you have done. If you skip days, don't get discouraged. Resolve to do better the next day, week, and so forth.

- If you have fallen out of the practice of exercising, **don't give up!**

- There are **no strike outs** in exercising. No matter how long it's been since you last exercised, no matter how many times you have promised yourself you would exercise and then didn't, **you can improve your health and get back into the habit of exercising.**

- If you haven't exercised in a while, **take it slow at first** so that you don't hurt yourself.

Week 10 News

NEWSLETTER FOR THE EXERCISE AND NUTRITION HEALTH EDUCATION CLASS

Exercise and Illness

- If you are ill, stay away from exercising.

- Your lack of concentration can put you at risk of injury. It's better to wait until you feel better so you can exercise safely.

- Physical activity and exercise build your immune system so you will not get sick.

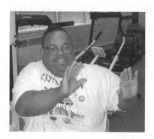

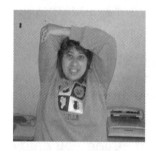

This week, we took a field trip to reward ourselves on doing a great job with making healthy choices.

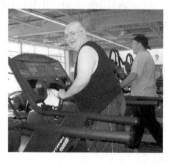

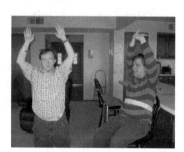

How Can We Reward Ourselves When We Exercise?

We have talked about ways to reward ourselves for exercising regulary.

Some of the things that we could do include dancing, fishing, eating pizza or a piece of cake, going to the movies and dinner, listening to the radio, going on vacation, going to church, and cleaning the house.

How Am I Doing?

1. Did I stick with my exercise plan for the whole week?

   _____

2. If yes, what helped?

   _____

3. If no, what prevented me from doing so?

   _____

4. Did family members and/or friends encourage or discourage me from participating?

   _____

5. Are my muscles firmer?

   _____

6. Is there a change in the way my clothes fit?

   _____

7. **Aerobic assessment:** Is it easier to breathe when I exercise? Can I exercise longer (e.g., ride a bike longer and breathe easier)?

   _____

Restructuring My Environment

How Am I Doing?

8. **Flexibility assessment**: Can I move and bend easier now that I've been exercising?

_____

9. **Strength assessment**: Is there any difference in my muscle tone? Am I any stronger?

_____

10. **Endurance assessment**: Can I do more activities during the day? Do I have more energy?

_____

11. Will I continue with my exercises? If no, why not?

_____

12. What is my fitness plan for the upcoming week?

_____

13. What did I learn from this activity?

_____

Health Matters: The Exercise and Nutrition Health Education Curriculum for People with Developmental Disabilities
by Beth Marks, Jasmina Sisirak, and Tamar Heller

Getting Back on Track

<table>
<tr><td>

Objectives

Participants will

- Identify feelings that will motivate them to start exercising again
- Describe ways to get back on track
- Discuss the benefits of walking as a way to begin an exercise program

</td><td>

HANDOUTS

also on CD-ROM

Participant Handout(s):

   Six Rules to Stay on Track

   Walking Your Way Back to Fitness

MATERIALS

Blackboard and chalk

Pens or pencils

Personal Notebooks for handouts and pictures

</td></tr>
</table>

Suggested Activities

INSTRUCTOR ACTIVITY	INSTRUCTOR SCRIPT/DIRECTIONS
REVIEW	*In our last class, we discussed ways that we could change our environment to support us in doing our exercise program. What were some things that we discussed?*
	Review barriers and ways that people can address these barriers.
INTRODUCE LESSON	*Today, we are going to talk about ways to get back on track if we get out of the habit of exercising.*
DISCUSS	*When we start an exercise program, it's normal to get off track and stop our program. We are going to talk about how we may feel if this happens and what we can do about it so that we can exercise again.*
CONTINUE	Discuss the following:
	• When we stop exercising, we may feel frustrated.
	• Identify feelings that might help us start exercising again (e.g., feeling more confident, active, happy, healthy).
DISTRIBUTE AND DISCUSS PARTICIPANT HANDOUT: Six Rules to Stay on Track	Distribute the **Six Rules to Stay on Track** handout. Discuss ways to start exercising again. You may use problem-solving methods with participants.
	• Make a plan that is realistic and simple.
	• Pick a person who you can call (e.g., friend, boy- or girlfriend, support person, family member) or have someone call you.

INSTRUCTOR ACTIVITY	INSTRUCTOR SCRIPT/DIRECTIONS
	• Exercise with a partner.
	• Look for things that you need to continue the activity (e.g., money, transportation, time).
	• Buy new shoes or new exercise clothes.
	• Change your activity.
	• Chart and share your progress.
	• Think about ways of getting started again.
	• **Keep it fun!**
DISTRIBUTE AND DISCUSS PARTICIPANT HANDOUT: Walking Your Way Back to Fitness	*Walking is a great way to get back on track if you stop exercising.* Review the **Walking Your Way Back to Fitness** handout.
SUMMARIZE	Have participants summarize different ways to get back on track if they stop exercising.

EVALUATION

- Did participants identify feelings that will motivate them to start exercising again?
- Did participants identify ways to get back on track?
- Did participants identify the benefits of walking as a way to start exercising again?

Six Rules to Stay on Track

1. **THE ONE-MINUTE RULE.** If you don't feel like exercising, put your shoes on and exercise for at least **one minute.** You'll probably exercise for 30 minutes and feel great.

2. **THE STOP RULE. Stop** exercising if you have any chest tightness or chest pain, severe shortness of breath, or feel dizzy, faint, or sick to your stomach. If you continue to feel this way, contact your health care provider.

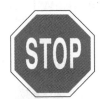

3. **THE WRENCH RULE.** If you have **muscle pain or cramping** during any exercise, stop that exercise. Relax the affected muscle by rubbing it gently with your hands. Start exercising again with slower and easier movements.

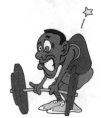

4. **THE TALK TEST.** If you can carry on a normal conversation while doing your exercises, you are probably working at a safe level. If you become out of breath and find it difficult to talk to someone while walking or doing your exercises, you are walking or exercising too fast.

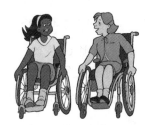

5. **THE TWO-HOUR PAIN RULE.** If your exercises cause pain that continues **two hours** after exercising, don't do as many as you were doing and don't do them as strong. If this does not help, choose a different exercise that will give the same result but that is better for you.

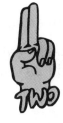

6. **MY BODY, MY FRIEND RULE.** Exercises that seem easy one day **may be too hard** the next. When this happens, cut back on the number of times that you do the exercise and then return to your amount when you can. If you notice a big change in what you are able to do, contact your health care provider for advice.

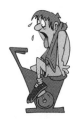

Walking Your Way Back to Fitness

Walking is one of the most natural physical activities and the least likely to cause an injury.

A walking program is an excellent form of exercise for people because it combines stretching, strengthening, and endurance exercises.

Walking briskly while swinging your arms can almost give you all of the benefits of jogging without the strain on your body.

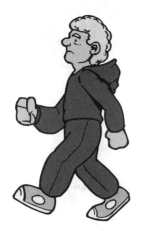

THE BENEFITS OF WALKING

Walking can be **done anywhere, any season** of the year, at **no cost.**

You can **walk alone** or **with others.**

You **don't need any special equipment** or clothing, just comfortable shoes.

Walking is something you **can usually do for the rest of your life.**

Walking has a positive effect in the following areas:

- Strengthens muscles (including the heart), ligaments, tendons, and cartilage and tones leg muscles.

- Improves the body's ability to deal with sugar.

- Strengthens the bones to prevent them from breaking, and it may slow down osteoporosis, a thinning of the bones.

- Improves self-image and makes you happier.

- Increases caloric expenditure, controls appetite, and burns fat—you can lose weight as well as inches.

STEP RIGHT THIS WAY

Find a route.

Put on your walking shoes.

Warm-up and stretch.

Walk 15–20 minutes between 3–5 times per week.

You'll feel great!

Creating an Exercise Video

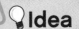

Objectives

Participants will

- Review what they should do before they exercise
- Identify different types of exercises
- Create a group exercise video

HANDOUTS

None

MATERIALS

VCR/DVD player, television, and video camera

Blank video or DVD to make exercise video

Personal Notebooks for handouts and pictures

💡Idea

Field Trip: Participants can choose to go to someone's house to make an exercise video.

Suggested Activities

INSTRUCTOR ACTIVITY	INSTRUCTOR SCRIPT/DIRECTIONS
REVIEW	*We have been talking about ways to get back on track with our exercise program. We have also been talking about things we can do to get past barriers that may prevent us from exercising and eating healthy foods. What are some things that may prevent us from exercising? What are some things that we can do to help us stick with our exercise and nutrition plans?*
INTRODUCE LESSON	*Today, we are going to begin making our own Group Exercise Video that we can use at home when this program is over.*
SELECT A GROUP LEADER	Have participants gather into a single group and select a group leader for the second part of the video.
DISCUSS	Review the types of clothing that should be worn for exercising. *What types of exercises would you like to do on the tape (e.g., stretches, warm-ups, aerobics, cool-downs)?* You can incorporate various exercises that they have done throughout the program (e.g., working out in gym with equipment, using exercise bands, walking, doing various exercise videos, stretching, warming up). You can also review the **Warm-Ups and Stretches** and **What to Wear** handouts (Lesson 3).

INSTRUCTOR ACTIVITY	INSTRUCTOR SCRIPT/DIRECTIONS
TAKE A FIELD TRIP *(OPTIONAL)*	Participants can choose whose home they would like to use to make the video. The goal of this field trip is to encourage participants to think about exercising and physical activity in a variety of places and to encourage them to make choices and support each other outside of class. Also, it can give participants an opportunity to take leadership roles in producing the video. Everyone should have a role to play.
BEGIN EXERCISE ACTIVITIES AND TAPING	Have the group leader introduce him- or herself. The group leader should instruct the class through the exercise program. Then, begin filming exercise activities.
SUMMARIZE	Compliment participants on their video production. Summarize the components of their exercise program.

EVALUATION

- Did participants describe the things they need to do before they exercise on a regular basis?

- Did participants participate with the class to create an exercise video?

HELPFUL HINTS

The field trips are designed to give participants opportunities to experience being physically active and making healthy choices in their community. Units that have field trip activities may be taught with or without the field trip.

Reviewing Our Goals to Stay Connected

Objectives

Participants will

- Review their individual goals
- Discuss their individual concepts of health
- State what they should do before they exercise
- Describe the benefits of exercise and good nutrition
- Discuss their rights and responsibilities in maintaining an exercise program
- Review the exercise and nutrition plan that they will follow after the program is completed
- Describe ways that they can stay connected with their support people to help them meet their exercise and nutrition goals

HANDOUTS

also on CD-ROM

Participant Handout(s):

Week 11 News

MATERIALS

Blackboard and chalk

Personal Notebooks for handouts and pictures

Suggested Activities

INSTRUCTOR ACTIVITY	INSTRUCTOR SCRIPT/DIRECTIONS
DISTRIBUTE AND DISCUSS NEWSLETTER: Week 11 News	Give participants the **Week 11 News** handout. Discuss the newsletter.
REVIEW	*In our last class, we started making our own exercise video. We have been talking about things we need to wear while we exercise. And we have been talking about ways to stick with our exercise program. Does anyone want to say who they are going to rely on to support them with their program? What can you do if you don't feel like exercising?*
INTRODUCE LESSON	*Today, we are going to talk about things we learned in our health education classes.*
	We are going to begin by reviewing our exercise goals.

INSTRUCTOR ACTIVITY	INSTRUCTOR SCRIPT/DIRECTIONS
CONTINUE	*We are also going to talk about ways we can stay connected with each other, our friends, and our family. This helps maintain a healthy lifestyle.*
DISCUSS	Discuss ways of connecting with friends and family members: • Have a regular **workout partner**. Schedule a time that you always meet with this person. Make the commitment. • Find someone who **encourages you to exercise** (e.g., family member, workout partner, close friend, support person). • Consider being a **role model** for friends, family members, or coworkers. • **Advocate for yourself** at work. Talk to your employer about creating a fitness/exercise center or walking clubs during breaks or before and after work.
SUMMARIZE	Review the following areas: • Review the individual concepts of health. • Discuss what they should do before they exercise. • Review the benefits of exercise and good nutrition. • Review their rights and responsibilities in maintaining an exercise program. Discuss participants' exercise and nutrition plans that will be followed after the program is completed
ASK	Ask participants if they would like to do anything different or change anything in the **health education/promotion classes.** *What were some things that you liked in the classes? What were some things that you did not like in the classes?*
PREPARE FOR NEXT CLASS	*During our next class, we will talk about the things we have learned and begin to make plans for our graduation ceremony and party.*

EVALUATION

• Did participants discuss how they plan on staying connected with people to keep exercising?

• Did participants identify the benefits of having friends or family members encourage them to exercise, especially when they do not feel like exercising?

• Did participants identify ways to build connections with people to sustain their exercise goals?

• Did participants review their individual concepts of health?

• Did participants review the benefits of exercise and good nutrition?

• Did participants review their rights and responsibilities in maintaining an exercise program?

• Did participants review their exercise and nutrition plan that they will follow after the program is completed?

Week 11 News

NEWSLETTER FOR THE EXERCISE AND NUTRITION HEALTH EDUCATION CLASS

Getting Past Barriers

This week, we talked about ways to get past barriers so that we can keep with our exercise program.

- Keep exercising fun.

- Set reachable goals.

- Keep a log of how much you exercise.

- Exercise with a friend.

- Use the One-Minute Rule: if you do not want to exercise, walk for one minute, and you'll probably walk for 30 minutes.

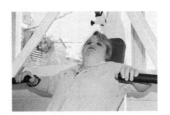

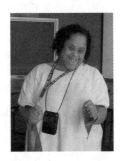

We started working on our own exercise video. At the end of the program, we will have a video of ourselves doing aerobic exercises, stretches and warm-ups, and strength exercises that we can do at home.

Rules to Stay on Track

1. **THE ONE-MINUTE RULE.** If you don't feel like exercising, put your shoes on and go outside and walk for 1 minute. You'll probably exercise for 30 minutes and feel great!

2. **THE STOP RULE. Stop exercising** if you have any chest tightness or chest pain, severe shortness of breath, or feel dizzy, faint, or sick to your stomach. Call your doctor if you continue to have these problems.

3. **THE WRENCH RULE.** If you have muscle pain or cramping during any exercise, stop that exercise. Gently rub the sore muscle with your hands and continue exercising with slower and easier movements.

4. **THE TALK TEST.** If you can talk while doing your exercises, you are probably working at a safe level. If you can't talk, you are probably walking or exercising too fast.

5. **THE TWO-HOUR PAIN RULE.** If your exercise causes pain that continues 2 hours after exercising, decrease the number of repetitions and be less forceful. If this doesn't help, pick another exercise to do.

Putting It All Together

Objectives

Participants will

- Review the benefits of an exercise and nutritional program
- Discuss their exercise goals

HANDOUTS

also on
CD-ROM

Instructor Reference(s):

Putting It All Together: Revisiting Our Goals

MATERIALS

Blackboard and chalk

Personal Notebooks for handouts and pictures

Suggested Activities

INSTRUCTOR ACTIVITY	INSTRUCTOR SCRIPT/DIRECTIONS
INTRODUCTION	*Today, we are going to talk about what we have learned about health during our classes.*
REVIEW	*As a refresher, can anyone describe how people look if they are getting ready to exercise? What type of clothes should they be wearing?*
	What are different types of exercises we should be doing?
DISCUSS	*Each one of us can take responsibility to help keep our body healthy. How can we do that?* Write responses on the board.
ASK	*How can we keep our bodies in good working order?*
	Briefly review concepts of how participants can keep their bodies healthy. Make sure to talk about exercising, eating healthy foods, resting, not smoking, having check-ups, drinking water, and following your health care provider's recommendations.
	When we do these things, we are making healthy choices and taking responsibility for our own health.
CONTINUE	*We can help keep our bodies from getting really stiff and keep our muscles strong. We do that by* **stretching and exercising.**
	We have been exercising regularly in class and in our free time. Have the group talk about what they have been doing.

Exercising helps our bodies in several ways. If we exercise, our bodies will get stronger. We can lose fat and gain muscle.

Have participants identify different muscle groups by tightening and then relaxing them (e.g., arms, legs). Ask them to describe how tightening and relaxing feels.

Our blood flows more smoothly around our bodies and our hearts do a better job pumping our blood. Exercise can help our body work better. We often feel better when we exercise.

REFER TO
INSTRUCTOR REFERENCE:
   Putting It All Together:
     Revisiting Our Goals

Use the **Putting It All Together: Revisiting Our Goals** reference to review participants' plans for an active lifestyle.

PREPARE FOR GRADUATION

Ask participants to think about what they would like to do for their graduation party. Provide different alternatives, such as going to different types of restaurants and doing different types of activities.

EVALUATION

- Can participants describe the things they need to do before they exercise on a regular basis?

- Do participants understand the benefits of good nutrition and exercise on health?

- Did participants review their goals for exercising?

Putting It All Together: Revisiting Our Goals

We have learned about the benefits of exercise and how to exercise safely and at our own pace. Now we need to think about our goals after the class ends. Here are some things to consider when developing individual goals and commitment plans for continuing to lead an active lifestyle.

Review the class goals identified at the beginning of the exercise program and see what progress has been made toward those goals.

- We have made progress toward our goals. How can we keep going?

- Do we need to change our goals so that we can realistically reach them?

- Are there *other* goals that we have for being healthy?

- Can anyone think of other steps that can help you reach your goals?

Look at PROS and CONS and Tips to Change for Healthy Lifestyles.

(You may refer back to the Positive Things Related to Exercise and Negative Things Related to Exercise references from Lesson 13)

- Are there any PROS that we can add to our plans?

- Are there any CONS that we need to think about and find ways to handle things that are problems for us?

- Consider the following tips for our plans:

  Make a plan

  Use our time wisely

  Start with a small change

  Vary our activity routine

  Keep it fun

  Pick a partner

  Share your fitness news

  Balance your energy

  Chart your progress

  Reward your achievements

Finishing Touches on Our Video

Objectives

Participants will

- Review what they should do before they exercise
- Finish their group exercise video
- Create a flyer advertising an exercise group they would like to offer

HANDOUTS

also on CD-ROM

Participant Handout(s):

Sample Advertisement Flyer

MATERIALS

DVD/VCR, TV, and video camera

Blank videotape or DVD

Exercise bands

Camera to take pictures of participants creating an advertisement for their exercise group

Personal Notebooks for handouts and pictures

💡 Idea

Field Trip: Participants can choose whose home they would like to go to continue taping an exercise video.

Suggested Activities

INSTRUCTOR ACTIVITY	INSTRUCTOR SCRIPT/DIRECTIONS
REVIEW	*In our last class, we talked about ideas for our graduation party. Would anyone like to make any other suggestions for the party?*
	We also talked about the things that we learned about staying healthy. Review things that people can do to stay healthy (e.g., eat nutritious foods, exercise regularly).
INTRODUCE LESSON	*Today, we are going to finish making our own Group Exercise Video that we can use at home when this program is over.*
	When we finish with our exercises, we are going to create a flyer to advertise an exercise group we would like to have during our lunch break or downtime at work.
TAKE A FIELD TRIP *(OPTIONAL)*	Participants can choose someone's house to continue taping an exercise video. They may decide to continue taping at the same home that was chosen in Lesson 33.

INSTRUCTOR ACTIVITY	INSTRUCTOR SCRIPT/DIRECTIONS
	Again, the idea is to encourage participants to think about exercising and physical activity in a variety of places and to encourage people to make choices and support each other outside of class.
SELECT A GROUP LEADER	Have group members select a group leader to finish the video.
DISCUSS	Review the types of clothing that should be worn for exercising and what they should do before they exercise (stretches and warm-ups).
	Decide what exercises they would like to do to finish the group video. You can incorporate various exercises that they have done throughout the program (e.g., working out in the gym with equipment, using exercise bands, walking, doing various exercise videos, stretching, warming up).
BEGIN EXERCISE ACTIVITIES AND TAPING	Have the group leader introduce him- or herself on the video. The group leader should instruct the class through the exercise program. Begin filming exercise activities.
CREATE FLYER	Have participants decide on the type of group they would like to lead at work with their friends and coworkers. You may suggest the following: using exercise bands, doing aerobic videos, walking groups and so forth.
	Discuss the ways in which participants could start a group at work. Take pictures of each participant advertising his or her group activity.
DISTRIBUTE PARTICIPANT HANDOUT: Sample Advertisement Flyer	Give participants the **Sample Advertisement Flyer** handout an example of a flyer.
SUMMARIZE	Compliment participants on their video production. Summarize the components of their exercise program.
	For our next class, we will have our graduation party. Come to class ready to celebrate and have a great time. We will also watch our Group Exercise Video.

EVALUATION

- Did participants participate with the class to create an exercise video tape?

- Did participants identify an exercise group they would like to form at work?

- Did participants discuss the steps they might take to start an exercise group?

HELPFUL HINTS

The field trips are designed to give participants opportunities to experience being physically active and making healthy choices in their community. Units that have field trip activities may be taught with or without the field trip.

Sample Advertisement Flyer

COME JOIN OUR GROUP!

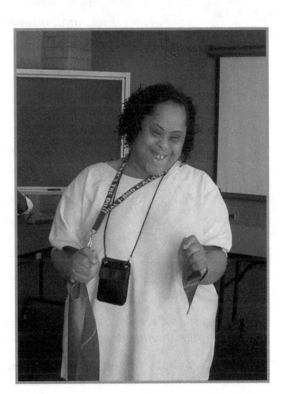

We Are Doing Exercise Bands

Days: Monday, Wednesday, and Friday

Time: 12:00pm

Place: Community Center

Graduation Party

also on
CD-ROM

Objectives

Participants will

- Celebrate their successes
- Receive their Certificates of Achievement
- Receive the Group Exercise video that students previously created

HANDOUTS

Participant Handout(s):

Week 12 News

Program Summary

Certificate of Achievement

Individual Progress Report

MATERIALS

Blackboard and chalk

TV and VCR/DVD player

Group Exercise Video from previous lesson

Personal Notebooks for handouts and pictures

Suggested Activities

INSTRUCTOR ACTIVITY	INSTRUCTOR SCRIPT/DIRECTIONS
DISTRIBUTE AND DISCUSS NEWSLETTER: Week 12 News	Give participants the **Week 12 News** handout. Discuss the newsletter.
INTRODUCE	*Today, we are celebrating your accomplishments in the health education/promotion classes.*
DISTRIBUTE AND DISCUSS PARTICIPANT HANDOUTS: Program Summary Certificate of Achievement	*We hope that you have enjoyed the classes and learned things about yourself and how to lead healthy lifestyles.* Give participants the **Program Summary** handout and their **Certificates of Achievement**. Invite each participant to report to the group what they learned through their classes.
DISTRIBUTE PARTICIPANT HANDOUT *(OPTIONAL):* Individual Progress Report	You may want to give participants an **Individual Progress Report** that shows changes in their fitness level and body composition over time.
WATCH GROUP EXERCISE VIDEO	Watch the video with participants and support persons.
SUMMARIZE	Thank participants for their active involvement in the health education/promotion classes. Also, thank each of the support persons for their involvement.

Week 12 News

NEWSLETTER FOR THE EXERCISE AND NUTRITION HEALTH EDUCATION CLASS

Congratulations on your accomplishments!

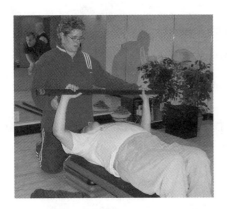
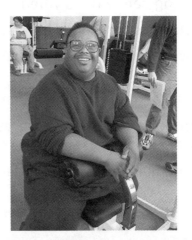
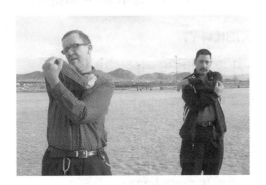
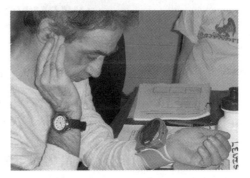
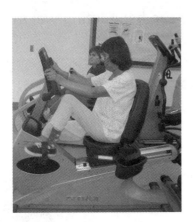
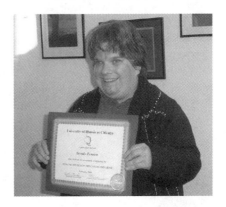

Keep up the good work!

Program Summary

We have talked about the following topics in our health education classes:

- Breathing correctly while exercising
- Exercising in our target heart rate zone using heart rate monitors
- Drinking plenty of water every day
- Following safety rules when exercising
- Knowing the difference between good and bad pain
- Identifying things that influence our food choices

We have also learned the following:

- The importance of carbohydrates (energy), protein (muscle building), and fat (energy storage)
- How medications make us feel

As a part of our exercise program, we have focused on four different areas:

WARMING UP (FLEXIBILITY)

To get ready to exercise, we have been doing stretches.

HEALTHY HEART (AEROBIC ENDURANCE)

To keep our heart healthy and strong, we have been doing such aerobic exercises as walking on the treadmill and doing exercise videos.

STRONG MUSCLES AND BONES (STRENGTH)

To keep our muscles and bones strong, we have been lifting weights.

BALANCE

To keep us from falling, we have been doing balance exercises.

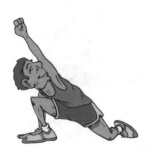 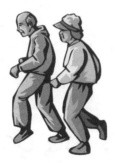 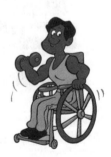

Health Matters: The Exercise and Nutrition Health Education Curriculum for People with Developmental Disabilities
by Beth Marks, Jasmina Sisirak, and Tamar Heller

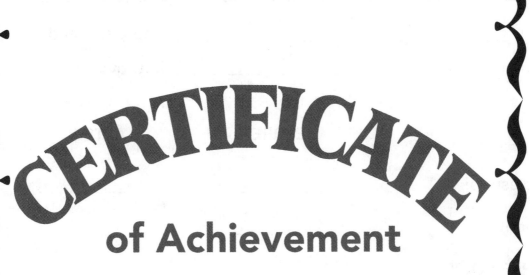

CERTIFICATE

of Achievement

Presented to

_____

In recognition of completion of the Exercise and Nutrition Health Education Curriculum.

PARTICIPANT HANDOUT

Individual Progress Report

Your _____ improved, and

your _____ improved!

	BEFORE	AFTER
Cholesterol	_____	_____
Weight	_____	_____
UPPER BODY		
Bench Press	_____	_____
LOWER BODY		
Sit to Stand	_____	_____

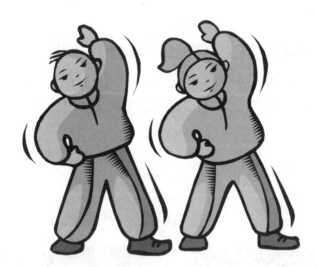

CONGRATULATIONS!

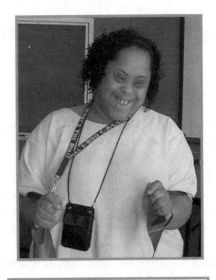

Section III

Appendixes

Description of the Appendixes

Appendix A—the Lifelong Learning Series—includes 22 lessons. These lessons were designed to complement the 36 lessons in the 12-week program to sustain long-term adoption of healthy lifestyles. Specifically, the aim of the classes is to reinforce the information presented during the 12-week program and to provide ongoing support for people to continue developing new skills and greater confidence to engage in regular physical activity and make healthy food choices. These themes include advocacy and social support, exercise and physical activity, nutrition, and general health information. In addition, similar to the teaching strategies used in the core modules, the concepts of choice, self-determination, self-efficacy, self-advocacy, and rights and responsibilities should be used as a foundation for all of the classes.

Appendix B contains a glossary of health and exercise–related terminology.

Appendix C contains sample exercise workouts for flexibility, aerobic, balance, and strength (FABS) exercises. These exercises can be used to train people for the physical portion of the program. This section contains three sample workouts: circuit training sampler, inexpensive and portable equipment: using exercise bands, and inexpensive and portable equipment: using weighted bars.

Appendix D contains universal design strategies for health promotion. Universal design aims to design communication, products, and environments to be usable by all people, to the greatest extent possible, without adaptation or specialized design. This concept is also referred to as *inclusive design, design-for-all, lifespan design, barrier-free design,* or *human-centered design.* The underlying premise is that if universal design works well for people across the spectrum of functional ability, universal design will work better for everyone. The usability of a communication strategy, product, or environment can be enhanced by including designs for a broad range of users that incorporate the five senses: seeing, touching, smelling, tasting, and hearing. Including universal design strategies from the beginning can be done without significantly increasing the expense.

Appendix E contains a testing procedure manual; that is, procedures and directions for evaluating the success of your program using a variety of assessments with your participants.

Lifelong Learning Lessons

Appendix A

Self-Advocacy

Rights and Responsibilities

Objectives

Participants will

- Discuss rights and responsibilities
- Identify that their rights include responsibilities
- Choose a right that is important to them
- Practice, during the week, taking responsibility for what they have chosen
- Speak up about the right they have chosen

HANDOUTS

also on
CD-ROM

Instructor Reference(s):
    The Americans with Disabilities
        Act (ADA) and Your Rights
Participant Handout(s):
    Rights and Responsibilities[1]

MATERIALS

Guest speaker/self-advocate (e.g., SABE or People First).[2] Or revisit the video *Self-Advocacy: Freedom, Equality, and Justice for All*[3]

Blackboard and chalk

Paper and pencil

Reminder Envelope

Personal Notebooks for handouts and pictures

HOMEWORK

Have participants work on one of their rights and the responsibilities that go with it.

Suggested Activities

INSTRUCTOR ACTIVITY	INSTRUCTOR SCRIPT/DIRECTIONS
REVIEW	*In previous classes, we talked about how our thoughts, feelings, and actions affect our health and our behaviors. We also talked about how our family and friends can also affect our health and behaviors.*
	Have people identify some influences that affect their behaviors.
INTRODUCE LESSON	*Today, we are going to talk about your rights and responsibilities.*[4] *Rights are choices that you can make.*

---

[1]Heller, T., Preston, L., Nelis, T., Pederson, E., & Brown, A. (1995). *Making choices as we age: A peer training program.* Chicago: University of Illinois at Chicago and University of Cincinnati.

[2]Ask if the self-advocate would like to lead the discussion by him- or herself. If a self-advocate is not available, instructors can lead the discussion.

[3]Advocating Change Together (ACT). *Self-advocacy: Freedom, equality, and justive for all* [Video]. St. Paul, MN: Author. Available online at http://www.selfadvocacy.com

[4]Heller et al. (1995).

INSTRUCTOR ACTIVITY	INSTRUCTOR SCRIPT/DIRECTIONS
REVIEW RIGHTS AND RESPONSIBILITIES	*With rights, you also have responsibilities. For example, you have a right to choose to have a job. If you decide to have a job, you have a responsibility to be at work on time.*
ASK AND RECORD RESPONSES	*Did you make some choices during this past week?* You may probe by asking, *How did you spend your money? Who came to see you? What movie did your see?* Have the group talk about the choices they made in the last week. Record participants' responses.
ASK	*Did anyone make some choices during this past week? What choices did you make?* You may probe by asking, *Did you buy anything? Did you visit with a friend? Did you do something fun (e.g., bowling, dancing)?*
RECORD RESPONSES	Discuss the choices made by participants during the last week. Record participants' responses.
ASK	*Is there anyone who didn't make any choices? What prevented you from being able to make those choices? Is there some way we could help?*
ASK	*Did anyone make a choice that went badly?*
DISCUSS	*Let's talk about what rights you have. I mentioned having a job and going to church. I'm going to put those up on our board. What other rights do you have (e.g., right to ride the bus, have a relationship with someone, have friends)?*
RECORD RESPONSES	As participants discuss what rights they have, list these rights on the board and put up a picture for each one (if there is an available picture).
DISTRIBUTE AND DISCUSS PARTICIPANT HANDOUT: Rights and Responsibilities	After the participants have listed everything they can think of, add other rights they may have forgotten. Refer to the **Rights and Responsibilities** handout.
REVIEW AND DISCUSS INSTRUCTOR REFERENCE: The Americans with Disabilities Act (ADA)	*Some of the rights we have put on our list are human rights and some of them are rights that the law gives you.* Review **The Americans with Disabilities Act** reference.
REVIEW	Review the rights that mean the most to participants. Work with the group to list the responsibilities that go with those rights. For example: *We mentioned that you have the right to have a job. What responsibilities (or things that you need to do) do you have if you have a job?*
	Make a separate column on the board, opposite the "rights" column, for "responsibilities." List the responsibilities that go with having a job in that column on the board. (If you have appropriate pictures, use them to illustrate the responsibilities as people list them.)

INSTRUCTOR ACTIVITY	INSTRUCTOR SCRIPT
PROVIDE EXAMPLES OF RIGHTS AND RESPONSIBILITIES	*Another example is that you have the right to walk by yourself in your neighborhood. If you choose to walk in the neighborhood, what responsibilities do you have?* Give other examples of exercises. *You have the responsibility to keep yourself safe by walking alone only during the middle of the day, by staying away from places you know are dangerous, and so forth.* List the responsibilities in the proper column on the board and use pictures to illustrate them as needed.
PROVIDE MORE EXAMPLES OF RIGHTS	*What other rights did we list?* If participants need help recalling the rights they listed, go back to the list on the board and begin with the rights that are most important to them. Ask them to think about what responsibilities they have if they make these choices. Write the responsibilities they bring up. Add any responsibilities they do not mention that you want them to be aware of. (See the list of rights and responsibilities from the participant handout).
ROLE-PLAY	*Let's role-play with some of the things that you have listed as rights that you would like to have for yourself. I will tell you what happened, and you can show us what you would do.* Use examples that relate to the class discussion. See Helpful Hints for more information.
GIVE OUT HOMEWORK	*Today, we talked about the **rights** you have; that is, some of the **choices** you should be able to make. We also talked about the **responsibilities** you have; that is, what **you** have to do for yourself and for other people after you make your choice.* *During the coming week, I would like you to work on one of your rights and the responsibilities that go with it. For example, you have the right to speak up for yourself. The responsibility that goes with that is knowing exactly what you want and speaking up for what you want instead of complaining.* *You might decide to work on this right by practicing the skill of knowing what you want and speaking up for what you want instead of complaining.* Give participants paper and pens or pencils to write down their goal(s) for the session. *Remember, when you make a choice about something you want to do, you are making a goal for yourself.* Assist participants as needed in writing down their goals. Take time to work with participants as they choose and write down their goals. *When you are finished, we will all discuss the goals you have written.*

INSTRUCTOR ACTIVITY	INSTRUCTOR SCRIPT/DIRECTIONS
SAY	*We are putting a copy of your goal in a Reminder Envelope to help you remember to work on your goal. During the week, be sure to share your goal sheet with your support person.*
SUMMARIZE	*Let's summarize the list of rights we talked about today. Decide which one is most important to you. Think about what responsibilities go with that right.*

EVALUATION

- Did participants verbalize their rights?

- Can participants state their rights and include responsibilities?

- Did participants list the rights that are especially important to them?

- Did participants list the responsibilities that go along with the rights?

- Did participants choose one right to practice during the week?

- Did participants and support people identify how to let staff and community people know about choices they would like to make?

HELPFUL HINTS

It might be helpful to make up role plays that are about the rights the participants have listed or about additional rights you think they need to know about (related to exercise, nutrition, or other healthy behaviors).

In the Reminder Envelope, send a definition of rights and responsibilities in general, as well as the specific right that the participant chooses to work on. Ask the support person to work on this during the week whenever the opportunity comes up. Put a note in the Reminder Envelope asking the support person to look at the goal sheet with the participant. Ask that the participant and support person work together on that goal during the week whenever the opportunity comes up.

You may also consider showing the film *Self-Advocacy: Freedom, Equality, and Justice for All* [5] to discuss the self-advocacy movement.

[5] Advocating Change Together (ACT). *Self-advocacy: Freedom, equality, and justice for all* [Video]. St. Paul, MN: Author. Available online at http://www.selfadvocacy.com

The Americans with Disabilities Act and Your Rights

The Americans with Disabilities Act (ADA) talks about some of the rights you have in the community and at a job.

- The ADA talks about *discrimination.*

- *Discrimination* means treating someone differently or unfairly just because of some group the person belongs to.

- The ADA talks about discrimination against people *because* they have a disability.

- The ADA says discrimination based on disability is wrong.

- The ADA says people with disabilities should be able to go to the same places in the community as people who do not have a disability—places like shopping malls, restaurants, community centers, and on buses and trains.

- The ADA says people with disabilities should have the same chance for a job that people without disabilities have.

- The ADA says your boss cannot discriminate against you while you are working.

- The ADA says you have rights if you are arrested.

- The ADA helps you know what you can do if you think discrimination is happening to you because of your disability.

Where to get information about ADA:

Disability and Business
Technical Assistance Center
www.adata.org
1-800-949-4232

The Arc National Headquarters
1010 Wayne Avenue, Suite 650
Silver Spring, MD 20910
1-800-433-5255
www.thearc.org

_____

Source: This information is adapted from draft copies of the "The ADA Training Program for Self-Advocates," "Know Your Rights If You Get Arrested," and "ADA Help Checklist" written by The Arc (National Headquarters) and from "The Americans with Disabilities Act (ADA) and Working" and "The Road to Opportunity" published by The Arc and The Great Lakes Disability and Business Technical Assistance Center.

Self-Advocacy: Rights and Responsibilities

Rights and Responsibilities

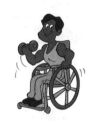

RIGHT: To choose when and what type of exercise to do

RESPONSIBILITY: *Participate in developing a plan as to what you are going to do and when.*

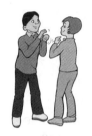

RIGHT: To speak up and express your own ideas

RESPONSIBILITY: *Know what you want. Speak up for yourself instead of complaining.*

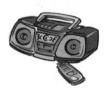

RIGHT: To own your own things

RESPONSIBILITY: *Keep your things in a safe place and in good condition.*

RIGHT: To have privacy

RESPONSIBILITY: *Respect the rights of others while you are alone.*

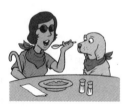

RIGHT: To make your own food choices and express what you like.

RESPONSIBILITY: *Understand the pros and cons of your choices. Understand how your choices affect other people and respect their rights.*

Sutton, E., Heller, T., Sterns, H.L, Factor, A., & Miklos, S. (1993). *Person-centered planning for later life: A curriculum for adults with mental retardation.* Akron, Ohio: Rehabilitation Research and Training Center on Aging with Mental Retardations, the University of Illinois at Chicago and the University of Akron.

In *Health Matters: The Exercise and Nutrition Health Education Curriculum for People with Developmental Disabilities*
by Beth Marks, Jasmina Sisirak, and Tamar Heller

Rights and Responsibilities

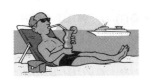

RIGHT: To do things in the community

RESPONSIBILITY: *Act according to the rules and dress appropriately.*

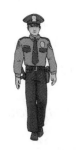

RIGHT: To be safe

RESPONSIBILITY: *Know how to stay safe. Don't harm other people.*

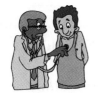

RIGHT: To choose your health care provider

RESPONSIBILITY: *Participate in choosing health care providers you like to see.*

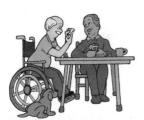

RIGHT: To visit and spend time with your family and friends

RESPONSIBILITY: *Respect the rules of other people's homes. Help out when needed.*

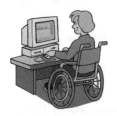

RIGHT: To have a job

RESPONSIBILITY: ***If you don't have a job,*** *prepare for the job you want by finding the support you need to look for a job.*

If you have a job, *be on time, do not be absent, do good work, and dress professionally.*

Rights and Responsibilities

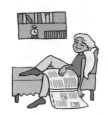

RIGHT:

To have your own room or your own space

RESPONSIBILITY:

Take care of your room or your space yourself.

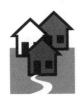

RIGHT:

To live in a neighborhood

RESPONSIBILITY:

Take care of the place where you live.

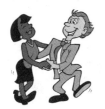

RIGHT:

To have intimate relationships

RESPONSIBILITY:

Make sure you know the other person, you are both safe, and you both agree.

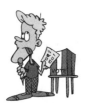

RIGHT:

To vote

RESPONSIBILITY:

Know as much as you can about the people who are running for office.

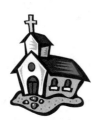

RIGHT:

To go to a church, synagogue, or temple

RESPONSIBILITY:

Find out when the services are. Commit yourself to spending time going to services. Act according to the rules.

Supports to Keep Us Healthy

Objectives
Participants will
• Differentiate among different types of friends
• Identify two behaviors that describe how to be a friend
• Describe their own friends/circles of friends and support networks who will encourage them to exercise when they do not feel up to it
• Identify ways they can help each other to exercise or have healthy behaviors
• Discuss the pros and cons of having a workout partner

HANDOUTS
Instructor Reference(s):
Friendships and Supports
Participant Handout(s):
Circle of Support

also on
CD-ROM

MATERIALS
Blackboard and chalk
Reminder Envelope
Video on friends and friendships (e.g., *Benny and Joon*)
Small plant or flower
Personal Notebooks for handouts and pictures

Suggested Activities

INSTRUCTOR ACTIVITY	INSTRUCTOR SCRIPT/DIRECTIONS
REVIEW	*In our last class, we talked about rights and responsibilities for being more physically active and making healthy food choices. We also talked about making choices and ways that we can let people know about the choices that we want to make.*
	Ask participants if they worked on their goals from the last class (rights and responsibilities).
INTRODUCE LESSON	*Today, we're going to talk about friends and how they can help us exercise and eat good foods. What is a friend? How would you describe a friend?*
CONTINUE	Discuss the qualities of a friend. *A friend is someone who likes you and who enjoys doing things with you. A friend is someone you know very well and can count on being there to help you. A friend is fair, understanding, and willing to share with you and listen to you.*
DISCUSS	Discuss characteristics and qualities of a friend: someone who likes you, you can enjoy doing things with, you know a good bit about, you can count on, who is fair and understanding, who shares, and who will listen to you.

INSTRUCTOR ACTIVITY	INSTRUCTOR SCRIPT/DIRECTIONS
SAY	*Friends help each other.*
RECORD RESPONSES	Record the characteristics and qualities of a friend on the board.
CONTINUE	*What about relatives, brothers, sisters, parents, and cousins? Can they be your friends? Of course. We need all the friends we can get. Why are friends and relatives important to us? Sometimes we need people to help us.*
CONTINUE	Discuss the benefits of having encouragement from friends and/or family members when participants do not feel like exercising. Prompt by saying: *Friends and family can remind us to exercise and give us positive feedback.*
CONTINUE	*Being willing to help each other is one of the most important things about friendships. How do we help each other in this group? Can someone give me an example?*
DISCUSS DIFFERENT TYPES OF SUPPORTS	• **Good friends:** Not necessarily your best friend or someone you are close to, but someone you like and trust and enjoy being with from time to time • **People who are friendly:** You see them at work, church, next door, or a senior center • **Neighbors:** People with whom you are acquainted who live next door or across the street • **New friends:** A person you have just met and would, perhaps, like to know better • **Staff friends:** Professionals whose job it is to help you at work or home, such as case managers, resident managers, team leaders, instructors, physical therapists, and so forth • **People we know a little bit:** People you know enough to say "hi" to (e.g., people at Laundromats or check-out counters)
DISTRIBUTE PARTICIPANT HANDOUT: Circle of Supports	Distribute and review the **Circle of Supports** handout. *Draw a picture of friendships—yours, mine, anyone's.* *Here is the **person** in the middle. That could be you or me. Let's draw the circles of friends— different kinds of friends.* Typically, circle members come from the family, school, workplace, church, or neighborhood. Service providers may be included in the mix, but the emphasis is on people who share common interests with the person. *The first circle is the one closest to the person—**best friends** or very special friends. Old friends might go in that circle, too. Knowing someone for a long time sometimes makes that person very special. These people who are closest to you are the ones you can turn to for help or advice when you need it. You can count on them. We'll make this circle thicker and darker to represent how special they are.*

INSTRUCTOR ACTIVITY	INSTRUCTOR SCRIPT
ASK QUESTIONS WHILE COMPLETING THE CIRCLE OF FRIENDS	*Name a friend that you have had for a long time. What's the name of a new friend? Who is someone who will really talk with you? Who is someone who you can go to for help? What can you tell me about this person?*
CONTINUE WITH THE SECOND CIRCLE	*Who should we put in the second circle? We could put in staff friends, your family doctor and nurse, and neighbors. Include those who aren't our special best friends but who are **good friends**—people we like and may see at work or at home. These could also be people we don't see very often but we like and trust.*
CONTINUE WITH THE THIRD CIRCLE	*The last circle can just be people we say "hi" to or other people we happen to know, just a little bit. Let's also put in that circle **new friends**—people we've just met.*
	Can someone in this farthest circle move up to this closest circle? Wait for responses. *That would be possible, but it would take a little doing on your part. You need to be a friend to have a friend. In order to grow, friendships have to be cared for, just like plants or flowers.*
WORK IN SMALL GROUPS	Work with participants in small groups to draw their own **Circle of Friends** and then put in names. Tell participants to first put themselves in the middle of the page (draw a stick figure or print name).
	Now, we will help you put names of your friends in the circles. Put at least one name on each circle. Not everyone has lots of special friends or good friends. Having one, two, or three is good for most people.
DISCUSS INSTRUCTOR REFERENCE: Friendships and Support	Have participants return to the large group. Ask questions from the **Friendships and Support** reference.
	Record responses on the board.
WATCH VIDEO ABOUT FRIENDS	*We're going to see a clip of a video that is about special friends. Be sure to notice the things they do and the places they go together.*
	What were some things that the friends did together? Where did they go together? Did they ever get into arguments? How did they resolve their arguments? What did you like about their friendship? Spending time with a friend is a wonderful way to use your free time.
SUMMARIZE	*We want to give each of you a little flower (plant) to remind you that keeping friends is like making a flower or plant grow. You have to take care of it.*
	Review the **Circle of Friends** handout with participants.

EVALUATION

- Can participants differentiate among different types of friends?

- Can participants identify two behaviors that describe how to be a friend?

- Can participants describe their own friends/Circle of Friends and support networks who will encourage them to exercise when they do not feel up to it?

- Can participants identify ways they can help each other to exercise or engage in healthy behaviors?

- Can participants discuss the pros and cons of having a workout partner from their Circle of Friends?

Friendships and Support

What are some things that good friends do to stay friends? How do we keep from losing our friends?

There is an old saying that to have a friend, you must be a friend. To be a good friend, we need to be interested in our friend. Know what he or she does, what he or she likes, and how he or she feels. We also need to keep in touch with our friend. We can can keep in touch by phone, sending cards (can make the cards), going places and doing things together, having a good time together, sharing secrets, giving gifts, having respect for each other, acting your best and looking your best when you are with that person, having something interesting to talk about, doing nice things for your friends, always be interested in what that person has been doing, or wants to do, or what that person thinks, and so forth.

What types of things do you like to do with your friends?

When your friend suggests that you go somewhere or do something, and you don't think it's a good idea, what should you do? Should you follow your friend's lead just because he or she is a good or special friend?

Reinforce the concept of self-advocacy, standing up for your own ideas, and so forth. Role-play a situation that illustrates this idea.

How can you make more friends? Where can you meet people who might become your friends?

We don't usually meet people who could become our friends out on the street or just in passing at the mall. We really need to meet new friends in a place where we are going to see them again and again, so we can become real friends. Elicit such answers as neighborhood, workplace, church, classes, and recreational centers.

How can your friends help you be more physically active and make healthier food choices?

Focus on exercise and nutrition goals. Have a workout partner. Friends can remind us to exercise and eat healthy foods.

Circle of Support

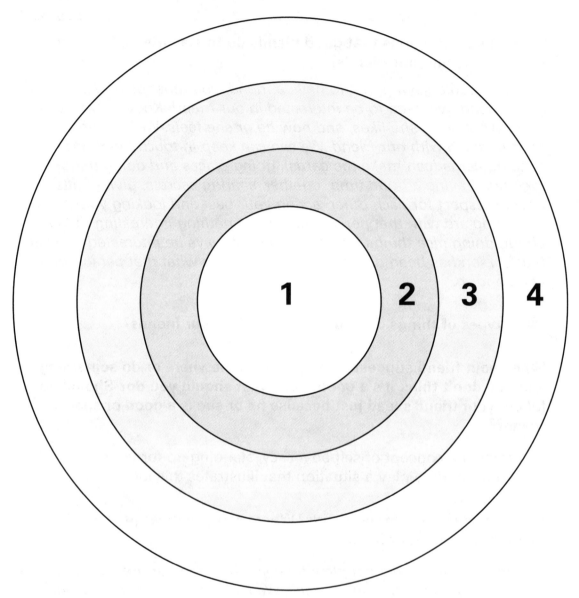

CIRCLE OF SUPPORT

1. **You**
2. **Best friends, close family**
3. **Staff, neighbors, family**
4. **People we do not know very well, new friends**

Write the names of your friends or family
in the circle with the corresponding number.

Source: Pearpoint, J. (1994). *From behind the piano: Building Judith Snow's unique circle of friends.* Inclusion Press.

Lesson C

Aerobic Exercise Tape of Choice

Objectives

Participants will

- Describe the benefits of aerobic exercise
- Discuss the benefits of the exercise video as an aerobic exercise option
- State whether the exercise video is an exercise option for themselves

HANDOUTS

also on CD-ROM

Participant Handout(s):

Tips: Warm-Ups *(see Lesson 3 for handout)*

Tips: Stretching *(see Lesson 3 for handout)*

Tips: Aerobic Exercises *(see Lesson 3 for handout)*

Tips: Cool-Downs *(see Lesson 3 for handout)*

Warm-Ups *(see Lesson 3 for handout)*

Stretches*(see Lesson 3 for handout)*

MATERIALS

Aerobic exercise video (e.g., Richard Simmons's aerobic video, National Association on Down Syndrome video, Tai Chi dancing tape)

TV and DVD player/VCR

Camera (to take participants' photos while doing the video for their newsletter)

Personal Notebooks for handouts and pictures

Suggested Activities

INSTRUCTOR ACTIVITY	INSTRUCTOR SCRIPT/DIRECTIONS
REVIEW	*In our last class, we talked about our friends and people who provide us with support to stay healthy. Our friends can help us meet our goals and support us when we make choices. For example, they can encourage us as we make changes in our diets and increase our physical activities.* Ask participants to describe their own Circle of Friends.
INTRODUCE LESSON	*Today, we are going to do an aerobic exercise video. You might like to do this at home with your family or friends or by yourself.*
ASK	*Before we do the video, let's review what we know about aerobic exercises.*

INSTRUCTOR ACTIVITY	INSTRUCTOR SCRIPT/DIRECTIONS
	• *Why do we need to do aerobic exercises?*
	• *What are some aerobic exercises?*
	• *How often should we do aerobic exercises?*
	• *What do we do before we begin an aerobic exercise?*
	Supplement participants' responses with information from the participant handouts.

REVIEW
PARTICIPANT HANDOUTS:
  Tips: Warm-Ups
  Tips: Stretching
  Tips: Aerobic Exercises
  Tips: Cool-Downs
  Warm-Ups
  Stretches
	Review the **Tips: Warm-ups, Tips: Stretching, Tips: Aerobic Exercises, Tips: Cool-Downs, Warm-Ups,** and **Stretches** handouts.
	
	Lead the group with a participant co-leader through warm-ups and stretches using the **Warm-Ups** and **Stretches** handouts.

ASK	*Have any of you tried this aerobic exercise video (name the tape that you are using)?*
ASK	*Who would like to co-lead the group today?* If more than one person wants to lead, work with participants to make an equitable decision (e.g., compromise or draw straws).
BEGIN VIDEO	Have the co-leader introduce the video and instruct the class during the tape.
ASK	At the end of the class, ask participants if they enjoyed doing the aerobic exercise video. Ask them if this is something they would like to do. Ask what an aerobic exercise means.
SUMMARIZE	Review and summarize the benefits of an aerobic exercise. Solicit responses from participants (e.g., health benefits, being with friends, having fun).

EVALUATION

- Are participants able to identify the benefits of aerobic exercise?

- Did participants identify the aerobic exercise video as an activity for exercise?

- Did participants express whether they would like to use the video as a regular activity?

Alternatives to the Gym

Objectives

Participants will
- Identify different options to getting exercise outside of the gym
- Practice using the exercise bands

HANDOUTS

also on CD-ROM

Participant Handout(s):
- Exercise Band Bench Press
- Exercise Band Tricep Extension
- Exercise Band Shoulder Press
- Exercise Band Leg Press

MATERIALS

Exercise bands (e.g., Dynabands) *(See Resources for ordering information.)*

Digital camera to take pictures of participants using exercise bands for the weekly newsletter

Personal Notebooks for handouts and pictures

Suggested Activities

INSTRUCTOR ACTIVITY	INSTRUCTOR SCRIPT/DIRECTIONS
REVIEW	*We have been talking about types of exercises we like to do and the foods we like to eat.*
	Briefly review the kinds of exercises people like to do and the types of foods people enjoy.
	Again, it's important to figure out what we like to do and the foods we like to eat. We are more likely to do exercises if we have fun with them. We are also more likely to stick with a balanced diet if we can find foods that are tasty to us. We all have our own foods we like to eat.
INTRODUCE LESSON	*Today, we are going to talk about another way that we can exercise when we are not at the gym. We are going to learn how to use **exercise bands** instead of the machines in the gym.*
DISCUSS	Discuss the use of exercise bands as a replacement for using equipment in the gym.
	Exercise bands can be done anywhere. You can use them in a group or you can use them by yourself in your home or in your bedroom.
	Exercise bands are also very inexpensive to use and can increase your strength and flexibility.

INSTRUCTOR ACTIVITY	INSTRUCTOR SCRIPT/DIRECTIONS

DISTRIBUTE AND DISCUSS PARTICIPANT HANDOUTS:
   Exercise Band Bench Press
   Exercise Band Triceps Extension
   Exercise Band Shoulder Press
   Exercise Band Leg Press
	Show participants how to use the **exercise bands** by reviewing the participant handouts. Discuss the benefits of the exercise bands. For example, exercise bands are inexpensive, easy to use, can be used anywhere, and can be used by yourself or with your friends.

TAKE PICTURES	Have participants demonstrate the exercises using the exercise bands. Take pictures of this activity to put in their Personal Notebooks.
SUMMARIZE	Summarize the use of exercise bands as an alternative to working out in a gym.

EVALUATION

- Do participants understand the benefits of using exercise bands as another way to exercise either by themselves or in a group?

- Are participants able to demonstrate how to use the exercise bands?

Exercise Band Bench Press

START

Place the band around your back and under your arms. Grab the band close to your body.

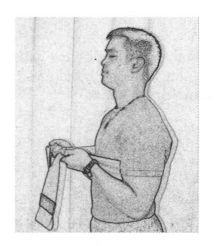

HALFWAY THERE

Slowly push out.

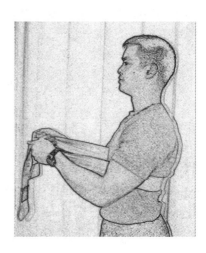

DONE

Keep pushing until your arms are straight. Then, bring your arms back to the starting position. This is one repetition.

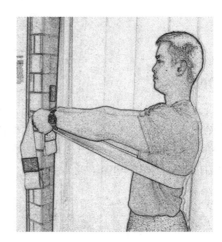

Exercise Band Tricep Extension

GRIP

Sit at the end of a bench with your back straight. Grab the band as shown in the picture on the right.

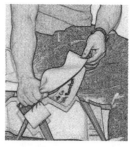

START

Put the band under your legs. Hold the band in your right hand. Raise your hand overhead.

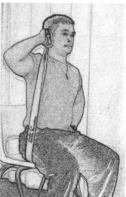

HALFWAY THERE

Keep raising your hand. Keep your upper arm close to your head.

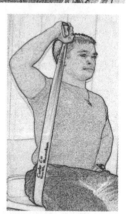

DONE

Raise your hand overhead to arm's length. Then, bring your arms back to the starting position. This is one repetition. Repeat with your left arm.

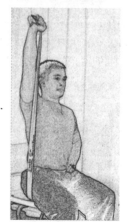

Exercise Band Shoulder Press

START

Place the band under your legs. Grab the band with your hands. Place your hands next to your shoulders.

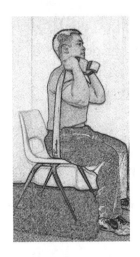

HALFWAY THERE

Slowly push up above your head.

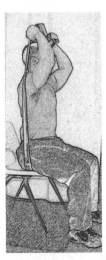

DONE

Keep pushing until your arms are almost straight. Then, bring your arms back to the starting position. This is one repetition.

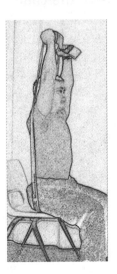

In *Health Matters: The Exercise and Nutrition Health Education Curriculum for People with Developmental Disabilities* by Beth Marks, Jasmina Sisirak, and Tamar Heller

237

Exercise Band Leg Press

BEFORE YOU START

Sit on the edge of a chair.

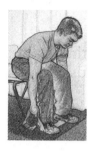

START

Slowly stand while you hold the band.

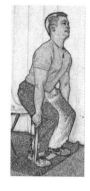

HALFWAY THERE

Continue standing until you are standing straight up.

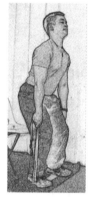

DONE

Lower yourself slowly back to a sitting position on the edge of the chair—GO SLOWLY! This is one repetition.

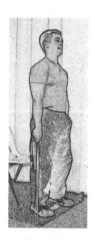

DON'T DO THE FOLLOWING!

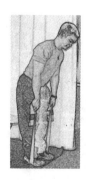

BEND

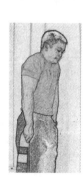

SHRUG

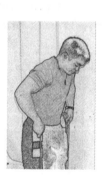

BEND ELBOWS

Lesson E

Joining a Community Fitness Center

Objectives

Participants will

- Visit a neighborhood community fitness center (e.g., YMCA, YWCA, Park District)
- Identify and discuss activities that they would be interested in doing
- Arrange a visit with the director of a fitness center (discuss any specific supports, adaptations needed, and accommodations to make this a viable community option for participants)

HANDOUTS

May obtain informational brochures from local fitness centers

MATERIALS

Transportation

Personal Notebooks for handouts and pictures

Suggested Activities

INSTRUCTOR ACTIVITY	INSTRUCTOR SCRIPT/DIRECTIONS
REVIEW	*We have talked about different types of exercises that we do and would like to do.* Have participants review different activities.
INTRODUCE LESSON	*Today, we are going to talk about different places that we can go to exercise.* *We are going to _____ (fitness center). When we are at the center, we will get a tour of the kinds of options for exercising and talk about how we can become members of the fitness center.*
DISCUSS	*In our community, there are different places that we can go for exercise, physical activity, and fun. The place (fitness center) that we are going to today is one place that you may like to go to exercise.*
TAKE A FIELD TRIP	At the fitness center, ask the director or an employee to give participants a tour of the facility. Allow time for participants to observe and possibly try out different activities (e.g., water aerobics, step aerobics, weight lifting). Talk about the membership plans.

INSTRUCTOR ACTIVITY	INSTRUCTOR SCRIPT/DIRECTIONS
SUMMARIZE	Summarize the different activities that were observed.
	Discuss ways that participants could become involved in the center. Talk about supports that are needed to join the fitness center.

EVALUATION

- Did participants see a new place that they could exercise at in their community?

- Are there activities of interest to participants?

- Do participants want to join the fitness center?

Dancing to Music

Objectives

Participants will

- Discuss the benefits of dancing as an aerobic exercise
- State whether dancing is an exercise option for themselves.

HANDOUTS

also on CD-ROM

Participant Handout(s):

Tips: Warm-Ups *(see Lesson 3 for handout)*

Tips: Stretching *(see Lesson 3 for handout)*

Tips: Aerobic Exercises *(see Lesson 3 for handout)*

Tips: Cool-Downs *(see Lesson 3 for handout)*

Warm-Ups *(see Lesson 3 for handout)*

Stretches *(see Lesson 3 for handout)*

MATERIALS

Music CD that participants have chosen

CD player

Camera to take photos of the participants while they dance to the music

Personal Notebooks for handouts and pictures

Suggested Activities

INSTRUCTOR ACTIVITY	INSTRUCTOR SCRIPT/DIRECTIONS
REVIEW	*In our last class, we talked about different places that we can go to exercise, and we visited a fitness (or recreational) center.*
	Ask participants if they are interested in becoming a member at a community fitness/recreation center or if they are interested in taking classes at the center.
INTRODUCE LESSON	*Today, we are going to dance to a music CD. Dancing is another type of aerobic exercise that many of us already do.*
ASK	*Who likes to dance?*
	Ask participants how often they dance, where they go dancing, and who goes dancing with them.
ASK	*Before we dance, let's review what we know about aerobic exercises.*
	• *Why do we need to do aerobic exercises?*
	• *What are some aerobic exercises?*
	• *How often should we do aerobic exercises?*
	• *What do we do before we begin an aerobic exercise?*

INSTRUCTOR ACTIVITY	INSTRUCTOR SCRIPT/DIRECTIONS
	Supplement participants' responses with information from the participant handouts.
REVIEW PARTICIPANT HANDOUTS: Tips: Warm-Ups Tips: Stretching Tips: Aerobic Exercises Tips: Cool-Downs Warm-Ups Stretches	Review the **Tips: Warm-ups, Tips: Stretching, Tips: Aerobic Exercises,** and **Tips: Cool Downs** handouts. Lead the group with a co-leader through warm-ups and stretches using the **Warm-Ups** and **Stretches** handouts.
ASK	*Have any of you danced to this CD?*
ASK	*Who would like to co-lead the group today?*
	If more than one person wants to lead, work with participants to make an equitable decision (e.g., compromise or draw straws).
BEGIN CD	Have the co-leader introduce the CD and instruct the class during the music.
ASK	At the end of the class, ask participants if they enjoyed dancing to the music. Ask participants if this is something they would like to do. Ask what an aerobic exercise means.
SUMMARIZE	Review and summarize the benefits of aerobic exercise. Solicit responses from participants (e.g., health benefits, being with friends, having fun).

EVALUATION

- Did participants identify the benefits of aerobic exercise?

- Did participants identify dancing as an activity for exercise?

- Did participants express whether they would like dancing as a regular activity?

Building My Self-Esteem with Exercise

Objectives

Participants will

- Identify factors that influence a person's self-esteem
- Explain the importance of self-esteem to health
- Describe the effects of self-esteem on how a person functions
- Clarify and develop strategies for the goal they hope to accomplish during the health class

HANDOUTS

Instructor Reference(s):
Self-Esteem

also on CD-ROM

MATERIALS

Blackboard and chalk
Paper and pencil
Personal Notebooks for handouts and pictures

Suggested Activities

INSTRUCTOR ACTIVITY	INSTRUCTOR SCRIPT/DIRECTIONS
REVIEW	Review with participants things that may help them exercise.
	We have talked about good and bad influences that can help us eat good foods and exercise or keep us from eating healthy foods and being active.
	Have participants identify some good and bad influences. Also, have them discuss some of the things they should do before they exercise.
	Review rights and responsibilities, along with being able to advocate for those rights. Have participants identify some rights and responsibilities.
INTRODUCE LESSON	*Today, we're going to talk about our self-esteem and how we feel about ourselves. We'll look at how high and low self-esteem affects our behavior and health.*
DISCUSS INSTRUCTOR REFERENCE: Self-Esteem	Discuss the **Self-Esteem** reference.

Source: McElmurry, B., Newcomb, B.J., Lowe, A., & Misner, S.M. (1995). *Primary Health Care Curriculum Grade K–8 for Urban School Children.* Chicago: University of Illinois at Chicago, College of Nursing, Global Halth Leadership Office.

INSTRUCTOR ACTIVITY	INSTRUCTOR SCRIPT/DIRECTIONS
	Our opinions of other people affect how they think and feel about themselves, and how they feel about us affects how we feel about ourselves. Sometimes people judge us based on our race or ethnic group, gender, or disability (personal characteristics), rather than treating us as individuals. This affects how we feel about ourselves. This is called self-esteem.
ASK AND RECORD RESPONSES	*Have people told you that you can't do something that you think you can?* Record participants' responses on the board.
COMPLETE PARTICIPANT EXERCISE	*Because our words and actions affect our self-esteem, it's important that we do what we can to increase each other's self-esteem. The exercise that we are going to do will help us feel better about ourselves and build our self-esteem.*
	Place everyone's name in a box or bag. Explain to participants that they will write notes to each other. Ask each participant to draw one name from the bag, and then spend 5 minutes writing something positive about that person. They may write positive attributes, compose a song, write a letter, and so forth. People will then read what they wrote. Provide assistance as needed.
SUMMARIZE	Summarize the positive attributes identified by participants.
	When we feel good about ourselves we are more likely to participate in activities and try new things.
	Learning new types of exercises and being able to succeed can help us feel better about ourselves.

EVALUATION

- Did participants describe personal characteristics that could influence self-esteem?
- Did participants practice behaviors that enhance the feelings of their classmate?

Self-Esteem

WHAT IS SELF-ESTEEM?

Self-esteem is the way we feel about ourselves most of the time. It is the degree to which we like and respect ourselves in spite of our human weaknesses and mistakes. It influences how we get along in the world. It involves our sense of self-respect, self-love, self-appreciation, self-acceptance, self-worth, self-competence, and self-confidence.

When we feel competent and loveable, we are said to have high self-esteem. When we feel incompetent and unlovable, our self-esteem is often low.

HOW DOES SELF-ESTEEM DEVELOP?

Our self-esteem is influenced by parents, relatives, peers, teachers, the media, churches, and the opportunities available to us in the society in which we live.

HOW DO SELF-IMAGE AND SELF-ESTEEM INFLUENCE OUR HEALTH?

Our feelings about ourselves influence the activities we might take part in to maintain or improve our health. With good self-esteem, we are more likely to exercise, eat correctly, and have good relationships. If our self-esteem is positive, we are more likely to try new things. When we are successful at doing something, we feel better about ourselves.

WHAT IS THE EFFECT OF LOW SELF-ESTEEM ON OUR HEALTH?

When we have low self-esteem, we may not take care of ourselves because we may not feel that we are worth it. We may actually do things to harm our health such as overeating or not eating good foods. With low self-esteem, our relationships may be poor. People with low self-esteem may be hostile or may withdraw from others and become loners.

HOW DO WE KNOW IF A PERSON HAS HIGH SELF-ESTEEM?

When we have high self-esteem, we are proud of our accomplishments, accept responsibility, tolerate frustration, are enthusiastic about new challenges, and feel capable of influencing others without bullying or threatening them. People may feel happy, loved, capable, and proud of their accomplishments.

HOW DO WE KNOW IF A PERSON HAS LOW SELF-ESTEEM?

People with low self-esteem avoid situations that are new, they feel unloved and unwanted, and they blame others when they fail. People may feel lonely, depressed or sad, scared, angry, or unworthy. They are overly influenced by others instead of making their own decisions.

Source: McElmurry, B., Newcomb, B.J., Lowe, A., & Misner, S.M. (1995). *Primary Health Care Curriculum Grade K–8 for Urban School Children.* Chicago: University of Illinois at Chicago, College of Nursing, Global Halth Leadership Office.

Lesson H

New Ideas for Exercising in My Community

Objectives

Participants will

- Discuss different options for exercising in their community
- State exercises that they would like to try
- Identify where they would like to exercise (e.g., home, work, community center)

HANDOUTS

also on
CD-ROM

Participant Handout(s):

Community Options for Exercising

MATERIALS

Blackboard and chalk

Personal Notebooks for handouts and pictures

Suggested Activities

INSTRUCTOR ACTIVITY	INSTRUCTOR SCRIPT/DIRECTIONS
REVIEW	*In the last class, we talked about how exercise can help us feel better about ourselves.* Summarize the positive attributes identified by participants.
	When we feel good about ourselves we are more likely to participate in activities and try new things. Learning new types of exercises and being able to succeed can help us feel better about ourselves.
INTRODUCE LESSON	*Today, we are going to talk about different types of exercise activities that we can do in our community.*
	We are also going to talk about activities that we like to do and activities we might like to try.
ASK	*Where can you exercise in your neighborhood?*
ASK	Ask participants to name different types of exercises that they can do at home, at work, or in their community.
	Ask each participant for his or her ideas, and supplement their replies with additional examples.
RECORD RESPONSES	Write responses on the board. Discuss responses with the class. See if other participants also like to do each of the examples.

INSTRUCTOR ACTIVITY	INSTRUCTOR SCRIPT/DIRECTIONS
DISTRIBUTE AND DISCUSS PARTICIPANT HANDOUT: Community Options for Exercising	Give participants the **Community Options for Exercising** handout.
	Show pictures of each activity and have participants identify the activities that they like, don't like, or want to try.
	This activity can be done as a group or individually.
ASK	Once participants have identified exercises that they want to do, ask where they would like to do these exercises.
	Would you like to do this activity with someone? If so, who would that person be?
	Have the class identify different places that exercises could be done.
	Can these exercises be done outside? Can they be done during the winter?
SUMMARIZE	Review the different types of exercises. Summarize where people can go to do exercises (e.g., home, community center, at work during breaks or down time).

EVALUATION

- Can participants identify exercise activities that they would like to do in their community?

- Can participants identify where they could do these exercises?

New Ideas for Exercising in My Community

Community Options for Exercising

Directions: State whether you like this activity, do not like the activity, or would like to try it. Put an "X" by the appropriate choice.

ACTIVITY	Like	Don't like	Want to try
1. Weight training/fitness training			
2. Walking/jogging/running			
3. Dancing/doing aerobics			
4. Bowling			
5. Snow skiing/water skiing			
6. Playing volleyball			
7. Playing baseball			
8. Golfing			

Community Options for Exercising

New Ideas for Exercising in My Community

Directions: State whether you like this activity, do not like the activity, or would like to try it. Put an "X" by the appropriate choice.

ACTIVITY	Like	Don't like	Want to try
9. Rollerblading/ice skating			
10. Riding a horse			
11. Bike riding (stationary bike/ outdoor riding)			
12. Recreational water sports			
13. Playing football/basketball			
14. Swimming/aerobic swimming			
Other:			
Other:			

Lesson I

Other Ways to Stay Physically Active

Objectives
Participants will • Identify other ways to become and stay physically active

HANDOUTS

also on CD-ROM

Participant Handout(s):

Exercises and Activities I Like *(see Lesson 12 for handout)*

MATERIALS

Magazines (select a variety of activities, including recreation and leisure magazines)

Scissors

Personal Notebooks for handouts and pictures

Suggested Activities

INSTRUCTOR ACTIVITY	INSTRUCTOR SCRIPT/DIRECTIONS
REVIEW	*In our last class, we talked about different types of exercises that we can do in our community.* Ask participants to idenitfy and discuss various places people can go to do exercises (e.g., home, community center, at work during breaks or down time)
INTRODUCE LESSON	*Today, we will be talking about ways that we can stay active.*
CONTINUE	*For example, some things that we need to do in our everyday lives like housekeeping, doing laundry, and gardening can be physically demanding. Sometimes these activities can be similar to aerobic exercises or strength training.* *At times, we can do these activities instead of our regular exercise program, for example, heavy housecleaning or gardening.*
MAGAZINE	Have participants cut out pictures from magazines that represent alternative forms of exercise.
RECORD RESPONSES	Write down the activities that participants identified.

INSTRUCTOR ACTIVITY	INSTRUCTOR SCRIPT/DIRECTIONS
CONSIDER A GARDENING ACTIVITY	Depending on the location of the health education class, consider a gardening activity (e.g., planting flowers or shrubs, mulching).
DISCUSS MAKING CHOICES	Discuss the importance of making choices and deciding what type of physical activity you want to do.
	Remember, a choice is something that you want for yourself. It's not something that someone else wants for you.
SUMMARIZE	Discuss the importance of adding alternative activities as a substitute for your regular exercise routine.
	Sometimes we get too busy to exercise, but our household chores (e.g., washing windows, raking leaves, mopping floors, shoveling snow) may actually be the same as aerobic exercise.
	Summarize the importance of making choices.

EVALUATION

- Did participants identify alternative types of physical activities that they would like to do instead of their regular exercise routines?

- If applicable, did participants enjoy the alternative activity (e.g., gardening)?

- Do participants understand the importance of making choices in the types of exercises and physical activities they would like to do?

Lesson J

Going Grocery Shopping

Objectives

Participants will

- Develop a menu
- Select items in the grocery store for their menu
- Purchase the foods for the menu
- Prepare a meal or snack from their menu plan. (*Note:* This depends on the time frame of the class. It may be done during another class.)

HANDOUTS

also on **CD-ROM**

Instructor Reference(s):
Shopping for Groceries *(see Lesson 23 handout)*
MyPlate *(see Lesson 6 handout)*

MATERIALS

Transportation

Pen and paper

Plates, cups, knives, forks, and spoons

Cutting board

Personal Notebooks for handouts and pictures

Suggested Activities

INSTRUCTOR ACTIVITY	INSTRUCTOR SCRIPT/DIRECTIONS
REVIEW	*In the last class, we talked about the importance of adding alternative activities as a substitute for your regular exercise routine. Can anyone remember what some of those things were?*
INTRODUCE LESSON	*Today, we are going to go to a grocery store to buy the food items for our meal.* Use the **Shopping for Groceries** reference to make a menu.
DIVIDE PARTICIPANTS INTO SMALL GROUPS	At the grocery store, divide participants into small groups.
SELECT FOOD ITEMS	Assist participants in finding food items in the grocery store.
DISCUSS	You may review the different costs for similar items. Compare the quality of meats, fruits, and vegetables. Compare low-fat items (e.g., milk, cheese) versus regular food products. You may also discuss organic versus nonorganic depending on the group and products being bought.
CHECK OUT	Have participants pay for their food items.
PREPARE A MEAL	Encourage participants to assist in preparing a meal or snack from their menu plan.
CLEAN HANDS AND FOOD	*Before we prepare food, it's important that we have clean hands so that we can have clean food. Food must be clean*

	or it will make us sick. We need to wash our hands with soap and water before touching any food.
ASK	*How can germs get on food?* List responses.
	What do you see when you handle meat that is not cooked? Elicit responses such as "hands and knife become dirty with blood." *Raw meat carries germs, and it should be cooked before eating it. Raw meat and cooked meat should never touch each other.*
	What happens to fruits and vegetables in stores? Elicit responses such as "people touch them without washing their hands." Encourage people to conclude that they should wash fruits and vegetables before they are eaten.
	What can happen to us if we eat food that is not clean? Encourage responses such as stomachache, diarrhea, vomiting, and headache.
PREPARE MEAL	Work with participants to prepare the meal or snack. Have participants set the table. Then have the hosts and hostesses serve the food after everyone has washed their hands.
ENJOY MEAL	Participants have the opportunity to enjoy the meal or snack that they prepared with the group.
CLEAN UP	After the meal or snack, have participants help wash the dishes and store leftover food.
SUMMARIZE	*Before we shop for food, we need to decide on menus that include balanced meals. We should compare food items based on cost and content (e.g., fat, calories, sodium).*
	When we prepare a meal, we must wash our hands along with the fruits and vegetables. Dirty fruits and vegetables and raw meat can make us sick.

EVALUATION

- Did participants select and buy the food items for their menu plans?
- Did participants explain why they should wash their hands and utensils when they are handling food?
- Did participants explain why raw food should be washed before it is eaten?
- Did participants explain why raw meat should be cooked before it is eaten?
- Did participants prepare or assist in the preparation of the food items for a meal or snack?

HELPFUL HINTS

Low-fat cooking techniques

Bake, broil, boil, or grill for lower fat options.

Use nonstick pans.

Trim all the visible fat from meats, poultry, and seafood.

Thicken sauces with cornstarch instead of flour.

Lesson K

Energy Balance

Objectives

Participants will

- Discuss various energy needs for different activities
- Identify which activities will give them high energy
- State which activities will help them maintain or lose weight

HANDOUTS

Participant Handout(s):

Activities and Energy Needs

MATERIALS

Blackboard and chalk

Pens or pencil

Personal Notebooks for handouts and pictures

Suggested Activities

INSTRUCTOR ACTIVITY	INSTRUCTOR SCRIPT/DIRECTIONS
INTRODUCE LESSON	*Today, we are going to talk about different types of activities and why some activities take more energy than others. Activities that use lots of energy may help us lose or control our weight, keep our heart healthy, and give us more energy.*
REVIEW	*We talked about what it means to have energy.*
	It is important to know what type of activities use lots of energy and what types use less energy.
ASK AND WAIT FOR RESPONSES	*What does activity mean to you? What are some activities that you like to do during the day?*
	Participants may say watching TV, exercising, playing ball, listening to the radio, and walking. Use these examples to discuss the energy needs for each activity.
	How much energy does _____ take? Give an example of an activity that a participant gave.
	How do you feel when you are done _____ ? Give an example that a participant used of a **high energy** activity such as walking, exercising, or vacuuming.
	How do you feel when you are done _____ ? Give an example that a participant used of a **low energy** activity such as watching TV or listening to the radio.
SAY AND THEN ASK	*Some activities use lots of energy. What are some examples of these activities?* Wait for responses.

INSTRUCTOR ACTIVITY	INSTRUCTOR SCRIPT/DIRECTIONS
	Some activities use less energy. What are some examples of these activities? Wait for responses.
DISTRIBUTE AND DISCUSS PARTICIPANT HANDOUT: Activities and Energy Needs	Distribute and review the **Activities and Energy Needs** handout. *Tell me which activities will help you be healthy (lose or control your weight, give you energy).*
	Discuss different energy levels for the different activities listed.
SUMMARIZE	*Today, we talked about different types of activities. Some activities take more energy, such as exercising, walking, and riding a bike. Some activities need less energy such as relaxing and sleeping. High-energy activities can help us lose or maintain our weight.*

EVALUATION

- Can participants identify high energy activities, such as exercising, walking, or riding a bike?

- Can participants identify activities that will help them lose or control their weight, such as running, hiking, exercising, walking, or riding a bike?

Activities and Energy Needs

Which of the following should you do if you want to lose or control your weight?

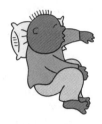

Sleep

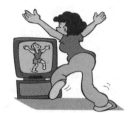

Exercise

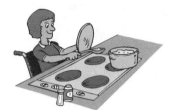

Cook

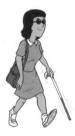

Walk

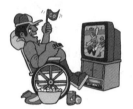

Watch TV

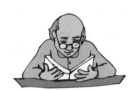

Read

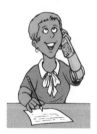

Talk on the phone

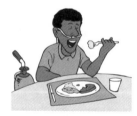

Eat

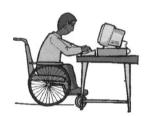

Use computer/study

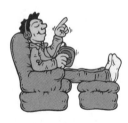

Relax

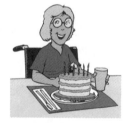

Eat cake

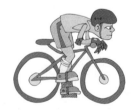

Ride a bike

From Illingworth, K., Moore, K., & McGillivray, J. (2003). The development of the Nutrition and Activity Knowledge Scale for use with people with an intellectual disability. *Journal of Applied Research on Intellectual Disabilities, 16,* 159–166; adapted by permission.

In *Health Matters: The Exercise and Nutrition Health Education Curriculum for People with Developmental Disabilities*
by Beth Marks, Jasmina Sisirak, and Tamar Heller

Activities and Energy Needs

Which activity do you think might help you to lose the most weight? Please circle.

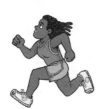

Running

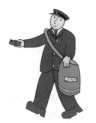

Mailing a letter

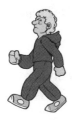

Walking

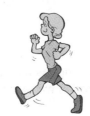

Speed walking

Which activity would help you lose the most weight? Please circle.

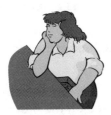

Relaxing

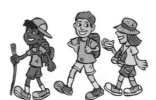

Hiking

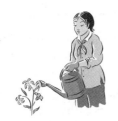

Watering plants

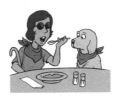

Eating

Lesson L

Healthy Food Choices

Objectives	HANDOUTS
Participants will	Participant Handout(s):
• Discuss how to choose healthy food choices for their meals	Healthy Food Choices
• Choose healthy snacks from vending machines	**MATERIALS**
• Identify foods that are heart-healthy	Blackboard and chalk
• State different food groups	Pens or pencils
	Personal Notebooks for handouts and pictures

also on CD-ROM

Note: This is a very long lesson. It could be broken up into two or three smaller sessions to cover different food groups in more detail.

Suggested Activities

INSTRUCTOR ACTIVITY	INSTRUCTOR SCRIPT/DIRECTIONS
INTRODUCE LESSON	*Today, we will talk about food choices during our meals. We will also talk about our favorite snacks and about some examples of snacks that are nutritious. We will talk about some foods that are good for your heart. We will also review activities that use lots of energy and activities that use less energy.*
DISTRIBUTE AND DISCUSS PARTICIPANT HANDOUT: Healthy Food Choices	Distribute the **Healthy Food Choices** handout. *Let's look at the handout.*
ASK AND WAIT FOR RESPONSES	Ask participants what they see on the first page of the handout. *Which is the healthiest breakfast?*
	Describe the three breakfasts pictured. *Which one is the healthiest one?* (Cereal with milk and orange juice) *Why?* (It is low in fat and high in vitamins and minerals.)
	Which breakfast is high in fat and cholesterol? (Bacon and eggs) *Which one do you think is high in sugar, calories, and fat?* (Pancakes with butter and syrup)
	Turn to the second page of the handout. Describe the three lunches pictured. *Which is the healthiest lunch?* (Turkey sandwich with cheese, a small green salad, and apple juice) *Why?* (It is lower in fat, has vegetables, and has fruit juice.)

Which lunch is high in fat and cholesterol? (Tacos with cheese and a regular soda, double cheeseburger with fries and a milkshake)

Turn to the third page of the handout. *What are healthy snacks?* (Grapes/raisins, pretzels, ice cream if it is low-fat frozen yogurt or sorbet, apple juice, fruit yogurt, apples, bananas, and strawberries)

Turn to the fourth page of the handout. Describe the foods pictured together with participants. *Which foods are best to keep your heart healthy? Can you tell me what some of them are?*

Which ones are high in fat? (Hamburgers, eggs, french fries, ice cream, popcorn, hot dogs, tacos, whole milk, and cheese) *Which ones are good for you and for your heart?* (Apples, pears, tomatoes, bananas, fish, strawberries, carrots, peas, and onions) *Why?* (They are low in fat and high in vitamins and minerals.)

Turn to the fifth page of the handout. *Which foods should you not have too often? Remember when we talked about nutrients in our food? What are the nutrients?* Wait for responses. *Nutrients are carbohydrates, proteins, and fat.*

Describe foods that are pictured and what nutrients they have. *Foods in the first square are high in protein. Foods in the second square are high in protein and fat and also rich in calcium for our bones. Foods in the third square are considered "junk" foods. They are high in sugar and fat. Foods in the fourth square are fruits and vegetables. They are rich in vitamins, minerals, and fiber. Foods in the third square should be eaten only once in a while.*

Another thing that we should know is that there are five different food groups. Can anyone tell me what they are? (Dairy/milk, meat, fruits, vegetables, and grain) *Also, there is another food group that contains sugary foods, such as candy bars, cakes, pies, and fatty foods, such as butter, chips, oils, and bacon.*

Look at the foods in the first square. What food group is that? Wait for responses. *The fish and meat group is high in protein. What does protein do?* (It helps us build tissue.)

Look at the foods in the second square. What food group is that? Wait for responses. *Milk and cheese belong to the dairy group, and they are high in calcium that makes our bones strong, and they are also high in fat.*

Look at the foods in the third square. What food group is that? (Candy and fast food) *What are they high in?* (Some are high in fat and sugar, and some are high just in fat.) *Should we eat these every day or just every once in a while?*

INSTRUCTOR ACTIVITY	INSTRUCTOR SCRIPT
	Look at the foods in the fourth square. What food group is that? (Fruits and vegetables) *What is good about them?* (Fruits and vegetables are full of vitamins.)
SUMMARIZE	*Today, we have talked about healthy choices for our meals. We have also talked about foods that are heart healthy. We also learned about different food groups, such as dairy, meat, fruit and vegetable, and grain.*

EVALUATION

- Can participants identify healthier alternatives for their meals?

- Can participants identify foods that are heart healthy?

- Can participants identify different food groups?

Healthy Food Choices

Which is the healthiest breakfast?

1.

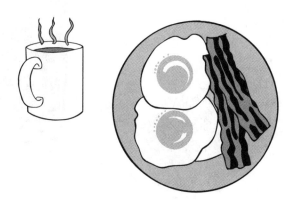

Coffee, two eggs, and two strips of bacon

2.

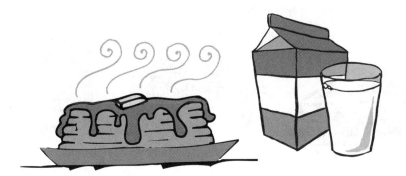

Pancakes with butter and syrup, and a glass of milk

3.

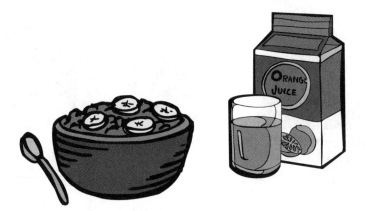

Cereal with milk and a glass of orange juice

From Illingworth, K., Moore, K., & McGillivray, J. (2003). The development of the Nutrition and Activity Knowledge Scale for use with people with an intellectual disability. *Journal of Applied Research on Intellectual Disabilities, 16,* 159–166, adapted by permission.

Healthy Food Choices

Which is the healthiest lunch?

1.

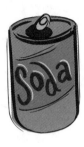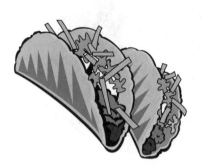

Two beef tacos with cheese and regular soda

2.

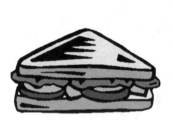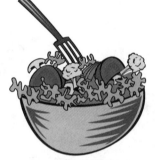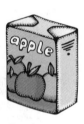

Turkey sandwich with cheese, a small green salad, and apple juice

3.

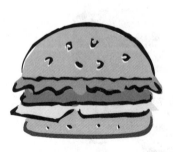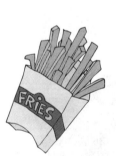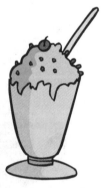

Double cheeseburger, fries, and strawberry milkshake

Healthy Food Choices

Circle all the foods that are healthy choices for a snack.

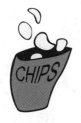

Potato chips

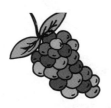

Grapes/raisins

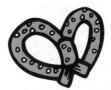

Pretzel

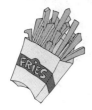

French fries

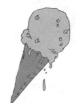

Ice cream

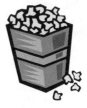

Popcorn without butter

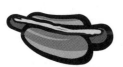

Hot dog

Apple juice

Fruit yogurt

Apple

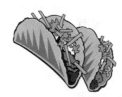

Taco

Regular soda

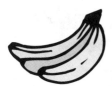

Bananas

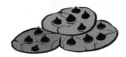

Cookies

Strawberries

Healthy Food Choices

Which foods are best to keep your heart healthy?

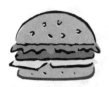
Hamburger

Eggs

Milk and cheese

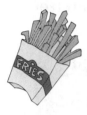
French fries

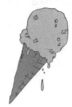
Ice cream

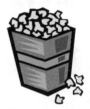
Popcorn

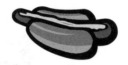
Hot dog

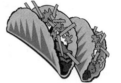
Tacos

Apple

Pear

Tomato

Bananas

Fish

Strawberries

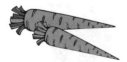
Carrots

Peas

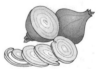
Onion

Healthy Food Choices

Which foods should you not have too often?

1.

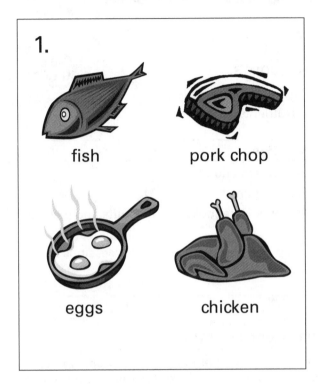

fish   pork chop

eggs   chicken

2.

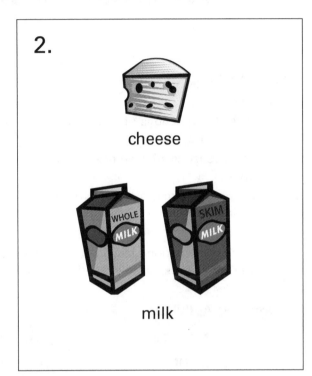

cheese

WHOLE MILK   SKIM MILK

milk

3.

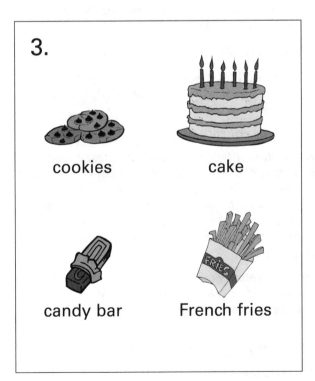

cookies   cake

candy bar   French fries

4.

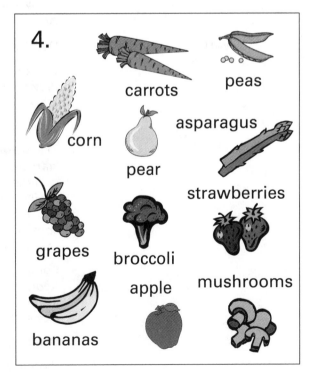

carrots   peas

corn   asparagus

pear

strawberries

grapes   broccoli

apple   mushrooms

bananas

In *Health Matters: The Exercise and Nutrition Health Education Curriculum for People with Developmental Disabilities*
by Beth Marks, Jasmina Sisirak, and Tamar Heller

265

Nutrients in Our Food

Objectives
Participants will • Discuss the functions of carbohydrates, proteins, and fats • Identify reasons why we need these nutrients • State good sources of carbohydrates, proteins, and fats

also on CD-ROM

HANDOUTS
Participant Handout(s): Nutrients in Our Food

MATERIALS
Blackboard and chalk Pens or pencils Personal Notebooks for handouts and pictures

Note: This is a very long lesson. It could be broken up into two or three smaller sessions to cover carbohydrates, proteins, and fats more extensively.

Suggested Activities

INSTRUCTOR ACTIVITY	INSTRUCTOR SCRIPT/DIRECTIONS
INTRODUCE LESSON	*Today, we will talk again about different nutrients in our food. Our food is made up of three different nutrients and many vitamins and minerals. These three nutrients are carbohydrates, fats, and proteins.*
ASK AND WAIT FOR RESPONSES	*What is a carbohydrate? Why do we need carbohydrates?* *Carbohydrates give all the cells in our bodies the energy they need. They let you run, jump, think, blink, breathe, and more.* *What are the sources of carbohydrates?* *There are two different types of carbohydrates: sugars and starches. Sugars are called simple carbohydrates. They are called simple because your body digests them quickly and easily. Simple carbohydrates are usually sweet tasting like cookies, candy, soda, and other sugary foods. There are some foods from nature, such as apples, bananas, grapes, raisins, and oranges.* *Complex carbohydrates are found in foods like bread, noodles, cereals, and rice, and in lots of tasty veggies such as corn, potatoes, and sweet potatoes. They take longer to digest.* *What is protein? Why do we need protein?* *Protein's biggest job is to build up, keep up, and replace the tissues in your body. Your muscles, your organs, even*

some of your hormones are made up mostly of protein. Making a big muscle? Taking a deep breath with your big lungs? Running down the street on your strong feet? You've got the power of protein!

CONTINUE

What are the sources of protein?

Sources of protein include meat, chicken, fish, eggs, cheese, yogurt, milk, beans (lentils and peas), and nuts. Some proteins are leaner than others. Choose lean protein, such as a chicken breast, fish, and skim milk.

What is fat? Why do we need fat?

Fat is the body's major form of energy storage. Our bodies can make fat. Fat insulates our bodies from the cold and provides some cushioning for our organs.

Fat sounds like it's always a bad thing that people avoid eating, but actually our bodies need some fat to work correctly.

Fat gives our bodies energy. Some fats help make up important hormones that we need to keep our bodies at the right temperature or keep our blood pressure at the right level. Fat helps us have healthy skin and hair. Fat is our bodies' very own storage and moving service. It helps Vitamins A, D, E, and K hang out and get transported through the bloodstream when our bodies needs them.

What are sources of fat?

Fats include oils, butter, and fried foods.

DISCUSS

Even though our bodies need some fat to work properly, they don't need as much as most people eat. It's a good idea to avoid eating a lot of fat because it can contribute to weight gain and obesity (when a person weighs too much for his or her height) and other health conditions that can occur when we get older, like heart disease or adult-onset diabetes. Foods with lots of fat in them taste good—like cookies, chocolate, fast-food hamburgers, and French fries. It is okay to eat these foods once in a while.

DISTRIBUTE AND DISCUSS PARTICIPANT HANDOUT:
  Nutrients in Our Foods

Distribute the **Nutrients in Our Foods** handout.

Which one of these foods has the most protein? Descibe the pictures. The answer is fish.

Which food has the most fat? Describe the pictures. The answer is baked potato with butter.

Turn to the second page of the handout. *Which group of foods has the most sugar?* Describe the pictures. The answer is Group 3.

Turn to the third page of the handout. *Which group of foods would cause you to put on the most weight?* Describe the pictures. The answer is Group 3.

INSTRUCTOR ACTIVITY	INSTRUCTOR SCRIPT
DISCUSS	*What type of nutrients does a cheeseburger have? A cheeseburger is high in protein and carbohydrates but also high in fat. Instead of a cheeseburger, we could have a grilled chicken sandwich. It is high in protein but low in fat.*
	How about doughnuts? Doughnuts are high in carbohydrates (sugar) but also high in fat. Instead of having doughnuts for breakfast, we could have cereal. Cereal is high in carbohydrates, fiber, vitamins, and minerals but low in fat.
	How about apple pie? Apple pie is high in carbohydrates (simple sugars) and fat. Instead of having apple pie for dessert, we could have fresh fruit and yogurt. Fresh fruit and yogurt are high in carbohydrates, fiber, vitamins, and minerals and low in fat.
SUMMARIZE	*Today, we have talked about different functions of carbohydrates, proteins, and fats. We have also learned about good sources of carbohydrates, proteins, and fats.*

EVALUATION

- Can participants identify functions of carbohydrates, proteins, and fats?
- Can participants identify good sources of carbohydrates, proteins, and fats?

Nutrients in Our Food

Which one of these foods has the most protein?

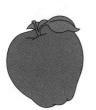

apple

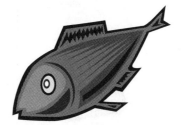

fish

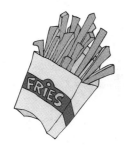

French fries

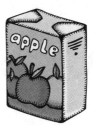

apple juice

Which one of these foods has the most fat?

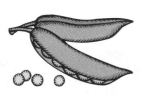

green peas

tomato

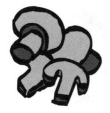

mushrooms

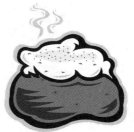

baked potato

From Illingworth, K., Moore, K., & McGillivray, J. (2003). The development of the Nutrition and Activity Knowledge Scale for use with people with an intellectual disability. *Journal of Applied Research on Intellectual Disabilities, 16,* 159–166; adapted by permission.

Nutrients in Our Food

Which group of foods has the most sugar?

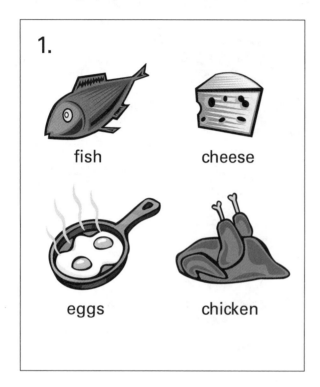

1.

fish   cheese

eggs   chicken

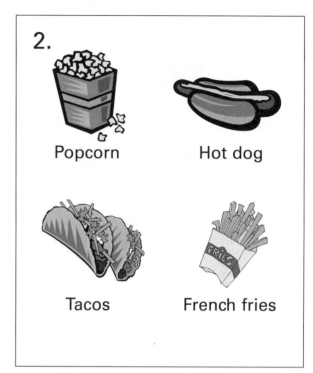

2.

Popcorn   Hot dog

Tacos   French fries

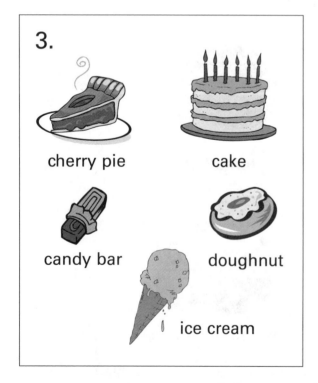

3.

cherry pie   cake

candy bar   doughnut

ice cream

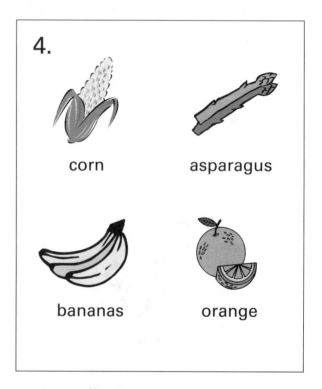

4.

corn   asparagus

bananas   orange

Nutrients in Our Food

Which group of foods would cause you to put on the most weight?

1.

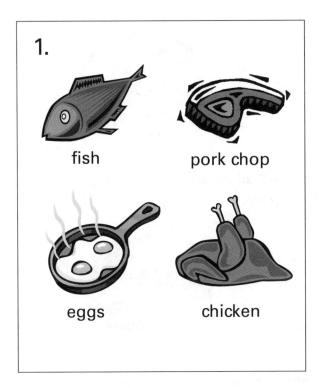

fish

pork chop

eggs

chicken

2.

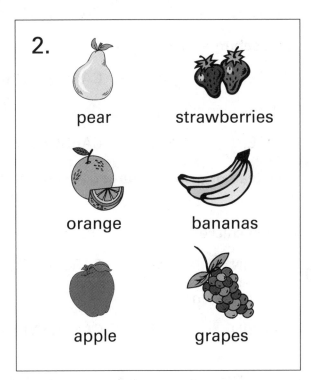

pear

strawberries

orange

bananas

apple

grapes

3.

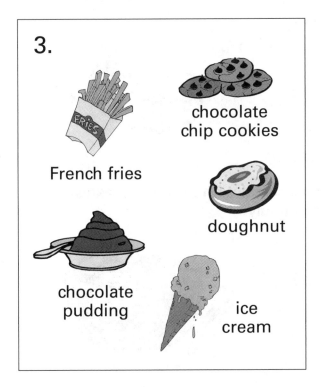

French fries

chocolate chip cookies

doughnut

chocolate pudding

ice cream

4.

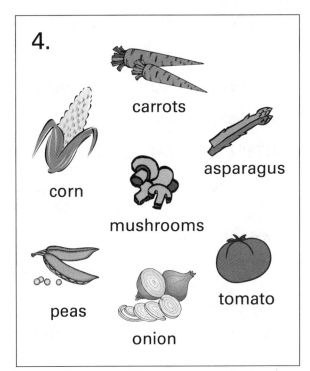

carrots

corn

asparagus

mushrooms

peas

onion

tomato

271

Nutrients in Our Food

What type of nutrients does a cheeseburger have? Circle all that apply.

PROTEIN   FAT   CARBOHYDRATES

Cheeseburger is high in

PROTEIN   FAT   CARBOHYDRATES

But it is also high in

PROTEIN   FAT   CARBOHYDRATES

Instead of a cheeseburger, we could have a grilled chicken sandwich for lunch.
Circle all that apply.

Grilled chicken sandwich is high in

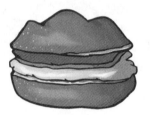

PROTEIN   FAT   CARBOHYDRATES

But it is low in

PROTEIN   FAT   CARBOHYDRATES

What type of nutrients does a doughnut have? Circle all that apply.

PROTEIN   FAT   CARBOHYDRATES

A doughnut is high in

PROTEIN   FAT   CARBOHYDRATES

But it is also high in

PROTEIN   FAT   CARBOHYDRATES

Instead of a doughnut, we could have cereal with milk for breakfast.
Circle all that apply.

Cereal is high in

PROTEIN   FAT   CARBOHYDRATES

But it is low in

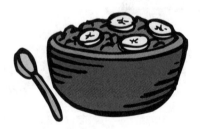

PROTEIN   FAT   CARBOHYDRATES

Nutrients in Our Food

What type of nutrients does cherry pie have? Circle all that apply.

PROTEIN   FAT   CARBOHYDRATES

Cherry pie is high in

PROTEIN   FAT   CARBOHYDRATES

But it is also high in

PROTEIN   FAT   CARBOHYDRATES

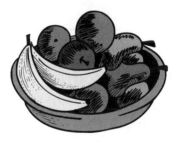

Instead of cherry pie, we could have fruit and yogurt for dessert.
Circle all that apply.

Fruit and yogurt is high in

PROTEIN   FAT   CARBOHYDRATES

But it is low in

PROTEIN   FAT   CARBOHYDRATES

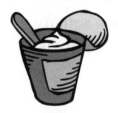

Lesson N

How Much Should I Eat?

Objectives
Participants will • Discuss how much food they should eat when doing different activities

also on
CD-ROM

HANDOUTS
Participant Handout(s):   Activities and Food We Need

MATERIALS
Blackboard and chalk Pens or pencils Personal Notebooks for handouts and pictures

Suggested Activities

INSTRUCTOR ACTIVITY	INSTRUCTOR SCRIPT/DIRECTIONS
INTRODUCE LESSSON	*Today, we will talk about how much food we should eat, depending on what we do during the day.*
DISCUSS	*Some activities use lots of energy. What are some examples of these activities?* Wait for responses. Review Lesson K.
	Some activities use less energy. What are some examples of these activities? Wait for responses.
DISTRIBUTE AND DISCUSS PARTICIPANT HANDOUT: Activities and Food We Need	Distribute the **Activities and Food We Need** handout. *Let's look at our handout. The first picture shows a man walking a dog. He is going for a long walk with his dog. Which breakfast should he eat?* Describe the breakfast choices.
	Why? Does walking take more energy that sitting down? Do you need to eat more if you will be going for a long walk?
	Let's look at the next page. What is the man doing? (Relaxing on the beach) *Does this take a lot of energy? What breakfast should he eat? Why?*
	What is the woman on the next page doing? (Reading a book) *What breakfast should she eat? Why?*
	Look at the man in the last picture. He is getting ready to take a long walk. What breakfast should he eat? Why?
SUMMARIZE	*What have we learned from these pictures? Some activities take more energy; therefore, we need to eat more food. Some activities take less energy, and we don't need to eat as much food.*

You can also talk about different nutrients in each breakfast. Nutrients in food are explained in the Lesson M. If you have extra time in this lesson, you may use it to introduce the basics of carbohydrates, fat, and protein.

EVALUATION

- Can participants identify how much one should eat when doing different activities?

Activities and Food We Need

This man is going for a long walk with his dog.

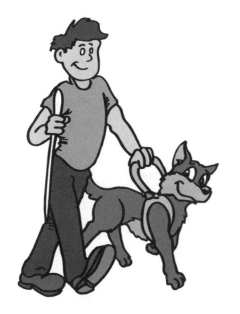

What breakfast should he eat?

1.

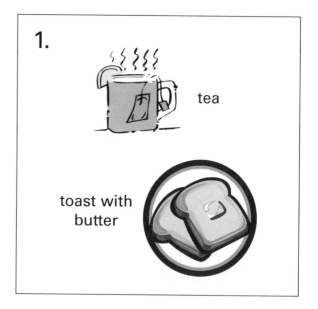

tea

toast with butter

2.

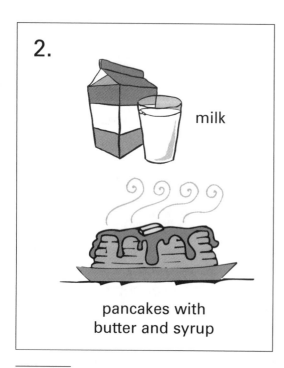

milk

pancakes with butter and syrup

3.

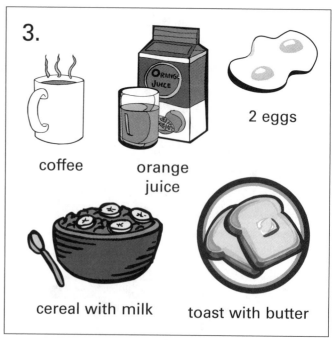

coffee

orange juice

2 eggs

cereal with milk

toast with butter

From Illingworth, K., Moore, K., & McGillivray, J. (2003). The development of the Nutrition and Activity Knowledge Scale for use with people with an intellectual disability. *Journal of Applied Research on Intellectual Disabilities, 16,* 159–166; adapted by permission.

Activities and Food We Need

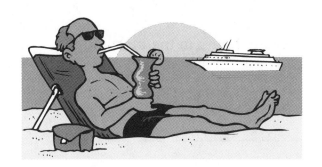

This man is going to relax on the beach this morning.

What breakfast should he eat?

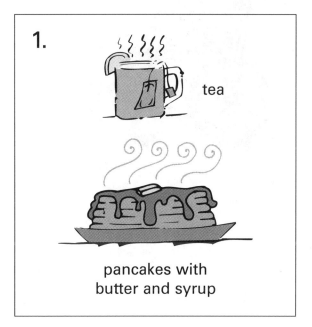

1. tea

pancakes with butter and syrup

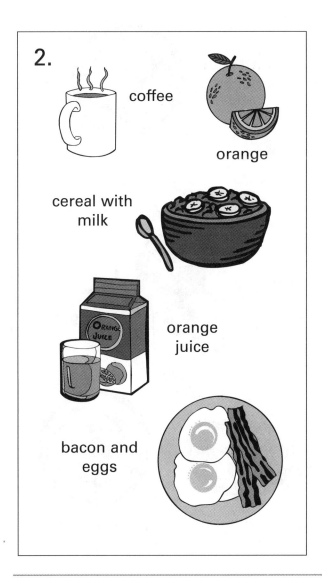

2. coffee

orange

cereal with milk

orange juice

bacon and eggs

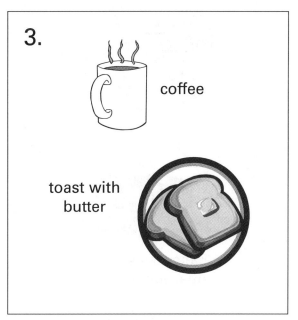

3. coffee

toast with butter

Activities and Food We Need

This woman is going to read for several hours in the morning.

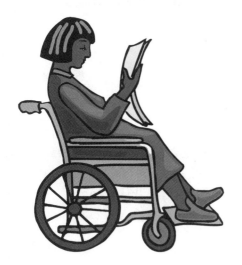

What breakfast should she eat?

1.

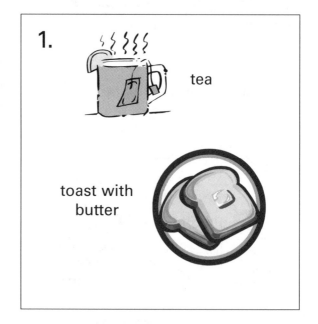

tea

toast with butter

2.

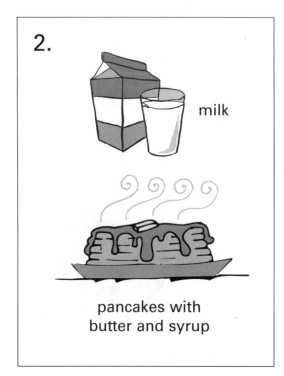

milk

pancakes with butter and syrup

3.

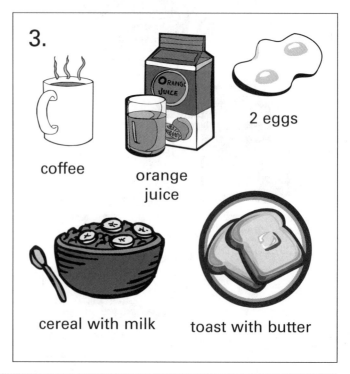

coffee

orange juice

2 eggs

cereal with milk

toast with butter

Activities and Food We Need

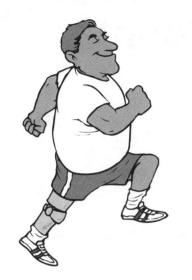

This man is going for a long walk.

What breakfast should he eat?

1.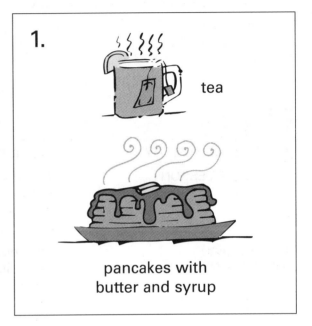

tea

pancakes with butter and syrup

2.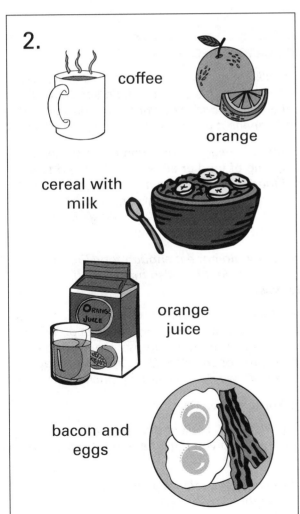

coffee

orange

cereal with milk

orange juice

bacon and eggs

3.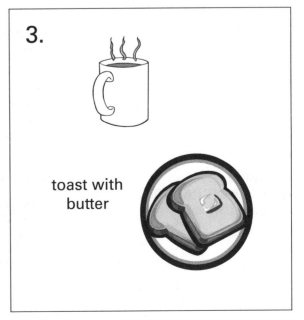

toast with butter

Portion Sizes Count

Objectives

Participants will

- Define a portion size
- Discuss the importance of portion sizes
- Talk about how much food is eaten during a meal

HANDOUTS

also on
CD-ROM

Participant Handout(s):
Portion Sizes

MATERIALS

Pens or pencils

Personal Notebooks for handouts and pictures

INSTRUCTOR ACTIVITY	INSTRUCTOR SCRIPT/DIRECTIONS
INTRODUCE LESSON	*Today, we will talk about how much food we eat. We will talk about portion sizes. This class will help you think about the amount of different foods you should eat during the day and what happens if you eat more or if you eat less.*
ASK AND WAIT FOR RESPONSES	*What does "portion" mean to you?* Participants may say things like a serving of food or amount of food. *Portion is the amount of food eaten during a meal or a snack. What happens if you eat too much food? You may gain weight. Gaining weight is hard on the heart. Weight gain can also make you tired and can slow you down.*
REVIEW	*What happens if you do not eat enough food? You may lose weight. Losing weight can also make you tired and can slow you down.*
	How much food we eat depends on what kind of activities we do during the day. If we are highly active (e.g., we walk most of the day), we need more energy—we need to eat more food. If we are not so active (e.g., if we sit or lay around watching TV), we do not need as much food.
DISTRIBUTE PARTICIPANT HANDOUT: Portion Sizes	Distribute the **Portion Sizes** Handout.
	Let's look at our handout. Look at the man at the top of the page. What sandwich do you think he might have been eating? Why?
	Look at the three men in business suits. Which one will gain the most weight? Why?

	How about the three women who are eating pizza? Which one will gain the most weight? Why?
	Look at the man with the milkshakes. Which milkshake do you think he has been drinking? Why?
SUMMARIZE	*Today, we learned about portion sizes. We discussed that if we eat too much we can gain weight. If we eat too little we may lose weight.*

EVALUATION

- Can participants define a portion size?

- Can participants identify the appropriate amount of food that should be eaten during meals?

Portion Sizes

What burger do you think this man might have been eating, a or b?

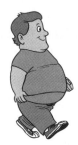 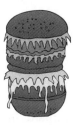

a   b

Which man will put on the most weight, a, b, or c?

 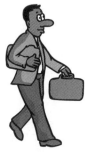 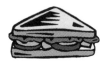

a

 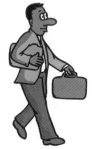 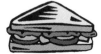 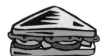 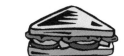

b

 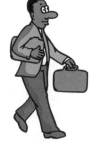 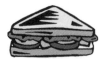 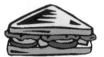

c

From Illingworth, K., Moore, K., & McGillivray, J. (2003). The development of the Nutrition and Activity Knowledge Scale for use with people with an intellectual disability. *Journal of Applied Research on Intellectual Disabilities, 16,* 159–166; adapted by permission.

Portion Sizes

Which woman will put on the most weight, a, b, or c?

a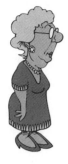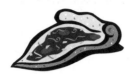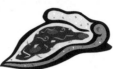

b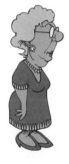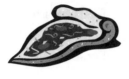

c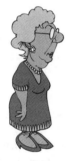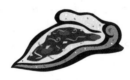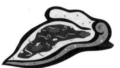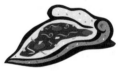

What milkshake do you think this man has been drinking, a, b, or c?

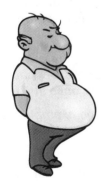 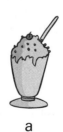 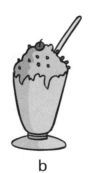 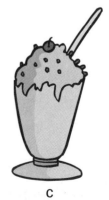

a   b   c

Snacking and Vending Machines

Objectives

Participants will

- Identify the importance of snacking
- Discuss what influences snacking choices
- Talk about reasons why we snack

HANDOUTS

also on CD-ROM

Participant Handout(s):

Snacking and Vending Machines

MATERIALS

Pens or pencils

Personal Notebooks for handouts and pictures

Suggested Activities

INSTRUCTOR ACTIVITY	INSTRUCTOR SCRIPT/DIRECTIONS
INTRODUCE LESSON	*Today, we will talk about snacking and eating snack food. We will discuss the reasons we snack and why we choose certain types of snack food. We will also talk about our favorite snacks and give some examples of nutritious snacks.*
ASK AND WAIT FOR RESPONSES	*Why do we snack? Snacking is good for us. Did you know that snacking keeps your weight in check, keeps your energy level high all day, and prevents you from getting too tired during the day? It also helps you think clearly during the day, gives you energy to exercise harder, and helps you sleep better.*
	It is important to choose the right snack. Some snacks are full of sugar and fat. These snacks are commonly called "junk foods." Can someone give me examples of junk foods?
	Chips, candy, cake, cookies, and doughnuts are all examples. These foods may not be the best snack choice all of the time, but they are okay to eat every once in a while.
	Snacks can be good for us. What are some examples of snacks that are good for you? Fruit, cereal, vegetables, and pretzels are all examples.
DISTRIBUTE PARTICIPANT HANDOUT: Snacking and Vending Machines	Distribute the **Snacking and Vending Machines** handout.

INSTRUCTOR ACTIVITY	INSTRUCTOR SCRIPT/DIRECTIONS
ASK AND WAIT FOR RESPONSES	*What are your favorite snacks? Look at the first page of the handout. What are some of your favorite snacks? What snacks are not shown in these pictures that you like to eat? What snack food would you like to try? Circle all of the snacks that you like. Add more snacks that are not on the sheet. How do you decide what kind of snack you will have?*

Look at the second page of your handout. What are some of the reasons you snack? Look at the pictures (boredom, hunger, nervousness, taste). Are there any other reasons that you snack?

What are some things that affect your snack choice? Answers can include advertising, TV commercials, size of the snack, cost, and craving sweet or salty snacks. |
| TAKE PARTICIPANTS TO A VENDING MACHINE | Take a trip to the vending machine in the building. Discuss different kinds of foods that are available in the vending machine.

Talk about which snacks are healthy and which ones are not so healthy. Discuss which snacks are okay to have more often and which snacks are okay to have every once in a while. Ask participants to identify their favorite snack.

Discuss how we decide what to have for a snack.

Label foods in your vending machine. If you have a vending machine on the premises, you may add a red heart to the snacks that are a healthier choice. Talk to your supervisor or vendor to add these stickers. |
| SUMMARIZE | *Today, we talked about what things influence our snacking choices. We also learned that snacking can be good for us depending on the snack that we choose.* |

EVALUATION

- Can participants identify what influences snacking choices?

- Can participants identify the importance of snacking?

Appendix A

Lesson P

Snacking and Vending Machines

Snacking and Vending Machines

What is your favorite snack? Please circle all that apply.

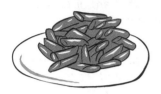 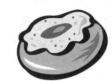 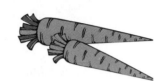 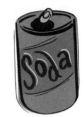

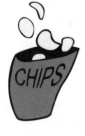 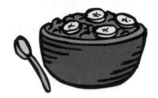 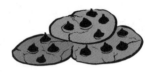 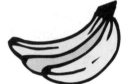

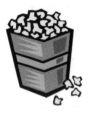 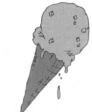

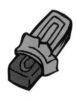 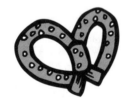 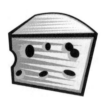 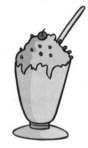

Other favorite snacks: _____

_____

_____

_____

In *Health Matters: The Exercise and Nutrition Health Education Curriculum for People with Developmental Disabilities*
by Beth Marks, Jasmina Sisirak, and Tamar Heller

Snacking and Vending Machines

Why do you snack? Circle responses.

Boredom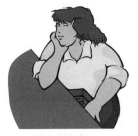

Nervousness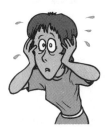

Hunger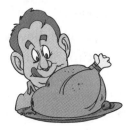

Taste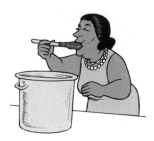

What are some things that affect your choices of snack foods? Circle responses.

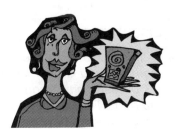

Advertising, TV commercials

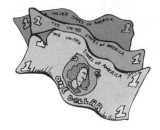

Cost

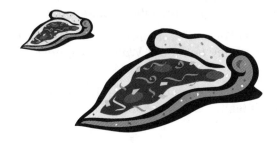

Size of snack

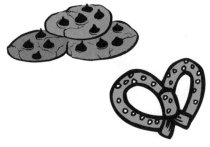

Craving sweet or salty

Taste, Texture, and Smell

Objectives
Participants will
• Identify different types of taste buds
• Discuss different food textures
• Describe the role their nose/smell plays in tasting food

also on CD-ROM

HANDOUTS
Participant Handout(s):
Taste, Texture, and Smell

MATERIALS
Pens or pencils
Small preparation bowls, spoons, and napkins
Activity 1: Ground coffee, lemon juice, sugar, and salt
Activity 2: Walnuts, gummy candy, animal crackers, pudding, and bananas
Activity 3: Small plastic cups and orange juice
Personal Notebooks for handouts and pictures

Suggested Activities	
INSTRUCTOR ACTIVITY	**INSTRUCTOR SCRIPT/DIRECTIONS**
INTRODUCTION	*Today we will talk about flavors we taste, the texture of the food we eat, and the smell. Did you know that our tongues can taste four basic types of taste: bitter, sour, salty, and sweet. We taste with taste buds. They are located in specific areas on our tongues. Texture means how food tastes in our mouths. Smell helps us taste the food we eat.*
COMPLETE ACTIVITY 1: TASTE	*Today we have three activities that we are going to do.*
	In four preparation bowls, pour some ground coffee beans, lemon juice, sugar, and salt. Distribute spoons to every participant. Each participant takes a sample of the four items. Everyone tastes ground coffee beans together.
	How does it taste? Yes, coffee is bitter. Have you tasted anything else that may be bitter? Wait for responses (e.g., burnt toast).
	Taste the remaining samples of lemon juice (sour), sugar (sweet), and salt (salty). Discuss some examples for each taste.
PREPARE FOR ACTIVITY 2: TEXTURE	Put some walnuts, gummy candy, animal crackers, pudding, and sliced bananas in preparation bowls.

INSTRUCTOR ACTIVITY	INSTRUCTOR SCRIPT/DIRECTIONS
DISTRIBUTE AND DISCUSS PARTICIPANT HANDOUT: Taste, Texture, and Smell	Distribute the **Taste, Texture, and Smell** handout. *In our new activity, we are going to taste some foods and try to describe the texture of these foods. Everyone will taste walnuts. What texture are the walnuts?* Wait for responses. Taste the remaining foods and fill out the texture section in the **Taste, Texture, and Smell** handout.
COMPLETE ACTIVITY 3: SMELL	Each participant should get a small serving of orange juice in a plastic cup. *Plug your nose with your hand. Take a sip of orange juice holding your nose. What do you taste?* Participants should not be able to taste anything.

Now take a sip of your orange juice without plugging your nose. What do you taste? Is there a difference? Our nose helps us taste the food that we eat. |
| SUMMARIZE | *Today, we talked about different types of taste buds. We also tried a variety of food textures and experimented with smell and taste.* |

EVALUATION

- Can participants identify different taste buds?

- Can participants identify food textures?

- Can participants understand how smell plays a role in tasting foods?

Taste, Texture, and Smell

Directions: Circle the texture that goes with each food.

Walnuts

Crispy/crunchy	Dry
Hard	Heavy
Gummy	Rough
Chewy	Slippery
Smooth	

Gummy bears

Crispy/crunchy	Dry
Hard	Heavy
Gummy	Rough
Chewy	Slippery
Smooth	

Banana

Crispy/crunchy	Dry
Hard	Heavy
Gummy	Rough
Chewy	Slippery
Smooth	

Crackers

Crispy/crunchy	Dry
Hard	Heavy
Gummy	Rough
Chewy	Slippery
Smooth	

Pudding

Crispy/crunchy	Dry
Hard	Heavy
Gummy	Rough
Chewy	Slippery
Smooth	

Your tongue has four basic types of taste buds. Your taste buds are located in specific areas on your tongue:

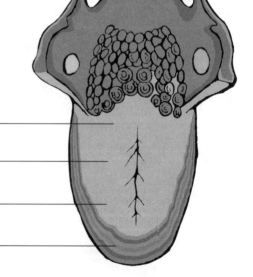

BITTER

SOUR

SALTY

SWEET

Taste, Texture, and Smell

Taste, Texture, and Smell

Examples of different types of taste

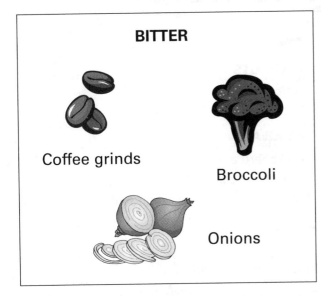

BITTER

Coffee grinds

Broccoli

Onions

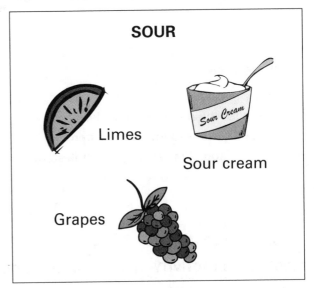

SOUR

Limes

Sour cream

Grapes

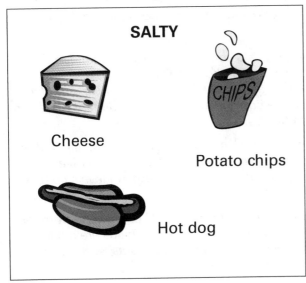

SALTY

Cheese

Potato chips

Hot dog

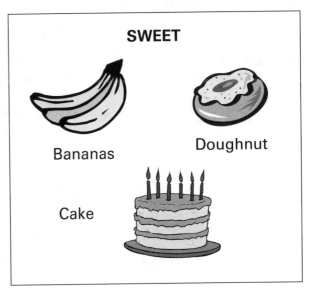

SWEET

Bananas

Doughnut

Cake

Your nose plays a major part in sensing the actual flavors of the foods you love.

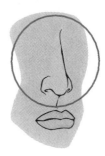

Lesson R

What Is Cholesterol?

also on
CD-ROM

Objectives

Participants will
- Discuss the meaning of cholesterol
- Identify ways to lower cholesterol
- Label foods that are high in cholesterol

HANDOUTS

Participant Handout(s):
   Cholesterol in Our Food

MATERIALS

Blackboard and chalk

Pens or pencils

Personal Notebooks for handouts and pictures

Suggested Activities

INSTRUCTOR ACTIVITY	INSTRUCTOR SCRIPT/DIRECTIONS
INTRODUCE LESSON	*Today, we will talk about cholesterol. We will also discuss ways to lower our cholesterol and list some foods that are high in cholesterol.*
ASK AND WAIT FOR RESPONSES	*What is cholesterol? It is a soft, waxy substance found in the blood and other parts of the body (cell walls of tissue). Cholesterol is a normal part of a healthy body. It is not bad to have cholesterol. The body needs a certain amount of cholesterol to build cell membranes.*
	Where do you get cholesterol? Your body (liver) usually makes enough cholesterol for your body. The food you eat gives you cholesterol. Your diet can make your cholesterol levels go up or down.
	What are the food sources of cholesterol? Cholesterol from food is only found in foods from animals. These foods are meats, cheese, and eggs. Foods that come from plants, such as fruits and vegetables, do not have any cholesterol.
	What if your blood cholesterol is good? You should still:

What if your blood cholesterol is good? You should still:

- *Eat lots of fruits and vegetables.*
- *Eat less foods that have a lot of saturated fat and cholesterol.*
- *Be physically active.*

What if you have too much cholesterol in your blood? You would be at a greater risk for heart disease:

- *Increased plaque (a thick, hard deposit) can plug your arteries.*
- *Arteries may become thicker, harder, and less flexible.*
- *Cholesterol slows down and sometimes blocks blood flow to the heart.*

* *You may have chest pain or a heart attack.*

How do you check your cholesterol?

* *You should have your cholesterol levels checked every five years—or more often if you're a man over 45 or a woman over 55.*
* *Cholesterol is checked to see your risk of having heart or any other health problems.*
* *Cholesterol is checked by taking some blood from your finger or your arm.*
* *This test is done in the morning before you have breakfast.*

DISCUSS

The following are values for cholesterol testing:

Total cholesterol (TC):	• Good (< 200) • A little high (200–239) • High (> 240)
Triglycerides (TRG):	• Good (< 150) • A little high (150–199) • High (200–499) • Very high (> 500)
High-density lipoprotein (HDL)—"good" cholesterol:	• Too low (< 40) • Good (40–59) • Very good (> 60)
Low-density lipoprotein (LDL)—"bad" cholesterol:	• Good (< 100) • Not so good (100–129) • A little high (130–159) • High (160–189) • Very high (> 190)
TC/HDL Ratio (risk of heart disease):	• Very good (< 3.8) • Average (3.9–4.7) • A little high (4.8–5.9) • High risk (> 6.0)

DISTRIBUTE AND DISCUSS PARTICIPANT HANDOUT:
  Cholesterol in Our Food

Distribute the **Cholesterol in Our Food** handout. Circle foods with cholesterol.

Foods with no cholesterol include peanut butter, apples, broccoli, ketchup, bananas, and vegetable oil. Foods with cholesterol include steak, cheese, butter, shrimp, mayonnaise, and eggs.

SUMMARIZE

Today, we talked about cholesterol. We also discussed which foods have cholesterol and which ones do not.

EVALUATION

* Can participants define cholesterol?

What Is Cholesterol?

Cholesterol in Our Food

Directions: Circle foods that are high in cholesterol.

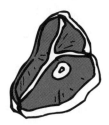

Steak

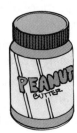

Peanut butter

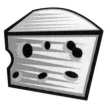

Cheese

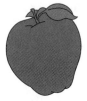

Apple

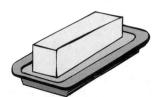

Butter

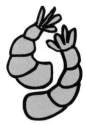

Shrimp

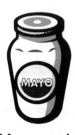

Mayonnaise

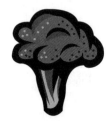

Broccoli

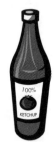

Ketchup

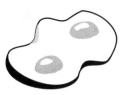

Eggs

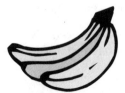

Banana

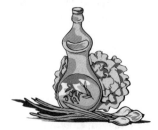

Vegetable oil

What Influences Our Food Choices?

Objectives

Participants will
- Discuss the reasons why they eat
- Identify factors that influence their food choices

HANDOUTS

also on
CD-ROM

Participant Handout(s):
  What Influences Our Food Choices?

MATERIALS

Blackboard and chalk

Pens or pencils

Personal Notebooks for handouts and pictures

Suggested Activities

INSTRUCTOR ACTIVITY	INSTRUCTOR SCRIPT/DIRECTIONS
INTRODUCE LESSON	*Today, we will discuss reasons why we eat and what influences our food choices. We will also review nutrients in our food that we discussed last class.*
ASK AND WAIT FOR RESPONSES	*What are some reasons we eat? We eat to make sure we are healthy. Food helps us breathe, move, think, and have more energy. This is the physical reason why we eat.*
	We also eat because we like the taste of food and we socialize around food. We can eat because we are nervous, bored, hungry, or are craving a particular food. Eating is enjoyable and satisfying to our appetites and our bodies.
DISTRIBUTE AND DISCUSS PARTICIPANT HANDOUT: What Influences Our Food Choices?	Distribute the **What Influences Our Food Choices?** handout. Ask participants how important the items on the list are to them when they choose foods.
SUMMARIZE	*Today, we talked about what influences our food choices. You probably see now that there are many different reasons why we choose to eat certain foods.*

EVALUATION

- Can participants identify factors that influence food choices?

What Influences Our Food Choices?

Directions: Circle what items influence your choice of food.

WEIGHT CONTROL	Important	Not important
HEALTH	Important	Not important
FOOD COSTS	Important	Not important
CONVENIENCE/TIME	Important	Not important
FAMILY BACKGROUND	Important	Not important
ADVERTISEMENTS (TV OR RADIO)	Important	Not important
EMOTIONS	Important	Not important
PEERS (FRIENDS, CO-WORKERS)	Important	Not important
CUSTOMS/ETHNIC BACKGROUND	Important	Not important
PHYSICAL ACTIVITY LEVEL	Important	Not important
TASTE	Important	Not important

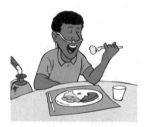

What are some things that
affect my choices of food?

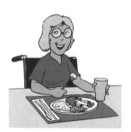

_____

_____

_____

_____

Lesson T

Blood Circulation

Objectives

Participants will

- Discuss how blood circulates in their body
- State the importance of exercise for their heart

HANDOUTS

Participant Handout(s):

Pieces of Albert's Body

Inside Albert's Body

MATERIALS

Blackboard and chalk

Scissors

Red, blue, green, and yellow colored paper

A copy of the pictures of the body parts: head, arms, legs, lungs, heart, and stomach

Heart rate monitor watch

Personal Notebooks for handouts and pictures

Suggested Activities

INSTRUCTOR ACTIVITY	INSTRUCTOR SCRIPT/DIRECTIONS
INTRODUCE LESSON	**Everyone keeps his or her heart rate monitor on.** *Today, we will talk about how our blood circulates in our bodies. We will also talk about how important it is to exercise our hearts.* *Make a fist. Cup your other hand around it. That is about the shape and size of your heart.* *What happens to your heart when you exercise? It beats faster so blood has extra food and oxygen.*
DISTRIBUTE PARTICIPANT HANDOUT: Pieces of Albert's Body 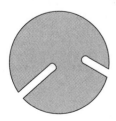	Prepare pictures of body parts from the **Pieces of Albert's Body** handout. These pieces include head (Albert), arms, legs, lungs, heart, and stomach. This handout can also be printed in color from the accompanying CD-ROM. You will need different colored papers: red (blood), blue (oxygen), and yellow (food). Cut the red paper in circles. Make two cuts in the circle (see picture on left). Cut the rest of the blue and yellow paper in smaller pieces. These will be used to attach them to the red (blood) piece as they travel through the body. Have everyone sit at a table or on the floor and help with the assembly of Albert's body.

INSTRUCTOR ACTIVITY	INSTRUCTOR SCRIPT/DIRECTIONS
ASK AND WAIT FOR RESPONSES	Place the blue pieces of paper (oxygen) around the head.
	Where does the air go when we breathe in? Wait for the correct response: lungs. Place some of the blue pieces in the lungs. Have someone else help.
	Where do we find our blood? Yes, our blood is all over our bodies. Blood keeps us alive by bringing food and oxygen to our bodies. Put blood pieces all over the body. *Blood picks up oxygen from the lungs.* Put some red and blue pieces together in the lungs. *The heart gives the blood a push.*
	Where does our food go when we eat it? Yes, it goes to the stomach. Put yellow pieces of paper in the stomach. *Blood picks up food from the stomach and our intestines.* Put together some red and yellow pieces in the stomach. *Blood goes around the body, giving food and oxygen to body parts.* Put red, blue, and yellow pieces together and put them around the body, legs, arms, and head.
	When blood gives food and oxygen to our muscles and body parts, it runs out of food and oxygen. Blood comes back to the heart for another push.
	What is the most important muscle in your body? The heart is the most important muscle in our bodies. What is your heart beat right now? Everyone checks his or her heart monitor. *What do you think happens to the heart when you do jumping jacks?*
	Let's do some jumping jacks. What happened to the heart beat? Yes, it is beating faster. What do you think will happen to the heart beat when you sleep or rest? Yes, it goes slower. Why do you think we exercise? It keeps our hearts strong and healthy.
DISTRIBUTE AND DISCUSS PARTICIPANT HANDOUTS: Inside Albert's Body	Distribute and review the **Inside Albert's Body** handout.
SUMMARIZE	*Today, we have talked about how our blood circulates in our bodies. We have learned that our hearts are muscles that pump our blood through our bodies. We have also learned that our blood picks up oxygen in our lungs and food in our stomach and intestines and carries them around to other body parts.*

EVALUATION

- Can participants identify how blood circulates in their body?

- Can participants identify that blood carries oxygen and food to the body parts?

- Can participants identify what happens to their heart when they exercise?

Pieces of Albert's Body

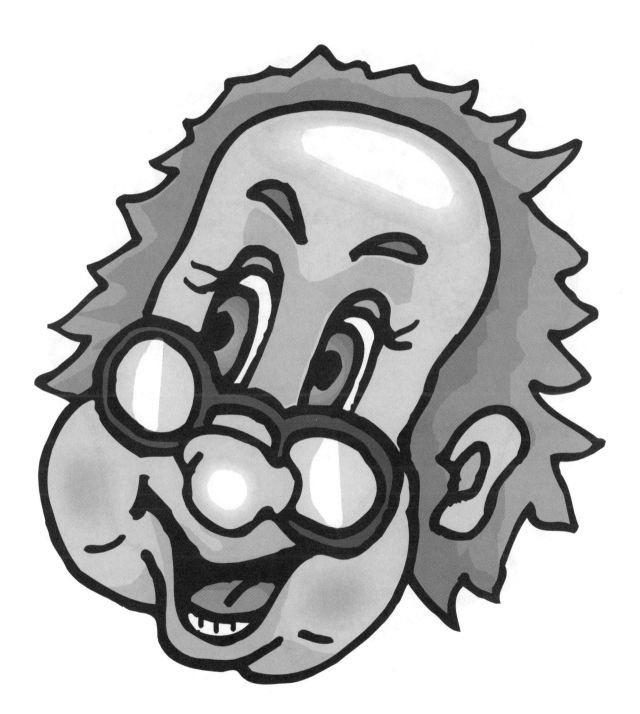

Head (Albert)

In *Health Matters: The Exercise and Nutrition Health Education Curriculum for People with Developmental Disabilities*
by Beth Marks, Jasmina Sisirak, and Tamar Heller

299

Pieces of Albert's Body

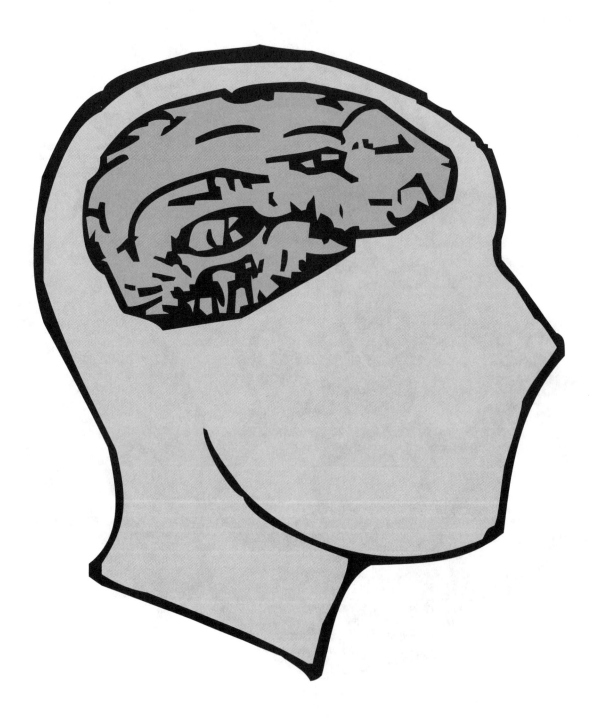

Brain

Pieces of Albert's Body

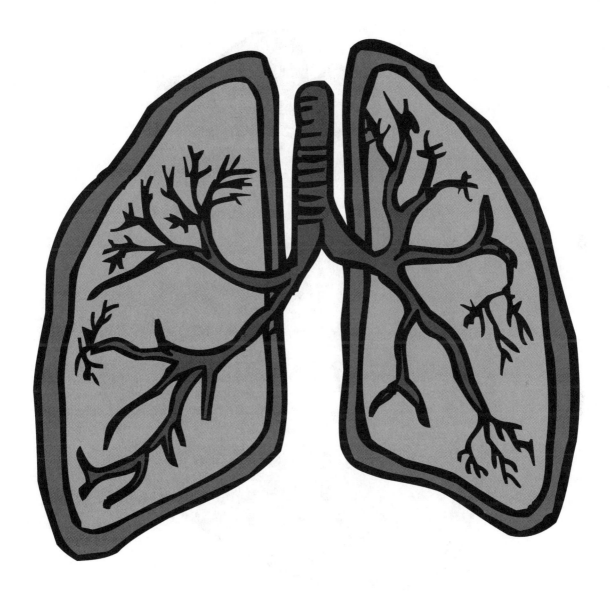

Lungs

Pieces of Albert's Body

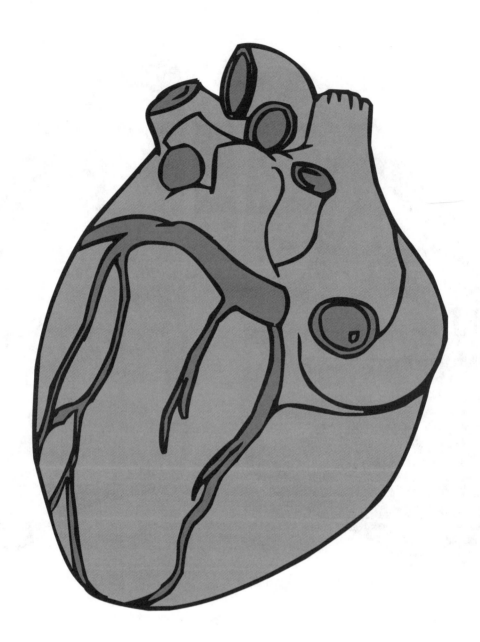

Heart

Pieces of Albert's Body

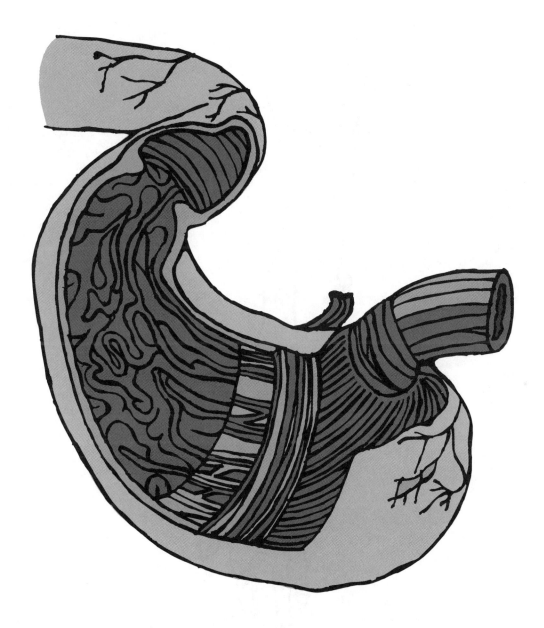

Stomach

Pieces of Albert's Body

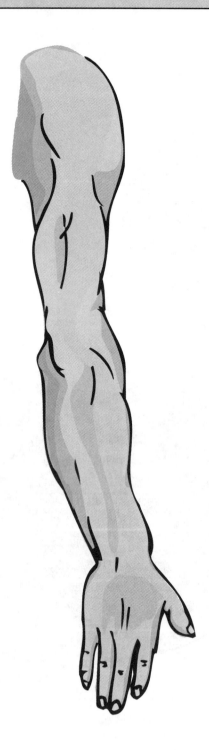

Arm

In *Health Matters: The Exercise and Nutrition Health Education Curriculum for People with Developmental Disabilities*
by Beth Marks, Jasmina Sisirak, and Tamar Heller

Pieces of Albert's Body

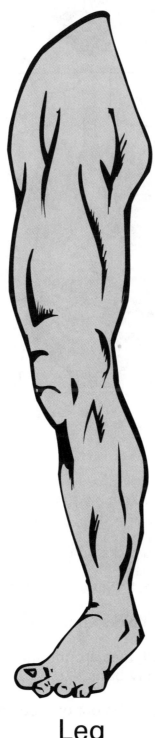

Leg

In *Health Matters: The Exercise and Nutrition Health Education Curriculum for People with Developmental Disabilities*
by Beth Marks, Jasmina Sisirak, and Tamar Heller
305

Inside Albert's Body

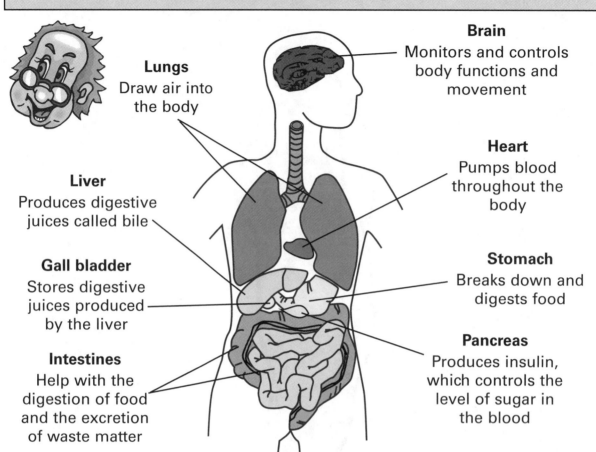

Brain
Monitors and controls body functions and movement

Lungs
Draw air into the body

Heart
Pumps blood throughout the body

Liver
Produces digestive juices called bile

Gall bladder
Stores digestive juices produced by the liver

Stomach
Breaks down and digests food

Pancreas
Produces insulin, which controls the level of sugar in the blood

Intestines
Help with the digestion of food and the excretion of waste matter

Blood

Oxygen

Food

1. Blood keeps you alive by bringing food and oxygen to your body.

2. Blood picks up oxygen from the lungs.

3. The heart gives the blood a push.

4. Blood picks up food from (or near) the stomach.

5. Blood goes around the body, giving food and oxygen to body parts.

6. Blood runs out of food and oxygen.

7. Blood comes back to the heart for another push.

What Is Diabetes?

Objectives

Participants will

- Discuss the meaning of diabetes
- Discuss the meaning of glucose
- Discuss the meaning of insulin
- State ways to prevent/control diabetes

HANDOUTS

also on
CD-ROM

Participant Handout(s):

You Have the Power to Prevent Diabetes!

MATERIALS

Blackboard and chalk

Pens or pencils

Participant Notebooks for handouts and pictures

Suggested Activities

INSTRUCTOR ACTIVITY	INSTRUCTOR SCRIPT/DIRECTIONS
INTRODUCE LESSON	*Today, we will talk about what it means to have diabetes.*
ASK AND WAIT FOR RESPONSES	*What is diabetes? Diabetes means that your blood sugar or glucose is too high.*
	Where do you find glucose? Glucose comes from the food you eat. Our bodies also make glucose in the liver and muscles. Our bodies need glucose for energy. There is always some glucose in our blood. Too much glucose in our blood is not good for our health.
	How does our body control blood glucose? The pancreas is an organ in our bodies that controls how much glucose is in our blood. The pancreas makes insulin, which helps glucose get from food into our cells. Our cells take the glucose and make it into energy that we need to live.
	What is insulin? Insulin is a hormone that is needed to convert sugar, starches, and other food into energy needed for daily life.
	In a person with diabetes, the pancreas does not make enough or makes no insulin. Sometimes the cells do not use insulin well. Glucose builds up in our blood. When our blood glucose gets too high it can damage our bodies.
	What is high blood sugar or glucose? A fasting plasma glucose test is used to check for blood glucose. A sample of blood is taken from a vein in the arm.
	*What are the types of diabetes? In **Type 1** diabetes, the pancreas stops making insulin. You will need to get insulin from a shot or a pump.*

Source: American Diabetes Association, http://www.diabetes.org

INSTRUCTOR ACTIVITY	INSTRUCTOR SCRIPT/DIRECTIONS
	*In **Type 2** diabetes the pancreas still makes some insulin but the cells can't use it very well.*
	The goal in managing diabetes is to keep the blood glucose as close to normal as possible. Your health care provider will tell you what you need to do. Some of the ways of keeping your blood sugar in check are to:
	• Eat healthy foods
	• Get exercise every day
	• Stay at a healthy weight
	• Take your medicine
	• Check your blood glucose
DISTRIBUTE AND DISCUSS PARTICIPANT HANDOUT: You Have the Power to Prevent Diabetes!	Distribute and discuss the **You Have the Power to Prevent Diabetes!** handout.
SUMMARIZE	*Today, we talked about diabetes and what it means to have high blood sugar. We also talked about how to prevent diabetes and how to control it if you already have diabetes.*

EVALUATION

- Can participants define diabetes?
- Can participants define glucose?
- Can participants define insulin?
- Can participants describe ways to prevent/control diabetes?

You Have the Power to Prevent Diabetes!

You can prevent diabetes if you lose as little as 10 pounds by walking 30 minutes a day 5 days a week and making healthy food choices!

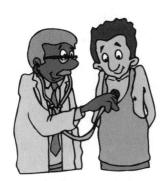

Get regular checkups

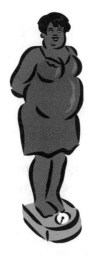

Lose weight if
you're overweight

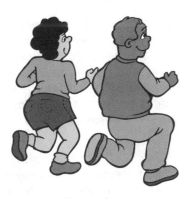

Exercise

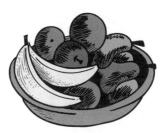

Eat healthy

Get help from your
family and friends

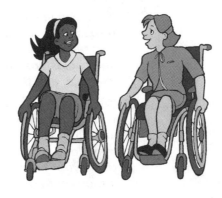

Lesson V

What Is Heart Disease?

Objectives

Participants will

- Define heart disease
- Discuss ways one can develop heart disease
- Identify ways to lower the risk of developing heart disease
- State different tests that check for heart disease

HANDOUTS

also on
CD-ROM

Participant Handout(s):

How Do I Prevent Heart Disease?

MATERIALS

Blackboard and chalk

Pens or pencils

Personal Notebooks for handouts and pictures

Suggested Activities

INSTRUCTOR ACTIVITY	INSTRUCTOR SCRIPT/DIRECTIONS
INTRODUCE LESSON	*Today, we will talk about heart disease.*
ASK AND WAIT FOR RESPONSES	*What is heart disease? Heart disease means that your heart is not getting enough blood and oxygen. This is caused by fatty materials (cholesterol) that build up in the arteries. Arteries carry blood and oxygen to your heart. Arteries can close up and become hard, which means less blood gets to your heart. If your heart does not get enough blood and oxygen, it begins to die. Heart disease develops over time and can start in childhood.*
	What can lead to heart disease? Cigarette smoking, high blood cholesterol, high blood pressure, being overweight, being over 45 years of age for men and over 55 for women, diabetes, and a family history of heart disease are all risk factors for developing heart disease.
	What can you do to lower your chances of getting heart disease? Do not smoke or quit smoking, eat foods with less fat, eat foods with less salt, get your blood pressure and cholesterol checked, lose weight if you are overweight, exercise, and take care of your diabetes.
	What are the tests to check for heart disease? Going to your health care provider does not mean that there is anything wrong with your heart. Your health care provider may do just one test or many of the following tests to check your heart. To maintain your good health, it is important to get your heart checked on a regular basis.

Source: American Heart Association, http://www.americanheart.org

	• Medical history and physical exam
	• Electrocardiogram (ECG or EKG) is a painless test that measures your heart's electrical activity.
	• Stress test or treadmill test is a painless test that measures your heart's electrical activity when you are exercising.
	• Echocardiography uses sound waves to show the size, shape, and movement of your heart.
	• Nuclear scan measures how your heart contracts as blood flows through it.
	• Coronary angiography or arteriography can show places where blood flow is slowed or blocked in your body.
DISTRIBUTE AND DISCUSS PARTICIPANT HANDOUT How Do I Prevent Heart Disease?	Distribute and review the **How Do I Prevent Heart Disease?** handout.
SUMMARIZE	*Today, we talked about heart disease and the ways we can prevent heart disease.*

EVALUATION

- Can participants identify heart disease?

- Can participants identify ways one develops heart disease?

- Can participants identify what actions lower the risk of developing heart disease?

How Do I Prevent Heart Disease?

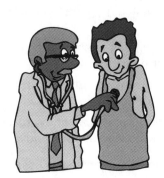

Get regular checkups

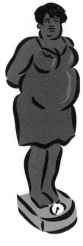

Lose weight if
you're overweight

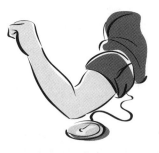

Get your blood
pressure and
cholesterol checked

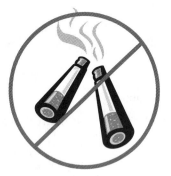

Do not smoke or
quit smoking

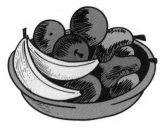

Eat foods with less fat

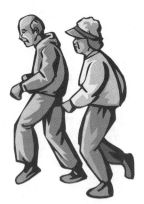

Exercise

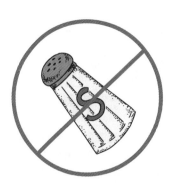

Eat foods with less salt

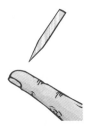

Take care of
your diabetes

Glossary

Note: This glossary includes an overview of common terms pertaining to exercise, health, medicine, nutrition, physiology, etc.

adherence Maintaining a lifestyle change. Used to describe a person's continuation in an exercise program.

aerobic Using oxygen.

aerobic activities Activities using large muscle groups at moderate to vigorous intensities that permit the body to use oxygen to supply energy and to maintain a steady state for more than a few minutes.

aerobic endurance The ability to continue aerobic activity over a period of time.

amino acids The building blocks of protein. Twenty different amino acids are required by the body.

anaerobic activities Activities using muscle groups at high intensities that exceed the body's capacity to use oxygen to supply energy and that create an oxygen debt by using energy produced without oxygen.

angina A gripping or suffocating pain or pressure in the chest (angina pectoris), most often caused by an insufficient flow of oxygen to the heart muscle during exercise or stress. Exercise should be stopped, and medical attention should be sought to clarify the reason for the symptoms.

arrhythmia Any abnormal rhythm of the heartbeat. Because some causes of arrthythmia may have threatening health consequences, exercisers experiencing irregular heartbeats should be referred for a medical evaluation.

asthma A pulmonary condition caused by constriction of the bronchial tubes from allergies, physical activity, or other irritants. It is characterized by wheezing, coughing, and labored breathing.

blood pressure The pressure exerted by the blood on the wall of the arteries. Maximum and minimum measures are used: Systolic pressure reaches a maximum just before the end of the pumping phase of the heart; diastolic pressure (minimum) occurs late in the refilling phase of the heart. Measures are in millimeters of mercury (as 120/80mm Hg).

body composition The proportions of fat, muscle, and bone that make up the body. It is usually expressed as the percent of body fat and the percent of lean body mass.

body mass index (BMI) The variable used to assess weight relative to height. Body mass index is calculated by dividing body weight in kilograms by height in meters squared (kg/m^2). A BMI of 25.0 to 29.9 kg/m^2 is considered overweight, and a BMI equal to or greater than 30.0 kg/m^2 is classified as obese.

calorie The calorie used as a unit of metabolism (as in diet and energy expenditure) equals 1,000 small calories and is often spelled with a capital C to make that distinction. It is the energy required to raise the temperature of 1 kg of water 1° C. Also called a *kilocalerie (kcal)*.

carbohydrate A chemical compound of carbon, oxygen, and hydrogen. Common forms are starches, sugars, cellulose, and gums. Carbohydrates are more readily used for energy production than are fats and proteins.

cardiac Pertaining to the heart and blood vessels.

cholesterol A substance in animal tissue that is an essential component of cell membranes and nerve fiber insulation. Cholesterol is important for the metabolism and transportation of fatty acids and in the production of hormones and Vitamin D. Cholesterol is manufactured by the liver and is also present in certain foods (e.g., eggs, shellfish). There are two types of cholesterol in the blood: high-density (HDL) and low-density (LDL) lipoproteins. Total blood cholesterol levels

From Bryant, Cedric X., Barry A. Franklin, and Sabrena Newton-Merrill. (2007). *ACE's Guide to Exercise Testing & Program Design: A Fitness Professional's Handbook, 2nd Edition.* Monterey, CA: Healthy Learning; and Bryant, C.X., Franklin, B.A., & Conviser, J.M. (2002). *Exercise Testing & Program Design: A Fitness Professional's Handbook.* Healthy Learning (pp. 187-212); adapted by permission.

above 240 mg/dL are considered high. Levels between 200–239 mg/dL are considered borderline high. Levels under 200 mg/dL are considered desirable.

chronic   Continuing over time.

circuit training   A series of exercises, performed one after the other, with little rest between. Resistance training in this manner increases strength while potentially providing some modest contribution to cardiovascular endurance as well.

conditioning   Long-term physical training.

cool-down   A gradual reduction of the intensity of exercise to allow physiological processes to return to normal. A cool-down avoids blood pooling in the legs and may reduce muscular soreness.

coronary heart disease (CHD)   Atherosclerosis of the coronary arteries.

dehydration   The condition resulting from the excessive loss of body water.

detraining   The process of losing the benefits of training by returning to a sedentary lifestyle.

diabetes mellitus   A metabolic disorder characterized by high blood sugar levels (hyperglycemia). The disease develops when there is insufficient production of insulin by the pancreas (type 1) or inadequate utlization of insulin cells (type 2).

diastolic blood pressure   The minimum blood pressure that occurs during the refilling of the heart.

diet   The food one eats. It may include a selection of foods to help accomplish a particular health or fitness objective.

diuretic   Any agent that increases the flow of urine. Sometimes used inadvisably for quick weight loss, diuretics can cause dehydration.

duration   The time spent in a single exercise session. Duration, along with frequency and intensity, is a factor influencing the effectiveness of exercise.

electrocardiogram (EKG, ECG)   A graph of the electrical activity cause by the stimulation of the heart muscle. The millivolts of electricity are detected by electrodes on the body surface and are recorded by an electrocardiograph.

endurance   The capacity to continue a physical performance over a period of time.

energy   The capacity to produce work.

exercise   Physical exertion of sufficient intensity, duration, and frequency to achieve or maintain fitness or other health or athletic objectives.

exercise prescription   A recommendation for a course of exercise to meet desirable individual objectives for fitness. It includes activity types, duration, intensity, and frequency of exercise.

extension   A movement that moves the two ends of a jointed body part away from each other, as in straightening the arm.

fat   1) A white or yellowish tissue that stores reserve energy, provides padding for organs, and smoothes body contours.
2) A compound of glycerol and various fatty acids. Dietary fat (fat coming from food sources) is not as readily converted to energy as are carbohydrates.

fatigue   A loss of power to continue a given level of physical performance.

fitness   The state of well-being consisting of optimum levels of strength, flexibility, weight control, cardiovascular capacity, and positive physical and mental health behaviors that prepare a person to participate fully in life, to be cognizant of controllable health risk factors, and to achieve physical objectives consistent with his or her potential.

fitness center   A place furnished with space and equipment, where professional leadership and supervision are offered to further the fitness objectives of individuals.

fitness testing   Measuring the indicators of various aspects of fitness.

flexibility   The range of motion around a joint.

flexion   A movement that moves the two ends of a jointed body part closer to each other, as in bending the arm.

frequency   How often a person repeats a complete exercise session (e.g. three times per week). Frequency, along with duration and intensity, affects the effectiveness of exercise.

glucose   Blood sugar. The transportable form of carbohydrate, which reaches the cells.

glycogen   The storage form of carbohydrate. Glycogen is used in muscles for the production of energy.

hamstrings   The group of muscles and their tendons at the back of the thigh.

heart attack   An acute manifestation of heart disease, associated with permanent tissue damage or necrosis.

heart rate   Number of heart beats per minute.

heat cramps   Muscle twitching or painful cramping, usually following heavy exercise with profuse sweating. The legs, arms, and abdominal muscles are most often affected.

heat exhaustion   Caused by dehydration (and sometimes salt loss). Symptoms include dry mouth, excessive thirst, loss of coordination, dizziness, headache, paleness, shakiness, and cool and clammy skin.

high blood pressure   See *hypertension.*

High-density lipoprotein   A type of lipoprotein that seems to provide protection against the buildup of atherosclerotic fat deposits in the arteries. Exercise seems to increase the HDL fraction of total cholesterol. HDL contains high levels of protein and low levels of triglycerides and cholesterol. An HDL above 60 mg/dL is considered a "negative" risk factor.

hormone   A chemical, secreted into the blood stream that specifically regulates the function of a certain organ of the body. Usually, but not always, secreted by an endocrine gland.

hyperglycemia   Abnormally high levels of glucose in the blood (high blood sugar). The clinical hallmark of diabetes mellitus. Usually defined as a blood-sugar value exceeding 100 mg/dL.

hypertension   Persistent high blood pressure. Readings of 140/90 mm/Hg are considered a threshold for high blood pressure by some authorities.

hypoglycemia   Abnormally low levels of glucose in the blood (low blood sugar). May lead to shaking, cold sweats, goosebumps, hypothermia, hallucinations, strange behavior, and, in extreme cases, convulsions and coma.

infarction   Death of a section of tissue from the total obstruction of blood flow (ischemia) to the area.

inflammation   The body's local response to an injury. Acute inflammation is characterized by pain, with heat, redness, swelling, and loss of function. Uncontrolled swelling may cause further damage to tissues at the injury site.

informed consent   A procedure for obtaining an individual's signed consent to a research project or a fitness center's prescription. It is a single document that includes a description of the objectives and procedures with associated benefits and risks that are stated in plain language with a consent statement and signature line.

intensity   The rate of performing work: power. It is a function of energy output per unit of time. Intensity, along with duration and frequency, determines the effectiveness of exercise.

ketosis   An elevated level of ketone bodies in the tissues. This condition may occur during periods of starvation or in persons with diabetes and is a common symptom among dieters on very low carbohydrate diets.

kilocalorie (kcal)   A measure of the heat required to raise the temperature of 1 kg of water 1° C. A large calorie (kcal) used in diet and metabolism measures equals 1,000 small calories.

kilogram (kg)   A unit of weight equal to 2.204623 pounds; 1,000 grams (g).

lipid   A number of body substances that are fat or fat-like.

low-density lipoprotein (LDL)   A lipoprotein carrying a high level of cholesterol, moderate levels of protein, and low levels of triglycerides. Associated with the buildup of artherosclerotic deposits in the arteries.

maximum heart rate   The highest heart rate that an individual can attain. A general rule for estimating the maximal heart rate is 226 (beats per minute for women) or 220 (beats per minute for men) minus the person's age (in years).

metabolism   The total of all of the chemical and physical processes by which the body builds and maintains itself (anabolism) and by which it breaks down its substances for the production of energy (catabolism).

monosaturated fat   Dietary fat whose molecules have one double bond open to receive more hydrogen. Found in many nuts, olive oil, and avocados.

muscle group   Specific muscles that act together at the same joint to produce movement.

myocardial infarction   A common form of heart attack in which the complete blockage of a coronary artery cases death or necrosis of a part of the heart muscle.

nutrients   Food and its specific elements and compounds that can be used by the body to build and maintain itself to produce energy.

nutrition   The processes involved in consuming and using food substances.

obesity   Excessive accumulation of body fat.

one repetition maximum (1 RM)   The maximum resistance at which a person can execute one repetition of an exercise movement.

osteoarthritis   A noninflammatory joint disease of older persons. The cartilage in the joint wears down, and there is bone growth at the edges of the joints. It results in pain and stiffness, especially after prolonged exercise.

osteoporosis   Decreased bone mineral content causing reduced bone density that results in an increased risk of fracture due to skeletal fragility and compromised bone micro-architecture.

peak heart rate The highest heart rate reached during an exercise or physical activity session.

physical activity Any form of exercise or movement.

physical fitness The physiological contribution to wellness through exercise and nutrition behaviors that maintain high aerobic capacity, optimal body composition, and adequate strength and flexibility to minimize the risk of chronic health problems and to enhance the quality of life.

polyunsaturated fat Dietary fat whose molecules have more than one double bond open to receive more hydrogen. Found in safflower oil, corn oil, soybeans, sesame seeds, and sunflower seeds.

protein Compounds of amino acids that make up most of the body's cells and perform other physiological functions.

pulmonary Pertaining to the lungs.

quadriceps A muscle group at the front of the thigh connected to a common tendon that surrounds the knee cap and attaches to the tibia (lower leg bone). Acts to extend the lower leg.

radial pulse The pulse at the wrist.

renal Pertaining to the kidneys.

repetition A single completed exercise movement. Repetitions are usually done in multiples.

resistance The force that a muscle is required to work against.

retest A repetition of a given test after the passage of time, usually to assess the progress made in an exercise program.

risk factor A behavior, characteristic, symptom, or sign that is associated with an increased risk of developing a health problem.

saturated fat Dietary fats of which the molecules are saturated with hydrogen. They are usually hard at room temperature and are readily converted into cholesterol in the body. Sources include animal products as well as hydrogenated vegetable oils.

sedentary Sitting a lot, being inactive or unfit, or not being involved in any regular physical activity that might produce significant fitness benefits.

set A group of repetitions of an exercise movement done consecutively, without rest, and until a given number, or volitional fatigue, is reached.

strength The amount of muscular force that can be exerted. Speed and distance are not factors of strength.

stretching Lengthening a muscle to its maximum extension, or moving a joint to the limits of its extension.

syndrome A group of related symptoms or signs of disease.

systolic blood pressure Blood pressure during the contraction of the heart muscle.

target heart rate (THR) The rate at which one aims to exercise to improve cardiorespiratory fitness.

unsaturated fat Dietary fat of which the molecules have one or more double bonds to receive more hydrogen atoms. Replacing saturated fats with unsaturated fats in the diet can help reduce cholesterol levels.

vital signs The measurable signs of essential bodily functions, such as respiration rate, heart rate, temperature, and blood pressure.

vitamins A number of unrelated organic substances that are required in trace amounts for the metabolic processes of the body and that occur in small amounts in many foods.

warm-up A gradual increase in the intensity of exercise to allow physiological processes to prepare for greater energy outputs. Changes include a rise in body temperature, cardiovascular and respiratory system changes, an increase in muscle elasticity and contractility, and so forth.

workout A complete exercise session, ideally consisting of a warm-up, moderate to vigorous aerobic and/or strength exercises, and a cool-down.

Appendix C

Sample Exercise Workouts

Flexibility, Aerobic,
Balance, and Strength Exercises

EXERCISE PROGRAM GOAL

The goal of the 12-week exercise program is to support participants to identify exercises that they like to do and encourage them to gain a) knowledge, b) skills, and c) confidence in being able to exercise 3 days a week at a level of intensity tailored to individual need.

The 12-week exercise program will consist of the following activities:

Warm-Ups (5 minutes) (e.g. jumping jacks, arm circles, seated leg circles)

FABS: **F**lexibility (5 minutes) (e.g., head tilts, shoulder stretch, trunk side bends, leg stretch, calf stretch)

Aerobic (30 minutes) (e.g., treadmill, bike, speed walk around gym)

Balance (5 minutes) (e.g., heal-to-toe walking, stand on one foot)

Strength (20 minutes) (e.g., wrist curls, bicep curls, arm raises, sit-to-stand, wall sits, plantar flexion)

Cool Downs (5 minutes) (e.g. walk around gym)

SAFETY AND PHYSICAL ACTIVITY

Safety can be an issue if you choose to use a lot of equipment (free weights, treadmills, and other fitness center equipment). If choosing to do physical training in this environment, be sure to plan to have enough staff to assist and "spot" athletes during the entire exercise session. For each exercise, demonstrate proper technique and, if necessary, break the exercise into basic components.

THREE SAMPLE WORKOUT PROGRAMS

The following are suggestions for activities that can be used to train people for the physical portion of the program. Frequency and order of such activities can be a mutual decision. You may choose to do a longer training session with participants who have no other physical activity in their schedules, or in some cases, have the physical activity portion of this program serve as a supplement to an exercise routine or schedule that is already in place.

Circuit Training Sampler

Circuit training can be done with six participants and two to three staff/trainers and requires no equipment.

- Start each participant on a different exercise and rotate after 1–2 minutes.
- Each exercise should be performed for about 1–2 minutes.
- Repeat the circuit two to three times in one session.

Warm-Up/Stretching (15 minutes)

Stations (20 minutes)

One participant will be at each station, using a prompt (e.g., a whistle). Participant will assume a ready position and begin their station's exercise for approximately 30 seconds to 1 minute. The level of performance of your group can help determine how long each rotation should be. You want to challenge the participants to work hard, but you also want most of the athletes to be able to perform each station for the entire duration of each rotation. At each interval (around 30 seconds), the participants will quickly go to the next station (a clockwise or counter clockwise system is effective) and begin the next exercise when the whistle blows.

Game (10–15 minutes)

Depending on what facilities/equipment you have available, a game is a very effective way to disguise additional exercise and can serve as a motivating factor for other portions of the physical training. Relay races and other team contests tend to work better and keep all participants more involved at this point in the session regardless of the varied levels of physical or social ability.

Cool-Down/Stretching (10–15 minutes)

Use as a review of activities done at the beginning of the session.

Cool-downs and stretches are good practice activities to try to get one or more of the participants to lead the group.

Suggested activities are best suited to be done in a preestablished order, either indoors or out as stations. Stations should be set up so that there are enough of them for each athlete to be active at the same time.

STATION IDEAS

- Jumping Jacks
- Arm Circles
- Leg Lifts or Sit-Ups
- Jump Rope
- Squats (bodyweight only or with hand weights/dumbbells)
- Arm Curls/Presses/Rows (with weights or weight alternatives, such as water bottles/sandbags/milk jugs filled with water)
- Others? BE CREATIVE!
- Modified Push-Ups
- Jog in Place
- Sit & Reach
- Bear Crawls and Crab Walks

DESCRIPTIONS OF EXERCISES

Arm Circles (Flexibility)

Purpose: Warms up and stretches your upper body

- Stand with arms straight out from your body.
- Circle your arms slowly clockwise for **15 seconds.**
- Relax your arms for **5 seconds.**
- Stand with arms straight out from your body.
- Circle your arms slowly counter clockwise for **15 seconds.**
- Relax your arms for **5 seconds.** Repeat.

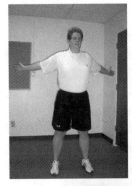
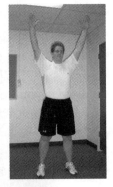
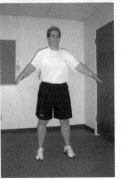

Seated "Y" Sit (Flexibility)

Purpose: Warms up your hamstrings and lower back

- Sit on the floor with both legs straight out in a "Y" position with your toes pointing towards ceiling.
- Keeping your knees straight, reach forward as far as you can (if possible, touch your right toe) with both hands.
- Hold for 10–15 seconds.
- Return to center.
- Repeat on left side.
- Return to center.
- Finally, reach both hands to center and hold for 10–15 seconds.
- Do this cycle two times.

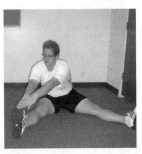
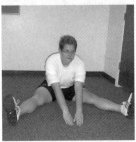
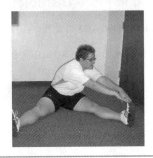

Wall Sits (Strength)

Purpose: Strengthens your buttocks, quadriceps, and hamstrings

- Stand with your back and palms flat against the wall.
- Slowly walk your feet out in front of you.
- Use your hands to slow your descent as your back slides down the wall.
- Lower yourself until you are in a sitting position, with your upper legs parallel to the floor, your knees at a 90-degree angle, and your feet directly below your knees.
- Do not let your knees extend beyond your toes.
- Hold as long as you can (1 minute or count to 60).

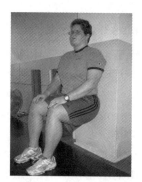

Jumping Jacks (Aerobics)

Purpose: Warms up your muscles

- Start with your feet together and stand at attention, with hands down by your side.
- Jump up, spread your feet apart, and clap your hands over your head.
- Jump up and land with your feet together and your hands at your sides.
- See if you can do 25 without stopping.

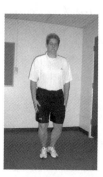
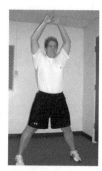

Sit-Ups (Strength)

Purpose: Strengthens your abdominal muscles

- Lie on your back with arms crossed on your chest or behind your head.
- Tighten your stomach muscles, and lift your head and shoulders off the floor.
- Do three sets of ten repetitions.

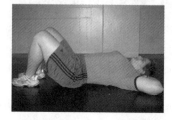
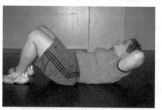

Jogging in Place or Marching in Place (Aerobic)

Purpose: Warms up your muscles

- Jog for about 1–2 minutes.

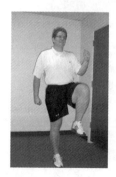
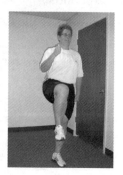

Modified Push-Up (Strength)

Purpose: Improves your upper body strength

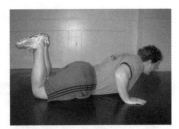

- Bend knees at **right** angles. To make sure that the knees are bent at right angles, you may want to use a large book and place it inside the knees.

- Place hands on the floor directly under the shoulders.

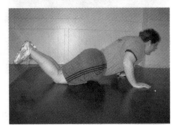

- Lower the body to the floor until the chest touches the floor. You may want to place a small folded towel or a sponge on the floor directly below the chest to serve as an indicator.

- Push back to the starting position, keeping your legs at 90 degrees.

- Repeat as many times for 1 minute.

- The body must not sag but maintain a straight line.

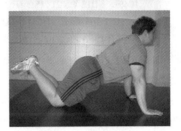

Anytime/Anywhere (Balance)

These types of exercises improve your balance. You can do them almost anytime, anywhere, and as often as you like, as long as you have something sturdy nearby to hold onto if you become unsteady.

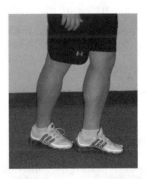

Purpose: Improves your overall balance

- Walk heel to toe. Position your heel just in front of the toes of the opposite foot each time you take a step. Your heel and toes should touch or almost touch.

- Stand on one foot. Alternate feet. You can do this while waiting in line at the grocery store or at the bus stop, for example.

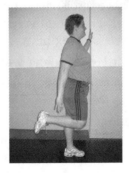

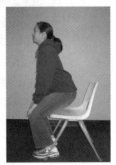

- Stand up, and sit down without using your hands.

Workout 2

Inexpensive and Portable Equipment

Using Exercise Bands

FLEXIBILITY

Sunshine Circles

Purpose: Warms up your core (shoulders to hip), back, and legs. This exercise incorporates a balance component and is a good overall warm-up exercise that increases flexibility.

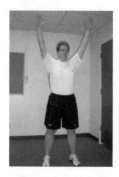
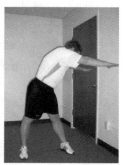
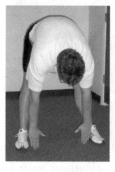
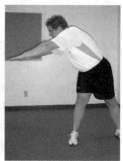

- Stand with your feet shoulder width apart.
- Extend both arms above your head.
- Slowly turn to your left side with your arms extended.
- Create a circle extending to the floor between your legs.
- Slowly complete the circle by extending both arms to the right side.
- Finish with your arms above your head.
- Do this five to eight times with one to two sets.

Diagonal Chop

Purpose: Warms up your core (shoulder to hip) back, and legs. This exercise incorporates a balance component. It is a good overall warmup exercise that increases flexibility.

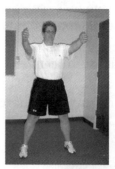
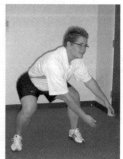
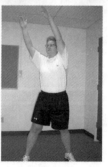

- Stand with your feet shoulder width apart.
- Hold your arms straight out in front of you with your arms parallel to the floor.
- With your head up and shoulders back, slowly lower your arms on a diagonal angle toward your right foot, then slowly return to starting position by keeping your head up and shoulders back. Follow the diagonal angle back up to parallel.
- Repeat on your left side.
- Do this five to eight times with one to two sets.

Arm Circles

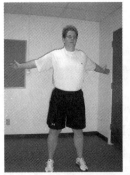
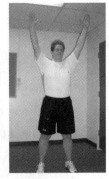

Purpose: Warms up your shoulders and chest

- Stand with your feet shoulder width apart.
- Standing shoulder width apart, make 10 big forward circles with your arms straight. Reverse and repeat backwards.
- Do this 10 times forward and 10 times backwards.

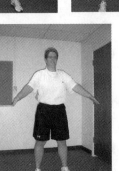

Seated "Y" Sit (Flexibility)

Purpose: Warms up your hamstrings and lower back

- Sit on the floor with both legs straight out in a "Y" position with your toes pointing toward the ceiling.
- Keeping your knees straight, reach forward as far as you can (if possible, touch your right toe) with both hands.
- Hold for 10–15 seconds (or as long as it takes you to hum the "Happy Birthday" song).
- Return to center.
- Repeat on left side.
- Return to center.
- Finally, reach both hands to center and hold for 10–15 seconds.
- Do this cycle two times.

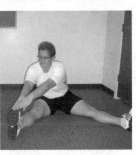

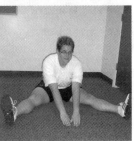

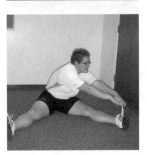

AEROBIC

Jumping Jacks

Purpose: Increases your heart rate

- Do jumping jacks in place.
- Do 20 jumping jacks.

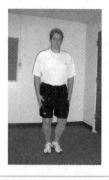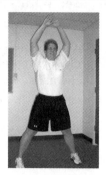

High Kicks

Purpose: Increases your heart rate

- Stand and kick each leg straight out individually.
- Do high kicks for 30 seconds.
- Do jumping jacks and high kicks in two cycles.

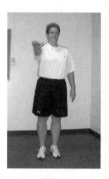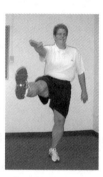

BALANCE

Stand on One Foot

Purpose: Increases your balance

- Stand with your head up, back straight, and feet shoulder width apart.
- Hold your arms out to your sides and parallel to the ground.
- Pick one foot up off the ground, and stand in that position until you lose your balance (have a chair close by to hang onto if necessary).
- Return foot to ground and repeat with opposite foot.
- Do each leg two times.

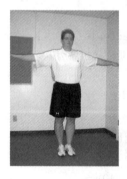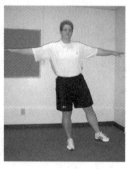

STRENGTH

Squat with Exercise Band

Purpose: Increases muscle strength in your legs

- Stand with your head up and back straight with your feet shoulder width apart.
- Place the middle of the exercise band under your feet.
- Put one handle in each hand, and raise your hands to your shoulders, palms facing out, with elbows tucked into your body.
- Bend your knees and squat down, like sitting in a chair, with your back straight.
- Stand back up into starting position while extending your arms above your head.
- Do 2 sets of 10 repetitions.

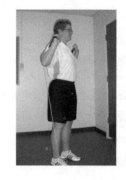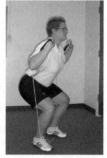

Chest Press

Purpose: Increases muscle strength in your chest

- Stand with your feet shoulder width apart with an exercise band handle in each hand.
- Have a partner stand one step behind you holding the middle of the exercise band.
- Extend your arms straight out from your body until your arms are extended out all the way and parallel to the ground.
- Return the band to your chest and repeat.
- Do 2 sets of 10 repetitions.

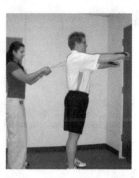

Shoulder Press

Purpose: Increases muscle strength in your shoulders

- Stand with your feet shoulder width apart.
- Place middle of exercise band under both feet.
- With a handle in each hand, press both arms over your head until your arms are fully extended.
- Slowly return your hands to your chest and repeat.
- Do 2 sets of 10 repetitions.

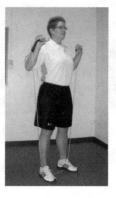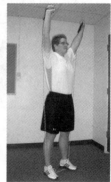

Using Exercise Bands

Two-Way Shoulder Raise

Purpose: Increases muscle strength in your shoulders

- Stand with your feet shoulder width apart (can be done sitting as well).
- Place the middle of the exercise band under both feet.
- With a handle in each hand, and with straight arms, raise your arms out from your sides to shoulder height, and return to starting position.
- Place arms in front of your body with palms facing in.
- Raise arms in front of your body to parallel.
- Repeat sequence.
- Do 2 sets of 10 repetitions.

Standing

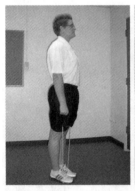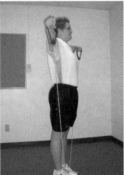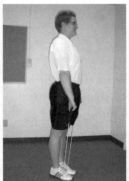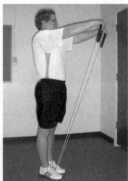

Sitting

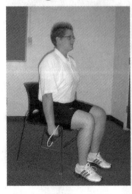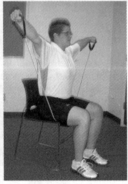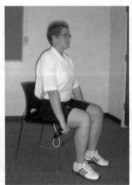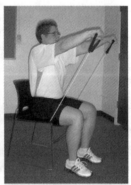

Workout 3

Inexpensive and Portable Equipment

Using Weighted Bars

(**Please note:** Use of weighted bars may be difficult for people who are just starting to exercise.)

FLEXIBILITY

Good Mornings

Purpose: Warms up your core (shoulders to hips), back, and legs. This exercise incorporates a balance component.

- Stand with your feet shoulder width apart.
- Hold your arms straight out in front of your body with your arms parallel to the floor.
- With your head up and shoulders back, bend your knees and lower your arms toward the ground.
- Slowly return to the starting position by keeping your head up and shoulders back, and stand straight up.
- Do this five to eight times in one to two sets.

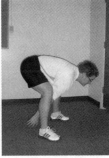
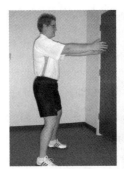

Arm Circles

Purpose: Warms up your shoulders and chest

- Stand with your feet shoulder width apart.
- Standing shoulder width apart, make 10 big forward circles with your arms straight. Reverse and repeat backward.
- Do this 10 times forward and 10 times backward.

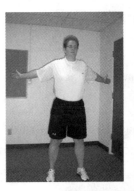
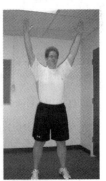
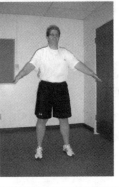

Toe Touches

Purpose: Warms up your lower back and hamstrings

- Stand shoulder width apart with knees slightly bent.
- Bend over and touch toes. Repeat 10 times.

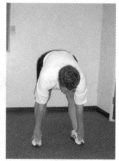 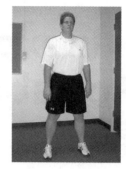

"Self-Hug"

Purpose: Warms up your upper body, including your arms

- With your arms parallel to the ground, wrap both arms around yourself, holding on at your shoulders.
- Maintain position for 10–15 seconds.

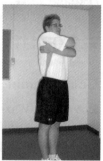 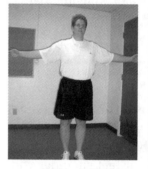

Seated Butterfly Stretch

Purpose: Warms up your hips and groin

- Sit on the floor and bend your legs into your body.
- Put the soles of your feet together.
- Let your knees fall down to either side.
- Using your elbows, slightly push your knees farther down.
- Maintain for 10–15 seconds.

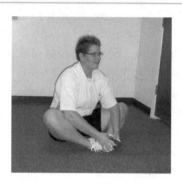

AEROBIC

March in Place

Purpose: Increases your heart rate

- March in place with high knees for 30 seconds.
- Marching in place is better for keeping form.

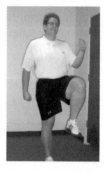 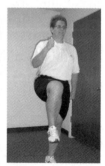

Walk Briskly

Purpose: Increases your heart rate

- Walk briskly around room for 1 minute, or walk with a "purpose."
- Repeat cycle two to three times.

BALANCE

Anytime/Anywhere

You can do these exercises almost anytime, anywhere (e.g., while waiting in line or at the bus stop), and as often as you like, as long as you have something sturdy nearby to hold onto if you become unsteady.

Purpose: Improves your balance

- Walk heel to toe. Position your heel just in front of the toes of the opposite foot each time you take a step. Your heel and toes should touch or almost touch.

- Stand on one foot. Alternate feet.

- Stand up and sit down without using your hands.

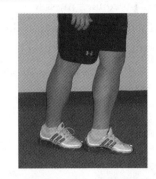

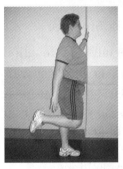

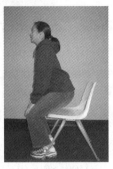

STRENGTH

Squat with Weighted Bar

Purpose: Increases your muscle strength

- Stand head up, back straight, with feet shoulder width apart.

- Place the middle of the weighted bar on your shoulders.

- Bend your knees and squat down, like sitting in a chair, with your back straight.

- Stand back up into starting position.

- Do 2 sets of 10 repetitions.

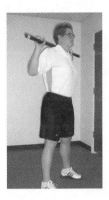

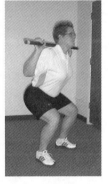

Chest Press

Purpose: Increases muscle strength in your chest

- Stand with your feet shoulder width apart with a weighted bar in your hands.

- Extend arms straight out from your body until your arms are extended out all the way and parallel to the ground.

- Return the bar to your chest and repeat.

- Make sure elbows are parallel to the ground.

- Do 2 sets of 10 repetitions.

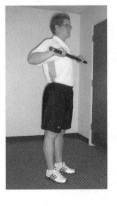

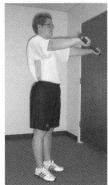

Shoulder Press

Purpose: Increases muscle strength in your shoulders

- Stand with your feet shoulder width apart.
- Place middle of weighted bar on your shoulders.
- Press both arms over your head until your arms are fully extended.
- Slowly return your hands to your chest and repeat.
- Do 2 sets of 10 repetitions.

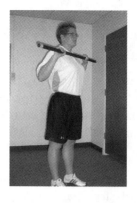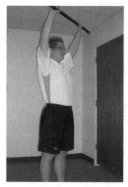

Bicep Curl with Weighted Bar

Purpose: Increases muscle strength in your biceps

- Stand with your feet shoulder width apart.
- Place middle of weighted bar in your hands with an underhand grip. Slowly curl bar up to chest. Make sure to keep elbows pinned to body. All movement should come from elbows, not shoulders.
- Do 2 sets of 10 repetitions.

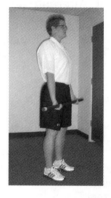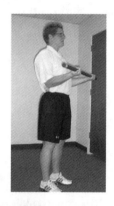

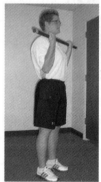

A Sampler of Exercises for Adults Aging with I/DD

HELPFUL TIPS

- Group warm-up session
- Group stretching session
- Divide group between strength and cardiovascular training areas.
- Alternate or switch groups: Strength goes to cardiovascular and cardiovascular goes to strength.
- Group cool-down session
- Group stretching session
- For the first 2 weeks of the program, start participants with 30 to 40 minutes per session and slowly increase their workout to 60–90 minutes.

FLEXIBILITY TRAINING

Set-up

- A comfortable space preferably with carpet or exercise mat.
- A chair, wall, or something for support if needed—a friend will work, too!

Health Benefits of Stretching

- Helps prevent muscle aches and pains.
- Improves posture and can reduce neck and lower back discomfort.
- Promotes greater flexibility so you can enjoy more activities with less fear of injury.
- Revitalizes the mind, reduces fatigue, and increases energy.
- Relieves stress and tension.

The Facts about Flexibility

Flexibility refers to how far and how easily you can move your joints. As you get older, your tendons and other connective tissues around your muscles begin to shorten and tighten, restricting the movement of your joints, you become less flexible. In many cases this loss of mobility/ flexibility is more related to inactivity than the aging process. The less you move, the less you're able to move.

Portions of this sampler are adapted from the National Institute on Aging. (2009, February 5). *Exercise & physical activity: Your everyday guide from the National Institute on Aging.* Available from U.S. National Institutes of Health at http://www.nia.nih.gov/HealthInformation/Publications/ExerciseGuide.

Floor Stretches

To get into a lying position:

1. Stand next to a very sturdy chair that won't tip over (put chair against wall for support if you need to).

2. Put your hands on the seat of the chair.

3. Lower yourself down on one knee.

4. Bring the other knee down.

5. Put your left hand on the floor and lean on it as you bring your left hip to the floor.

6. Your weight is now on your left hip.

7. Straighten your legs out.

8. Lie on your left side.

9. Roll onto your back.

Note: You don't have to use your left side. You can use your right side, if you prefer.

To get up from a lying position:

1. Roll onto your left side.

2. Use your right hand, placed on the floor at about the level of your ribs, to push your shoulders off the floor.

3. Your weight is on your left hip.

4. Roll forward, onto your knees, leaning on your hands for support.

5. Lean your hands on the seat of the chair you used to lie down.

6. Lift one of your knees so that one leg is bent, foot flat on the floor.

7. Leaning your hands on the seat of the chair for support, rise from this position.

Note: You don't have to use your left side; you can reverse positions, if you prefer.

Side Neck Stretch

Purpose: Stretches neck muscles

With shoulders relaxed, gently tilt your head toward your shoulder. Assist stretch with a gentle pull on the side of the head.

Hold for 5–10 seconds. Repeat 3 to 5 times.

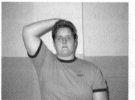 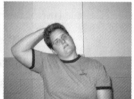

Neck Rotation (floor)

Purpose: Stretches neck muscles

Equipment: telephone book or thick book

Lie on the floor with a telephone book or other thick book under your head, then slowly turn your head from side to side, hold-

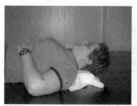 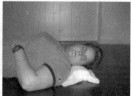

ing position for 10 to 30 seconds on each side. Your head should not be tipped forward or backward, but should be in a comfortable position. You can keep your knees bent to keep your back comfortable during this exercise. Repeat 3 to 5 times.

Summary:

1. Lie on your back.

2. Turn head from side to side, holding position each time.

Wrist Stretch

Purpose: Hand and arm flexibility

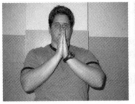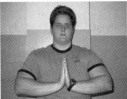

Press your hands together, elbows down. Raise your elbows as nearly parallel to the floor as possible, while keeping your hands together. Hold for 10 to 30 seconds. Repeat 3 to 5 times.

Summary:

1. Place hands together, in praying position.

2. Slowly raise elbows so arms are parallel to ground, keeping hands flat against each other.

3. Hold position for 10 to 30 seconds.

4. Repeat 3 to 5 times.

Triceps Stretch

Purpose: Stretches muscles in back of upper arm

Reach hand behind head as if to scratch your back. Grasp your elbow and gently push downward.

Hold for 10 to 30 seconds. Repeat 3 to 5 times.

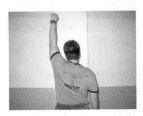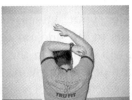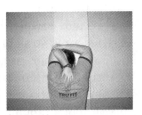

Triceps Stretch (modified)

Purpose: Stretches muscles in back of upper arm

Equipment: towel

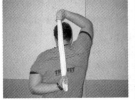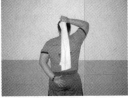

Hold one end of a towel in your right hand. Raise your left arm; then bend your left elbow so that the towel drapes down your back. Keep your left arm in this position, and continue holding onto the towel. With your right hand, reach behind your lower back and grasp the other end (the bottom end) of the towel. Gradually grasp higher and higher up the towel with your right hand, as high as you can. As you do this, you will find that it also pulls your left arm down. Continue until your hands touch, or as close to that as you can comfortably go. Reverse positions.

Summary:

1. Hold towel in left hand.
2. Raise and bend left arm to drape towel down back.
3. Grasp bottom end of towel with right hand.
4. Climb right hand progressively higher up towel, which also pulls your left arm down.
5. Reverse positions.

Shoulder Stretch

Purpose: Increases shoulder flexibility

Reach your left arm across your body and hold it straight. With the right hand, grasp the left elbow and pull it across the body toward the chest.

Hold each position 10 to 30 seconds. Repeat 3 to 5 times.

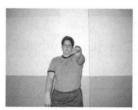 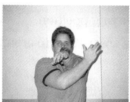 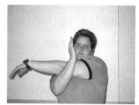

Shoulder Rotation (floor)

Purpose: Stretches shoulder muscles

Equipment: pillow, towel (optional)

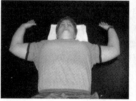 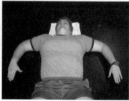

Lie on the floor with a pillow under your head, legs straight. If your back bothers you, place a rolled towel under your knees. Stretch your arms straight out to the side, on the floor. Your upper arms will remain on the floor throughout this exercise. Bend at the elbow so that your hands are pointing toward the ceiling. Let your arms slowly roll backwards from the elbow. Stop when you feel a stretch or slight discomfort, and stop immediately if you feel a pinching sensation or a sharp pain. Slowly raise your arms, still bent at the elbow, to point toward the ceiling again. Then let your arms slowly roll forward, remaining bent at the elbow, to point toward your hips. Stop when you feel a stretch or slight discomfort. Alternate pointing above your head, then toward the ceiling, then toward your hips in this manner. Begin and end with the pointing-above-the-head position. Hold each position 10 to 30 seconds. Keep your shoulders flat on the floor throughout. Repeat 3 to 5 times.

Summary:

1. Lie flat on floor, pillow under head.
2. Stretch arms out to side.
3. Bend elbows to crook lower arms downward, at right angle.
4. Hold position.

5. Bend elbows to crook lower arms upward, at right angle.

6. Hold position.

7. Keep shoulders flat on floor throughout.

Chest Stretch

Purpose: Improves posture

Place bent arm against a wall or doorway as shown. Slowly lean forward until a stretch is felt in the chest region.

Hold each position 10 to 30 seconds. Repeat 3 to 5 times.

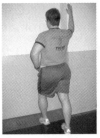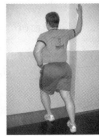

Upper Back Stretch

Purpose: Increases back flexibility

Clasp fingers together with thumbs pointing down; round your shoulders as you reach your hands forward.

Hold each position 10 to 30 seconds. Repeat 3 to 5 times.

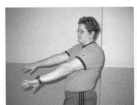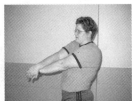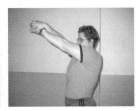

Low Back Stretch

Purpose: Relieves lower back tension

Lie on your back with knees bent. Slowly pull knees up to the chest until you feel a gentle stretch in the lower back.

Hold each position 10 to 30 seconds. Repeat 3 to 5 times.

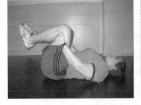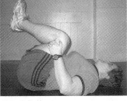

Glute Stretch

Purpose: Increases flexibility of hip and gluteal muscles

Lying on your back; cross legs, placing one ankle on the opposite knee as shown. Use the flexed leg to push the crossed leg back until you feel a stretch in the buttocks.

Hold each position 10 to 30 seconds. Repeat 3 to 5 times.

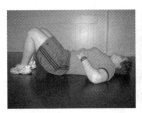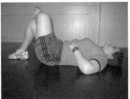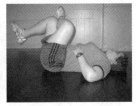

Butterfly Stretch

Purpose: Increases flexibility of leg muscles

Sit tall with the soles of your feet together. Allow your knees to ease down toward the floor until you feel a stretch along the groin region.

Hold each position 10 to 30 seconds. Repeat 3 to 5 times.

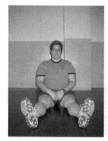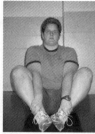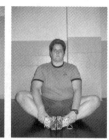

Hamstrings

Purpose: Stretches muscles in back of thigh

Lie flat on the floor with knees flexed to 90 degrees and back flat on the floor. Slowly raise and straighten one leg, grasping it loosely behind the thigh with both hands.

Hold each position 10 to 30 seconds. Repeat 3 to 5 times.

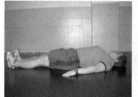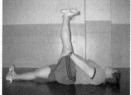

Hamstrings (modified)

Purpose: Stretches muscles in back of thigh

Equipment: bench or two chairs

Sit sideways on a bench or other hard surface (such as two chairs placed side by side) without leaning back against anything and with your back and shoulders straight. Start with your right leg on the bench (chair). Your right leg should be resting on the bench, toes pointing up. Your left leg should be resting over the side of the bench, with your left foot flat on the floor. If your right knee is bent, stretch to get it to lie flat on the bench. If you feel a stretch at this point, hold the position for 10 to 30 seconds. If your right leg is flat on the bench and you don't feel a stretch, lean forward slowly from the hips (not the waist) until you do, keeping your back and shoulders straight the entire time. (Note: Don't do this part if you have had a hip replacement. Don't lean forward, unless health professional has approved.) Stop and hold this position for 10 to 30 seconds. Reverse the position so that you stretch your left leg in the same way. Repeat 3 to 5 times on each side.

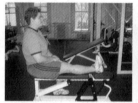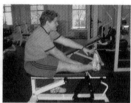

Summary:

1. Sit sideways on bench.

2. Keep one leg stretched out on bench, straight.

3. Keep other leg off of bench, with foot flat on floor.

4. Straighten back.

5. Lean forward from hips (not waist) till you feel stretching in leg on bench, keeping back and shoulders straight. Omit this step if you have had a hip replacement, unless surgeon/therapist approves.

6. Hold position.

7. Repeat with other leg.

Alternative Hamstring Stretch

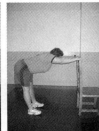
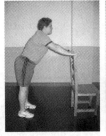

Purpose: Stretches muscles in the back of the thigh

Equipment: chair

Stand behind a chair, with your legs straight. Hold the back of the chair with both hands. Bend forward from your hips (not your waist), keeping your entire back and shoulders straight the whole time, until your upper body is parallel to the floor. Don't "hump" any part of your back or shoulders at any time. Hold position for 10 to 30 seconds. You should feel a stretch in the backs of your thighs. Repeat 3 to 5 times.

Summary:

1. Stand behind chair, holding the back of it with both hands.

2. Bend forward from the hips, keeping back and shoulders straight at all times.

3. When upper body is parallel to floor, hold position.

Standing Quadriceps Stretch

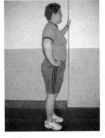
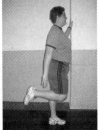
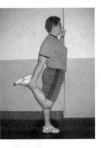

Purpose: Stretches muscles in front of thighs

Stand with one hand on wall for balance. Bring foot up to hand and grasp the ankle, gently pull up until stretch is felt. Keep knees side by side.

Hold each position 10 to 30 secnods. Repeat 3 to 5 times.

Quadriceps (floor)

Purpose: Stretches muscles in front of thighs

Equipment: pillow

Lie on your right side, on the floor. Your hips should be lined up so that the left one is directly above the right one. Rest your head on a pillow or your right hand. Bend your left knee, reach back with your left hand, and hold onto your left heel. If you can't reach your heel with your hand, loop a belt over your left foot. Pull slightly (with your hand or with the belt) until the front of your left thigh feels stretched. Hold the position for 10 to 30 seconds. Reverse position and repeat with other leg. Repeat 3 to 5 times on each side. If the back of your thigh cramps during this exercise, stretch your leg and try again, more slowly.

Summary:

1. Lie on your side.

2. Rest your head on your pillow or hand.

3. Bend the knee that is on top.

4. Grab the heel of that leg.

5. Gently pull that leg until front of thigh stretches.

6. Hold position.

7. Reverse position and repeat.

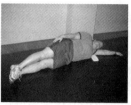

Knee Flexion Stretch

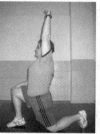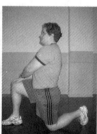

Purpose: Stretches muscles in the hip region

Kneel on the floor with your front knee bent at and back leg extended as shown. Keeping your back straight, slowly bend the lead leg until a stretch is felt. Do not lean forward or bend the lead leg more than 90 degrees.

Hold each position 10 to 30 seconds. Repeat 3 to 5 times.

Double Hip Rotation (floor)

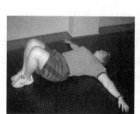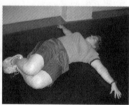

(Don't do this exercise if you have had a hip replacement, unless your surgeon approves.)

Purpose: Stretches outer muscles of hips and thighs

Equipment: pillow

Lie on your back, knees bent, and feet flat on floor. Keeping your shoulders on the floor, with your knees bent and together, gently lower both knees to one side as far as possible without forcing them. Hold the position for 10 to 30 seconds, then bring knees back to center and repeat on opposite side. Repeat 3 to 5 times on each side.

Summary:

1. Don't do this exercise if you have had a hip replacement, unless your surgeon approves.

2. Lie on floor, knees bent.

3. Keep shoulders on floor at all times.

4. Keeping knees together, lower legs to one side.

5. Hold position.

6. Return legs to upright position.

7. Repeat toward other side.

Single Hip Rotation (floor)

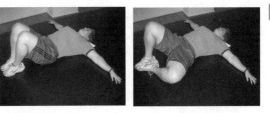

Purpose: Stretches muscles of pelvis and inner thigh

Equipment: pillow

Lie on your back and bend your knees. Let your right knee slowly lower to the right, keeping your left leg and your pelvis in place. Hold the position for 10 to 30 seconds. Bring your right knee slowly back to place. Repeat the exercise with your left leg. Repeat 3 to 5 times on each side. Keep your shoulders on the floor throughout the exercise.

Summary:

1. Lie on floor.

2. Bend knees.

3. Let one knee slowly lower to side.

4. Hold position.

5. Bring knee back up.

6. Keep shoulders on floor throughout exercise.

7. Repeat with other knee.

Calf Stretch

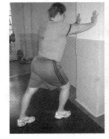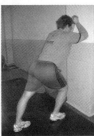

Purpose: Stretches lower leg muscles in two ways: with knee straight and knee bent

Stand 3–4 feet from wall with feet in the position shown and perpendicular to the wall. Lean against forearms, maintaining a straight line through the spine and back heel pressed to the ground.

Hold each position 10 to 30 seconds. Repeat 3 to 5 times.

Equipment: a clear wall area

While standing, place your hands on a wall, with arms outstretched, elbows straight. Keeping your left knee slightly bent, toes of right foot slightly turned inward, move your right foot back one or two feet, with your right heel and foot flat on the floor. You should feel a stretch in your right calf muscle, but you shouldn't feel uncomfortable. If you don't feel a stretch, move your right foot farther back until you do. Keep your right knee straight and hold that position for 10 to 30 seconds. Continuing to keep your right heel and foot on the floor, bend your right knee and hold for another 10 to 30 seconds. Repeat with opposite leg. Repeat 3 to 5 times on each side.

Summary:

1. Stand with hands against wall, arms straight.

2. Step back 1–2 feet with one leg, heel and foot flat on floor.

3. Hold position.

4. Bend knee of stepped-back leg, keeping heel and foot flat on floor.

5. Hold position.

6. Repeat with other leg.

Ankles

Purpose: Stretches front ankle muscles

Equipment: chair

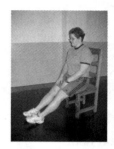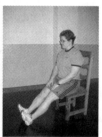

Remove your shoes. Sit toward the front edge of a chair and lean back, using pillows to support your back. Slide your feet away from the chair in front of you so that your legs are outstretched. With your heels still on the floor, point your toes away from you until you feel a stretch in the front part of your ankles. If you don't feel a stretch, lift your heels slightly off the floor while doing this exercise. Hold the position briefly. Repeat 3 to 5 times.

Summary:

1. Sit in chair.

2. Stretch legs out in front of you, feet off of floor.

3. Bend ankles to point feet toward you.

4. Bend ankles to point feet away from you.

5. If you don't feel the stretch, repeat with your feet slightly off the floor.

AEROBIC TRAINING

Set-up

- Find a comfortable space, preferably with carpet or exercise mat.

- Check each exercise for equipment that is needed.

Health Benefits of Aerobic Training

- Improves cholesterol

- Lowers blood pressure

- Lowers resting heart rate

- Helps decrease excess body fat

- Increases our capacity to do work

- Improves our immune system

- Revitalizes the mind, reduces fatigue, and increases energy

Jumping Jacks

Purpose: Warms up your muscles

1. Start with your feet together, stand at attention, hands down by your side.

2. Jump up and spread your feet apart and clap your hands over your head.

3. Jump up and land with your feet together hands at your sides again.

4. See if you can do 25 without stopping

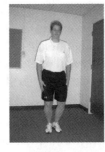
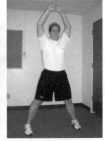

Jogging-in-Place

Purpose: Warms up your muscles

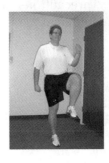
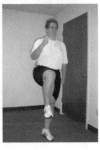

Swimming/Rowing Machine

Many times, people will mistime the action of their hands and knees.

- You should push with your legs and pull with your arms simultaneously on the stroke.

- On the return, straighten your arms first and then bend your knees.

- Keep your back straight and do not overreach.

- Keep your elbows in and pull the bar into your lower stomach.

Stepper

- Keep your heels down and take big steps, not little ones.

- Keep your arms relaxed.

- Don't lock them to support your body weight against the machine's handgrips.

Aerobic Steps (Step Aerobics)

Aerobic steps can provide a cardiovascular workout with continuous movements to elevate heart rate. Aerobic steps can allow people with higher skill levels to work harder and longer, and consequently burn more calories. The rate of energy expenditure will vary greatly depending on the person's performance ability. Steps can be used in early stages of conditioning if fitness is adequate.

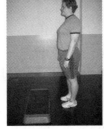
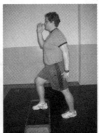
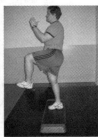

Cycling (indoor or outdoor)

A stationary bike provides lower body strength training and aerobic exercise. Bikes provide the ability to strengthen leg muscles. Cycling can be done at a consistent intensity and energy expenditure and is not dependent on the participant's skill level.

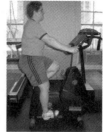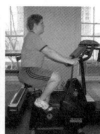

Consider using a standard upright bicycle or semi-recumbent (sitting) stationary bicycles, which may be more comfortable for some individuals. Review all of the safety precautions and ensure proper positioning with the equipment.

Stair Climbing

Stair climbing is an everyday task that involves the major muscle groups of the lower extremities and can improve cardiovascular endurance. Climbing stairs is one of the best ways to reduce body fat and burn calories.

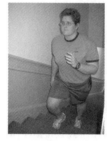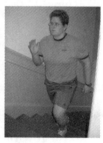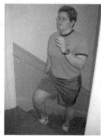

Cross-trainer

The cross-trainer is particularly good for stamina training. It mimics a running motion and reduces impact on your legs. This lessens the chances of injuries such as shin splints that may be caused by the repeated high impact of running on hard ground.

Keep your heels down and try moving the footplates forwards and backwards during different sessions.

Treadmill

Set the treadmill for a speed and duration that enables you to run within your training zone. Raising the incline on the treadmill increases the effort and varies the precise impact on your muscles. A 2% incline mimics road-running conditions.

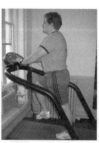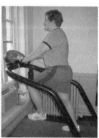

Safety

1. **Use those safety features.** Always use the safety key that allows the emergency shutoff. Attached to the key is a cord with a clip at the end that you attach to your clothing. When the key is pulled out of the slot, the treadmill immediately stops. If your treadmill has an automatic stop, the option to code out nonauthorized users, or some other safety feature, take advantage of it.

2. **Straddle the belt when you start out.** Always place one foot on either side of the belt as you turn on the machine. Then step on the belt only after you determine that

it's moving at the slow set-up speed. Most treadmills have safety features that prevent them from starting out at breakneck speeds, but don't take any chances.

3. **Use the handrails sparingly.** Holding on for balance is okay when you're finding out how to use the machine, but let go as soon as you feel comfortable. You move more naturally if you swing your arms freely. If you must hold on to the front rails to charge up a hill or maintain a speed, you have the treadmill set at too high an intensity. Over-reliance on the handrails can overstrain your elbows and shoulders and reduces the amount of calories you burn during a workout.

4. **Keep your eyes forward.** Your feet tend to follow your eyes, so if you focus on what's in front of you, you usually walk straight ahead instead of veering off to the side. Also, try to stay in the center of the belt rather than all the way toward the back or front. If you stay too close to the front, your foot can catch on the motor cover and trip you up; if you walk too close to the back, you may slide right off.

5. **Expect to feel disoriented.** The first few times you use a treadmill, you may feel dizzy when you get off. Your body is just wondering why the ground suddenly stopped moving. Most people experience this vertigo only once or twice, but be prepared to hold onto something for a few moments when you hop off so that you don't fall over.

BALANCE TRAINING

Set-up

- A comfortable space, preferably with carpet or exercise mat
- Check each exercise for equipment that is needed.

Health Benefits of Balance Training

Helps you stay independent by reducing the risk of falls

Plantar Flexion

Equipment: chair

Hold table with one hand, then one fingertip, then no hands; then do exercise with eyes closed, if steady.

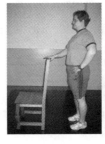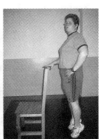

Summary:

1. Stand straight, holding onto a table or chair for balance.

2. Slowly stand on tiptoe, as high as possible.

3. Hold position.

4. Slowly lower heels all the way back down.

5. Repeat 8 to 15 times.

6. Rest a minute, then do another 8 to 15 repetitions.

7. Add modifications as you progress.

Knee Flexion

Equipment: chair

Hold table with one hand, then one fingertip, then no hands; then do exercise with eyes closed, if steady.

Summary:

1. Stand straight; hold onto table or chair for balance.

2. Slowly bend knee as far as possible, so foot lifts up behind you.

3. Hold position.

4. Slowly lower foot all the way back down.

5. Repeat with other leg.

6. Add modifications as you progress.

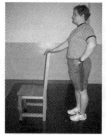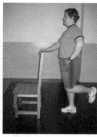

Hip Flexion

Equipment: chair

Hold table with one hand, then one fingertip, then no hands; then do exercise with eyes closed, if steady.

Summary:

1. Stand straight; holding onto a table or chair for balance.

2. Slowly bend one knee toward chest, without bending waist or hips.

3. Hold position.

4. Slowly lower leg all the way down.

5. Repeat with other leg.

6. Add modifications as you progress.

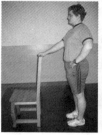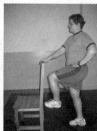

Hip Extension

Equipment: chair

Hold table with one hand, then one fingertip, then no hands; then do exercise with eyes closed, if steady.

Summary:

1. Stand 12–18 inches from table.

2. Bend at hips; hold onto table.

3. Slowly lift one leg straight backwards.

4. Hold position.

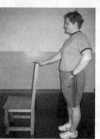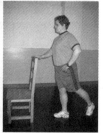

5. Slowly lower leg.

6. Repeat with other leg.

7. Add modifications as you progress.

Side Leg Raise

Equipment: chair

Hold table with one hand, then one fingertip, then no hands; then do exercise with eyes closed, if steady.

Summary:

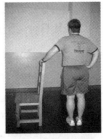

1. Stand straight, directly behind table or chair, feet slightly apart.

2. Hold table for balance.

3. Slowly lift one leg to side, 6–12 inches.

4. Hold position.

5. Slowly lower leg.

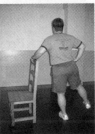

6. Repeat with other leg.

7. Keep back and knees straight throughout exercise.

8. Add modifications as you progress.

Anytime/Anywhere

These types of exercises also improve your balance. You can do them almost anytime, anywhere, and as often as you like, as long as you have something sturdy nearby to hold onto if you become unsteady.

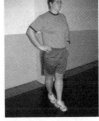

Examples:

- Walk heel-to-toe. Position your heel just in front of the toes of the opposite foot each time you take a step. Your heel and toes should touch or almost touch. (See Illustration.)

- Stand on one foot (while waiting in line at the grocery store or at the bus stop, for example). Alternate feet.

- Stand up and sit down without using your hands.

Balance Board

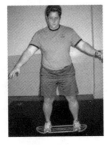

Excellent for improving balance. These exercises also help to condition all the muscles, tendons and ligaments.

Stand with your feet about shoulder-width apart and see-saw and pivot any way that feels good.

Balance Block

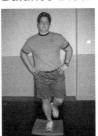

STRENGTH TRAINING

Set-up

- A comfortable space, preferably with carpet or exercise mat.
- Check each exercise for equipment that is needed.

Health Benefits of Strength Training

- Increases metabolism: Strength training increases the body's metabolic rate, causing the body to burn more calories throughout the day.
- Increases bone density and prevents bone loss: Inactivity and aging can lead to a decrease in bone density and brittleness. Studies have proven that consistent strength training can increase bone density and prevent osteoporosis.
- Increases lean muscle mass and muscle strength, power, and endurance.
- Prevents injury by strengthening our muscles.
- Improves balance, flexibility, mobility and stability. Stronger muscles improve our balance, which means more comfortable living and fewer falls or accidents.
- Decreases the risk of heart disease.
- Decreases cholesterol and lowers your blood pressure.
- Revitalizes the mind, reduces fatigue, and increases energy.

Side Arm Raises

Purpose: Strengthens shoulder muscles

Equipment: 3- to 5-pound dumbbells or food cans

Sit in a chair, with your back straight. Your feet should be flat on the floor, spaced apart so that they are even with your shoulders. Hold hand weights

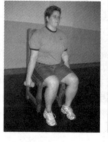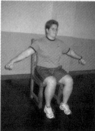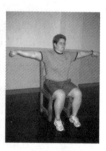

straight down at your sides, with your palms facing inward. Take 3 seconds to lift your arms straight out, sideways, until they are parallel to the ground. Hold the position for 1 second. Take 3 seconds to lower your arms so that they are straight down by your sides again. Pause. Repeat 8 to 15 times. Rest; do another set of 8 to 15 repetitions.

Summary:

1. Sit in chair.
2. Feet flat on floor; keep feet even with shoulders.
3. Arms straight down at sides, palms inward.
4. Raise both arms to side, shoulder height.
5. Hold position.
6. Slowly lower arms to sides.

Chair Stand

Purpose: Strengthens muscles in abdomen and thighs

Equipment: pillow for your back

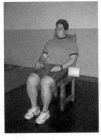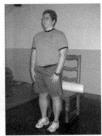

Sit toward the middle or front of a chair and lean back so that you are in a half-reclining position, with back and shoulders straight, knees bent, and feet flat on the floor. Be sure to place pillows against the lower back of the chair first, to support your back and keep it straight. Using your hands as little as possible (or not at all, if you can), bring your back forward so that you are sitting upright. Your back should no longer be leaning against the pillows. Keep your back straight as you come up, so that you feel your abdominal muscles do the work; don't lean forward with your shoulders as you rise. Next, with feet flat on the floor, take at least 3 seconds to stand up, using your hands as little as possible. As you bend slightly forward to stand up, keep your back and shoulders straight. Take at least 3 seconds to sit back down. Your goal is to do this exercise without using your hands as you become stronger. Repeat 8 to 15 times. Rest; then repeat 8 to 15 times more.

Summary:

1. Place pillows against back of chair.

2. Sit in middle or toward front of chair, knees bent, feet flat on floor.

3. Lean back on pillows, in half-reclining position, back and shoulders straight.

4. Raise upper body forward until sitting upright, using hands as little as possible.

5. Slowly stand up, using hands as little as possible.

6. Slowly sit back down.

7. Keep back and shoulders straight throughout exercise.

Biceps Curls

Purpose: Strengthens upper-arm muscles

Equipment: 3- to 5-pound dumbbells or food cans

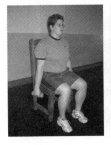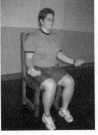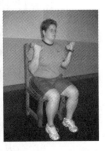

Sit in an armless chair, with your back supported by the back of the chair. Your feet should be flat on the floor, spaced apart so that they are even with your shoulders. Hold hand weights, with your arms straight down at your side, palms facing in toward your body. Take 3 seconds to lift your left hand weight toward your chest by bending your elbow. As you lift, turn your left hand so that your palm is facing your shoulder. Hold the position for 1 second. Take 3 seconds to lower your hand to the starting position. Pause, then repeat with right arm. Alternate until you have repeated the exercise 8 to 15 times on each side. Rest, then do another set of 8 to 15 alternating repetitions.

Summary:

1. Sit in armless chair, with your back supported by back of chair.

2. Feet flat on floor; keep feet even with shoulders.

3. Hold hand weights at sides, arms straight, palms in.

4. Slowly bend one elbow, lifting weight toward chest. (Rotate palm to face shoulder while lifting weight.)

5. Hold position.

6. Slowly lower arm to starting position.

7. Repeat with other arm.

Shoulder Press

Purpose: Strengthens upper-arm muscles

Equipment: 3- to 5-pound dumbbells or food cans

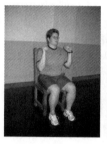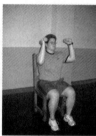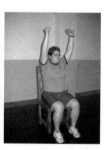

Sit in an armless chair, with your back supported by the back of the chair. Your feet should be flat on the floor, spaced apart so that they are even with your shoulders. Hold hand weights, with your arms straight down at your side, palms facing in toward your body. Take 3 seconds to lift your hand weights over head. Hold the position for 1 second. Take 3 seconds to lower your hand to the starting position. Repeat exercise 8 to 15 times on each side.

Summary:

1. Sit in armless chair, with your back supported by back of chair.

2. Feet flat on floor; keep feet even with shoulders.

3. Hold hand weights at sides, arms straight, palms in.

4. Slowly bend one elbow, lifting weight toward chest. (Rotate palm to face shoulder while lifting weight.)

5. Hold position.

6. Slowly lower arm to starting position.

7. Repeat with other arm.

Seated Row

Purpose: Strengthens upper-arm muscles

Equipment: 3- to 5-pound dumbbells or food cans

Sit in an armless chair, with your back supported by the back of the chair. Your feet should be flat on the floor, spaced apart so that they are even with your shoulders. Hold hand weights, with your arms straight down at your side, palms facing in toward your body. Take

3 seconds to lift your hand weights toward your chest by bending your elbow. Take 3 seconds to lower your hand to the starting position. Repeat the exercise 8 to 15 times side. Rest, then do another set of 8 to 15 alternating repetitions.

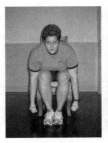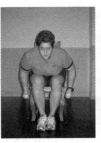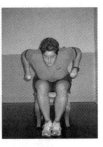

Summary:

1. Sit in armless chair, with your back supported by back of chair.

2. Feet flat on floor; keep feet even with shoulders.

3. Hold hand weights at sides, arms straight, palms in.

4. Slowly bend one elbow, lifting weight toward chest. (Rotate palm to face shoulder while lifting weight.)

5. Hold position.

6. Slowly lower arm to starting position.

7. Repeat with other arm.

Reverse Fly

Purpose: Strengthens upper-arm muscles

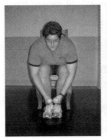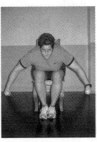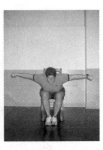

Equipment: 3- to 5-pound dumbbells or food cans

Sit in an armless chair, with your back supported by the back of the chair. Your feet should be flat on the floor, spaced apart so that they are even with your shoulders. Hold hand weights, with your arms straight down at your side, palms facing in toward your body. Take 3 seconds to lift your hand weights away from body by bending elbows. Take 3 seconds to lower your hand to the starting position. Repeat the exercise 8 to 15 times per side. Rest, then do another set of 8 to 15 alternating repetitions.

Summary:

1. Sit in armless chair, with your back supported by back of chair.

2. Feet flat on floor; keep feet even with shoulders.

3. Hold hand weights at sides, arms straight, palms in.

4. Slowly bend one elbow, lifting weight toward chest. (Rotate palm to face shoulder while lifting weight.)

5. Hold position.

6. Slowly lower arm to starting position.

7. Repeat with other arm.

Shoulder Flexion (Front Arm Raise)

Purpose: Strengthens shoulder muscles

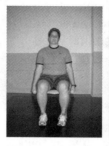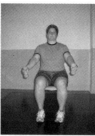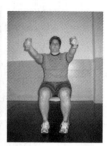

Equipment: 3- to 5-pound dumbbells or food cans

Sit in a chair, with your back straight. Your feet should be flat on the floor, spaced apart so that they are even with your shoulders. Hold hand weights straight down at your sides, with your palms facing inward. Take 3 seconds to lift your arms in front of you, keeping them straight and rotating them so that your palms are facing upward, until your arms are parallel to the ground. Hold the position for 1 second. Take 3 seconds to lower your arms so that they are straight down by your sides again. Pause. Repeat 8 to 15 times. Rest; do another set of 8 to 15 repetitions.

Summary:

1. Sit in chair.

2. Feet flat on floor; keep feet even with shoulders.

3. Arms straight down at sides, palms inward.

4. Raise both arms in front of you (keep them straight and rotate so palms face upward) to shoulder height.

5. Hold position.

6. Slowly lower arms to sides.

Plantar Flexion

Purpose: Strengthens ankle and calf muscles (also described in balance section)

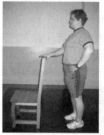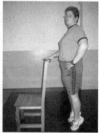

Equipment: ankle weights (optional)

Use ankle weights, if you are ready to. Stand straight, feet flat on the floor, holding onto the edge of a table or chair for balance. Take 3 seconds to stand as high up on tiptoe as you can; hold for 1 second, then take 3 seconds to slowly lower yourself back down. Do this exercise 8 to 15 times; rest a minute, then do another set of 8 to 15 repetitions. As you become stronger, do this exercise first on your right leg only, then on your left leg only, for a total of 8 to 15 times on each leg. Rest a minute, then do another set of 8 to 15 alternating repetitions.

Summary:

1. Stand straight, holding table or chair for balance.

2. Slowly stand on tiptoe, as high as possible.

3. Hold position.

4. Slowly lower heels all the way back down.

Variation, as strength increases: Do the exercise standing on one leg only, alternating legs.

Triceps Extension

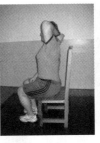
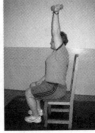

(If your shoulders aren't flexible enough to do this exercise, see alternative "Dip" exercise, below.)

Purpose: Strengthens muscles in back of upper arm

Equipment: 3- to 5-pound dumbbells or food cans

Sit in a chair, toward the front. Your feet should be flat on the floor, spaced apart so that they are even with your shoulders. Hold a weight in your left hand and raise your left arm all the way up so that it's pointing toward the ceiling, palm facing in. Support your left arm by holding it just below the elbow with your right hand. Slowly bend your left arm so that the weight in your left hand now rests behind your left shoulder. Take 3 seconds to straighten your left arm so that it's pointing toward the ceiling again. Hold the position for 1 second. Take 3 seconds to lower the weight back to your shoulder by bending your elbow. Keep supporting your left arm with your right hand throughout the exercise. Pause, then repeat the bending and straightening until you have done the exercise 8 to 15 times with your left arm. Reverse positions and repeat 8 to 15 times with your right arm. Rest; then repeat another set of 8 to 15 repetitions on each side.

Summary:

1. Sit in chair, near front edge.

2. Feet flat on floor; keep feet even with shoulders.

3. Raise one arm straight toward ceiling.

4. Support this arm, below elbow, with other hand.

5. Bend raised arm at elbow, bringing hand weight toward same shoulder.

6. Slowly re-straighten arm toward ceiling.

7. Hold position.

8. Slowly bend arm toward shoulder again.

Knee Flexion

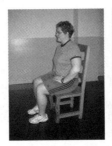
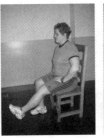
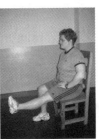

Purpose: Strengthens muscles in back of thigh

Equipment: ankle weights (optional)

Use ankle weights, if you are ready to. Stand straight, very close to a table or chair, holding it for balance. Take 3 seconds to bend your left knee so that your calf comes as far up toward the back of your thigh as possible. Don't move your upper leg at all; bend your knee only. Take 3 seconds to lower your left leg all the way back down. Repeat with right leg. Alternate legs until you have done 8 to 15 repetitions with each leg. Rest; then do another set of 8 to 15 alternating repetitions.

Summary:

1. Stand straight; hold onto table for balance.

2. Slowly bend knee as far as possible.

3. Hold position.

4. Slowly lower foot all the way back down.

5. Repeat with other leg.

Hip Flexion

Purpose: Strengthens thigh and hip muscles

Equipment: ankle weights (optional)

Use ankle weights, if you are ready to. Lay on the floor. Take 3 seconds to bend your left knee. Hold position for 1 second, then take 3 seconds to lower your left leg all the way down. Repeat with right leg; alternate legs until you have done 8 to 15 repetitions on each side. Rest; then do another set of 8 to 15 alternating repetitions.

Summary:

1. Stand straight, holding tall, stable object for balance.

2. Slowly bend one knee toward chest, without bending waist or hips.

3. Hold position.

4. Slowly lower leg all the way down.

5. Repeat with other leg.

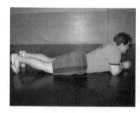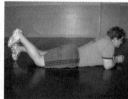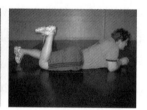

Knee Extension

Purpose: Strengthens muscles in front of thigh and shin

Equipment: ankle weights (optional)

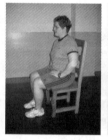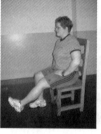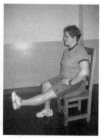

Use ankle weights, if you are ready to. Sit in a chair, with your back resting against the back of the chair. If your feet are flat on the floor in this position, you should place a rolled-up towel under your knees to lift them up. Only the balls of your feet and your toes should be resting on the floor. Rest your hands on your thighs or on the sides of the chair. Take 3 seconds to extend your right leg in front of you, parallel to the floor, until your knee is straight. With your right leg in this position, flex your foot so that your toes are pointing toward your head; hold your foot in this position for 1 to 2 seconds. Take 3 seconds to lower your right leg back to the starting position, so that the ball of your foot rests on the floor again.

Repeat with left leg. Alternate legs, until you have done the exercise 8 to 15 times with each leg. Rest; then do another set of 8 to 15 alternating repetitions.

Summary:

1. Sit in chair. Put rolled towel under knees, if needed.

2. Slowly extend one leg as straight as possible.

3. Hold position and flex foot to point toes toward head.

4. Slowly lower leg back down.

5. Repeat with other leg.

Hip Extension

Purpose: Strengthens buttock and lower-back muscles

Equipment: ankle weights (optional)

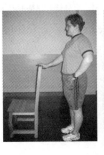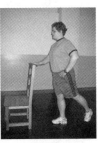

Use ankle weights, if you are ready to. Stand 12 to 18 inches away from a table or chair, feet slightly apart. Bend forward from the hips, at about a 45-degree angle, holding onto the table or chair for balance. In this position, take 3 seconds to lift your left leg straight behind you without bending your knee, pointing your toes, or bending your upper body any farther forward. Hold the position for 1 second. Take 3 seconds to lower your left leg back to the starting position. Repeat with right leg. Alternate legs, until you have repeated the exercise 8 to 15 times with each leg. Rest; then do another set of 8 to 15 alternating repetitions with each leg.

Summary:

1. Stand 12 to 18 inches from table.

2. Bend at hips; hold onto a table.

3. Slowly lift one leg straight backwards.

4. Hold position.

5. Slowly lower leg.

6. Repeat with other leg.

Side Leg Raise

Purpose: Strengthens muscles at sides of hips and thighs

Equipment: ankle weights (optional)

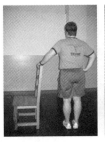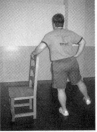

Use ankle weights, if you are ready to. Stand up straight, directly behind a table or chair, feet slightly apart. Hold onto the table to help keep your balance. Take 3 seconds to lift your right leg 6 to 12 inches out to the side. Keep your back and both legs straight. Don't point your toes outward; keep them facing forward.

Hold the position for 1 second. Take 3 seconds to lower your leg back to the starting position. Repeat with left leg. Alternate legs, until you have repeated the exercise 8 to 15 times with each leg. Rest; do another set of 8 to 15 alternating repetitions.

Summary:

1. Stand straight, directly behind table, feet slightly apart.

2. Hold table for balance.

3. Slowly lift one leg to side, 6–12 inches.

4. Hold position.

5. Slowly lower leg.

6. Repeat with other leg.

7. Back and both knees are straight throughout exercise.

Appendix D

Universal Design Strategies for Health Promotion

Developing Creative Solutions for People
Who Have Severe/Profound Intellectual Disabilities
and a Variety of Physical Disabilities

In the 1950s, universal design began to gain attention as a barrier-free design to remove obstacles in the environment for people with physical disabilities in Europe, Japan, and the United States. This corresponded with the social policy changes of moving people with disabilities from institutional settings to the community; however, barrier-free design was often segregated, special, and limited to people with serious physical limitations, primarily mobility impairments.

BACKGROUND OF UNIVERSAL DESIGN

Universal Design (UD) aims to design communication, products, and environments to be usable by all people, to the greatest extent possible, without adaptation or specialized design. This concept is also referred to as *Inclusive Design, Design-For-All, Lifespan Design, Barrier-Free Design*, or *Human-Centered Design*. The underlying premise is that if it works well for people across the spectrum of functional ability, it will work better for everyone. For example, medication labels that can be read by people with low vision are

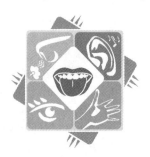

easier for everyone to read; minimizing external noises for classroom setting makes it easier for everyone to hear; and building entrances without stairs is useful for people who are pushing strollers, carrying groceries, or using a wheelchair.

The usability of a communication strategy, product, or environment can be enhanced by including designs for a broad range of users that incorporate the five sense: **seeing, touching, smelling, tasting, and hearing.** Including UD strategies from the beginning can be done without significantly increasing the expense of your program.

Normalization, Inclusion, and Civil Rights

Normalization and integration became ideals in the United States and parts of Europe by the 1970s. People were moving beyond the emphasis on special solutions tailored to individuals with disabilities and, increasingly, the terminology of choice was accessible design (Adaptive Environments, 2006). The 1970s also saw the disability rights movement in the

United States building upon the vision of civil rights articulated in the Civil Rights Act of 1964 (PL 88-352) for racial minorities. People with disabilities began arguing for equality of opportunities. For the first time, design was seen as a necessary condition for people with disabilities to achieve civil rights.

Beginning with Section 504 of the Rehabilitation Act of 1973 (PL 93-112) in the United States, entities receiving federal financial assistance were required to include accessible designs (Adaptive Environments, 2006). Although many Americans might overlook its significance, the effects of Section 504 are, today, visible everywhere—not only in the ramps and curb cuts that make our environment accessible to everyone but also in the greatly increased presence of people with disabilities in our communities. This legislation set the stage for the Americans with Disabilities Act (ADA) of 1990 (PL 101-336). Moreover, Section 504 obligates entities receiving federal funding to include universal design features in newly constructed and altered buildings (e.g., accessible bathrooms, ramps) and ensures that people with disabilities are not excluded from programs and activities on the basis of disability.

The ADA of 1990 significantly exceeded the requirements of Section 504 of the Rehabilitation Act by using much of its language from the Civil Rights Act of 1964, along with additional requirements for accessible design. The scope of responsible parties was expanded to include both public and private entities regardless of whether they received federal funds. The Act's Title II regulation covers "public entities," including any state or local government and any of its departments, agencies, or other instrumentalities. All activities, services, and programs of public entities are covered, including activities of state legislatures and courts, schools, town meetings, police and fire departments, motor vehicle licensing, and employment (Adaptive Environments, 2006).

Barrier Removal and Universal Design

Along with the philosophical paradigm shifts in the 1970s, American architect Michael Bednar introduced the idea that *everyone's functional capacity is enhanced when environmental barriers are removed* (Adaptive Environments, 2006). Bednar proposed the idea that a broader and more universal concept beyond accessibility was needed. Parallel to this shift in thinking about the impact of the environment on function, people with disabilities in many nations began organizing themselves in the 1980s and termed the *disability community*.

In the process of forming a community, people with disparate disabilities have discovered a common identity and a need to claim their human and civil rights. Like race and gender, disability came to be seen as a natural part of the human experience. In 1987, a group of Irish designers succeeded in getting a resolution passed at the World Design Congress that designers should include disability and aging into their work (Adaptive Environments, 2006). Progress toward universal design for people with disabilities has developed in the last few decades along three parallel tracks of activities: 1) legislation fueled by the disability rights movement, 2) the barrier-free design to universal design movement, and 3) advances in rehabilitation engineering and assistive technology.

SEVEN PRINCIPLES OF UNIVERSAL DESIGN

The seven principles of universal design establish a valuable language for explaining the characteristics of universal design and are commonly used around the world. The 10th anniversary of these principles of universal design took place in 2007 and is likely to evolve in response to experience with implementation and in order to incorporate insights and perspectives from the engagement of more diverse cultures. These principles are as follows:

1. *Equitable use:* The design does not disadvantage or stigmatize any group of users.
2. *Flexibility in use:* The design accommodates a wide range of individual preferences and abilities.
3. *Simple, intuitive use:* Use of the design is easy to understand regardless of the user's experience, knowledge, language skills, or current concentration level.
4. *Perceptible information:* The program design clearly communicates the necessary information to the user regardless of ambient conditions or the user's sensory abilities. Conveying information should include multimodal strategies that allow for redundancy.
5. *Tolerance for error:* The program design minimizes hazards. By considering the variety of ways that people function, the program design can include environmental and communication strategies that allow people to learn at their own pace and increase the success of participants.
6. *Low physical effort:* The program design can be used efficiently and comfortably and with a minimum of fatigue.
7. *Size and space for approach and use:* Appropriate size and space is provided for approach, reach, manipulation, and use regardless of the user's body size, posture, or mobility (Connell et al., 1997).

USING UNIVERSAL DESIGN TO DEVELOP CREATIVE SOLUTIONS

In working with people who have a variety of disabilities, several issues may require you to modify your teaching strategies. These areas may include the following:

- Communication/speech (e.g., people may use augmentative communication devices)
- Energy (or stamina)
- Hearing
- Learning/memory
- Mental health issues (e.g., mood, behavior)
- Mobility
- Vision

QUESTIONS TO CONSIDER REGARDING UNIVERSAL DESIGN WHEN USING THE HEALTH MATTERS CURRICULUM

These strategies may be particularly useful when working with people who have severe/profound intellectual disabilities and a variety of physical disabilities. Please review the curriculum to use the following ideas to adapt/modify modules for your clients/ consumers. Please think about the aforementioned characteristics that you may observe in people to whom you provide services. As you use the curriculum, you may consider the following questions:

- How will you **modify the content,** incorporating principles of universal design to include people with severe/profound intellectual disabilities and people with a variety of physical disabilities?

- What **physical/environmental modifications** will you need to make in the units to include principles of universal design?
- What **communication strategies** will you use to incorporate principles of universal design for participants with severe/profound intellectual disabilities and those with a variety of physical disabilities?

CONTENT MODIFICATIONS FOR UNIVERSAL DESIGN

Content modifications need to be made in the spirit of not disadvantaging, stigmatizing, or privileging any group of participants. Teaching strategies are aimed at providing the same means of use for all participants. Conversely, it is important to not segregate or stigmatize any group of participants and to make the exercise and health education program appealing for all participants.

For example, the following strategies can be used throughout the book to accommodate a wide range of individual preferences and participants' functional abilities:

- Increase the use of pictures throughout the curriculum. For example, in Unit 1 of the curriculum, you may include pictures of what *healthy* is as a way to increase visual examples and reduce verbal instruction.
- Decrease open-ended questions.
- Have pictures with words already cut out and available for participants to choose to describe.
- Use pictures from magazines (e.g., photos of people with disabilities doing health promoting activities).
- Include consistent reminders from the previous class.
- Giving participants too many choices can be confusing. Provide yes/no questions with pictures, or use either/or questions and provide two options in a question.
- Reduce the number of questions.
- Perform one to two healthy activities as examples for participants.
- Reduce the time of each session to 30 minutes.
- Use of "tabs" in the Personal Notebook for each participant can increase access for individuals, particularly for individuals who have motor control issues.
- Consider laminating handouts using sheet protectors.
- For participants who have a limited range of motion, consider getting a physical therapy evaluation before starting to stretch participants on any regular basis. For some participants who have a restricted range of motion, it may be helpful to have a physical therapist, parent, or doctor show you how to move participants through ranges of motion. Depending on the group, it may be useful to put participants together with similar physical abilities. This is especially useful if participants are trying to learn how to do certain exercises or activities, and other people who share their disability status can serve as role models. In addition, putting participants together with similar physical disabilities is also helpful during the health education classes when discussing specific issues related to certain types of disabilities (e.g., Down syndrome, spina bifida, cerebral palsy). For example, if the purpose of the class is to review common health concerns and related health promotion strategies, it can be helpful to have a group with similar types of disabilities or levels of functioning.

- Use content that is easy to understand regardless of the participant's experience, knowledge, language skills, or concentration level.
- Use more visual aids.
- Ask participants if they would like assistance to fill out forms or complete health education activities.
- Consistently ask participants if they would like assistance during the health education and fitness classes.
- Include more pictures of the foods. This is helpful for all participants.
- Expand the newsletter and put participants' pictures in it and modify it. Have them participate in developing the newsletter and make suggestions.
- Provide textbooks with step-by-step directions with specific cues, such as "First you do this, then you do this." You may consider using Velcro pictures that demonstrate how you do something first and then proceed to the next step.
- Use pictures from magazines or something that participants have seen on television as a way to reinforce educational messages related to health, nutrition, and physical activity. You may also obtain pictures from the Internet to include in the participants' optional Personal Notebooks.
- Incorporate sensory health messages (e.g., cut out pictures, paint grapes).
- Consider repeating one theme throughout the day in different programs aside from the health promotion classes. Have staff members be clear on their roles in promoting participants' health. Everyone has a role to play.
- Use real food products along with pictures.
- Reduce the number of pictures on a page.
- Cut down the curriculum if necessary. Units might take a long time to complete.
- Get a total "buy-in" from staff members. Staff members can benefit greatly from the curriculum. If you can identify key staff members who enjoy using/doing health promotion, buy-in is less critical.
- Clarify staff members' roles.
- Consider implementing a health promotion program with staff members first to see the results and to see how they have implemented this for themselves. The biggest revelation in looking at this curriculum is that some staff members would benefit from health education and physical activity classes.
- Consider the cultural appropriateness of food choices in the curriculum. Food choices may need modification for different cultural groups.
- Some staff members do not communicate well in these training logs. Develop a checklist, so communication logging can be easier for staff to use.
- Many of the units include activities based on discussions. Discussions are optional as many discussions may not occur for participants who are not verbal.
- Staff members may need training on using communication guides for participants.
- Make it clear that some groups of participants may not benefit from all parts of the health promotion program. Some ideas and strategies will work with some participants, whereas the same ideas may not be useful to others.
- Use pictures, verbal cues, and hand over hand. *Hand over hand* is a term used when someone shows a person how to do an activity by putting his or her hand over the participant's and simulating the action.

- The length of each unit, the suggested activities, and the handouts may need to be modified for participants with severe/profound intellectual disabilities and for participants with a variety of physical disabilities.
- You may consider using realistic models of different items, such as meats, vegetables, and cheeses, for participants to touch in order to increase retention.
- Develop alternative aerobic exercises for participants with physical disabilities.
- Develop alternative balance training exercises for participants with physical disabilities.
- You may modify what *being healthy* means for participants with different types of disabilities. For example, being physically healthy may be important to people who use wheelchairs as it can help them operate their wheelchairs.
- Video clips can be used to convey some of the many benefits physical activity can bring to a person with an intellectual or developmental disability including the following: 1) improved muscular strength and endurance, 2) improved flexibility, 3) improved cardiovascular health, and 4) improved functional ability to complete activities of daily life.
- Watch a video. The National Center on Physical Activity and Disability (NCPAD) presents an exercise video produced for persons with intellectual disabilities as an example of how to use exercise bands for strength training among adults with intellectual disabilities (NCPAD, 2004).

PHYSICAL AND ENVIRONMENTAL MODIFICATIONS

Universal access is the necessary first step toward effective accommodations in your health education and fitness program. Obstacles may include stairs, narrow entryways, desks at the wrong height, and inaccessible washrooms.

The following program modifications may be considered depending on your audience:

- The curriculum presents a 12-week program with three, 1-hour sessions per week. Depending on attention span, you may need to change sessions to the following: a 24-week program with three, 30-minute sessions per week. This could continue to be an extra schedule of three times per week exercise plan. If possible, add on an additional day every 2 weeks to eventually reach an exercise program ranging from 5–7 days per week.
- Use the curriculum as a resource instead of a series of lesson plans.
- Increase staff ratio to a 1:2 (one staff member per two participants) or a 1:1 ratio, depending on the group.
- For participants with visual disabilities, the health education materials may need to be translated and may include more information that uses texture.
- In advance, consider getting input from caregivers on individuals who are unable to share their information. Conversely, it may be important to share information with caregivers as to what is being done in the exercise and health education classes for reinforcement and feedback as to changes observed at home. Keep a communication book with caregivers because they can tell you if and what a participant has eaten, if he or she has slept well, and additional health-related information.
- Appropriate size and space is provided for approach, reach, manipulation, and use regardless of the participant's body size, posture, mobility, or functional abilities.

- Identify options for balance training among participants who are wheelchair users.
- Because of physical limitations due to disability, participants can be told to do the exercises to their best ability. Many participants may not be able to do some of the activities because their bodies do not move like the pictures in the curriculum. They may not be able to do everything the way it is written in the book. In addition, common health promoting activities such as "covering your mouth when you cough" may not be possible by everyone. You need to work with participants to develop health-promoting strategies that incorporate their abilities. Do warm-ups to the best of their abilities, particularly those with physical disabilities.
- Include wheelchair exercise videos in the list of resources for participants.
- Incorporate individual differences in baseline conditions. Measuring the energy level of someone who has a limited range may be different.
- Participants may also have pain caused by contractors and cerebral palsy.
- Adapt pain measures to include motions that are used by participants who use wheelchairs (e.g., lifting a leg onto the footrest, propelling, bearing weight, reaching for an object, putting a foot on a wheelchair).
- For participants who are on pureed diets, you may consider providing a food processor.
- Ensure that participants are hydrated. Include prompts to help them learn when to hydrate.
- Because passive and active ranges of motion are important components, staff members may need additional information on range of motion activities for participants with significant physical disabilities (e.g., what it means, how to do it).
- Participants may not be able to identify which healthy food they like. Consider allowing them to try different foods to see which one they respond to best. Use real foods to see how they do with it.
- Discuss positive things related to physical activity for participants who use wheelchairs. For example, physical activity can help participants propel their wheelchair.

COMMUNICATION STRATEGIES

Clear communication can include a dyad approach having support persons working together with persons with intellectual or developmental disorders.

- Culturally competent provider care (e.g., knowledge, attitudes, relevant practice)
- Adults with intellectual or developmental disorders and support persons working together
  To create accessible health materials you may include the following

1. *Multimodal formats* using multiple senses (e.g., sound, sight, touch, smell, taste)

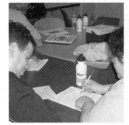 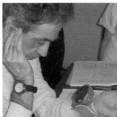 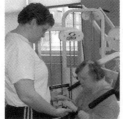 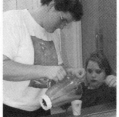 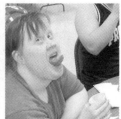

2. *Visual presentation* can include the following:
    - Simple backgrounds/high contrast
    - Simple, consistent page layout
    - Font size and style
    - Clear and uniform text

3. *Auditory presentation* can include one-on-one instructions on the following:
    - Monitoring health status
    - Learning how to use exercise machines
    - Preparing foods

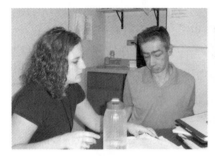 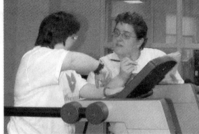 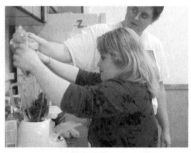

Monitoring health status   Using exercise machines   Preparing foods

4. *Auditory presentation* can include group instructions on the following:
    - Learning about our bodies
    - Learning about strength training
    - Preparing foods

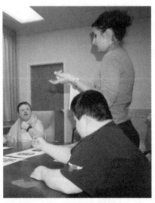 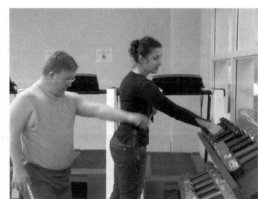

Learning about our bodies   Learning about strength training

5. *Tactile presentation* can include a variety of strategies ranging from using heart rate monitors to helping participants connect how they feel while watching their heart rate change on their watches.

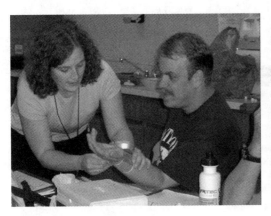

Learning about our blood pressure

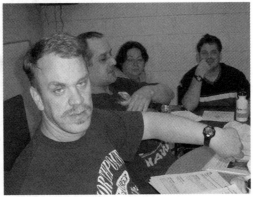

Learning about our heart rates

REFERENCES

Americans with Disabilities Act (ADA) of 1990, PL 101-336, 42 U.S.C. §§ 12101 *et seq.*

Adaptive Environments. (2006). *History of universal design.* Retrieved July 28, 2008, from http://www.adaptenv.org/index.php?option=Content&Itemid=26

Civil Rights Act of 1964, PL 88-352, 20 U.S.C. §§ 241 *et seq.*

Connell, B.R., Jones, M., Mace, R., Mueller, J., Mullick, A., & Ostroff, E. (1997). *Principles of universal design.* Raleigh, NC: Center for Universal Design, School of Design, State University of North Carolina at Raleigh.

National Center on Physical Activity and Disability (NCPAD). (2004). *Strength training video for people with intellectual disabilities: Upper body exercises.* Chicago: University of Illinois, Department of Disability and Human Development.

Rehabilitation Act of 1973, PL 93-112, 29 U.S.C. §§ 701 *et seq.*

Appendix E

Testing Procedure Manual

This appendix is in no way meant to substitute for a physician's advice or expert opinion; readers should consult a medical practitioner if they are interested in more information.
 Source: Marks and Sisirak (2009).

Before starting any physical activity testing, coaches, staff, and volunteers should be familiar with physical activity precautions and emergency procedures. Emergency procedures are the actions required to handle emergency situations. Please familiarize yourself with emergency procedures in your testing space.

CONSIDERATIONS PRIOR TO PHYSICAL ACTIVITY

Participants should not do any physical activity if

- Their blood glucose is > 240 mg/dL[1]
- Their systolic blood pressure (SBP) is > 200 and/or diastolic blood pressure (DBP) is > 110 at rest[2]
- Their SBP is > 170 (for those participants with hypertension and/or who had a stroke)
- Participants did not take their medications

Staff should know where the following items are located:

- Emergency phone numbers
- Emergency procedure signs
- Water cooler
- Refrigerator with juice boxes
- First-aid kit

SETTING UP FOR PHYSICAL ACTIVITY

When setting up, keep the following considerations in mind:

- Check the water cooler for ample water supply.
- Check for ample juice supply or for alternative sugar sources.
- Check that the first-aid kit is ready and accessible.
- Check that the room is clean, organized, and free of hazards.
- Encourage participants to wear loose, comfortable clothes.
- Have the same person do the pre- and posttesting for each test.

TESTING

Before Testing

Prior to testing, complete the following activities:
- Assess heart rate (HR) and blood pressure (BP).
- Assess arthritis pain, if applicable.
- If participant is diabetic, check blood glucose levels. In persons taking insulin, consideration should be given to the ingestion of 20–30 grams of additional carbohydrates before exercise when pre-exercise blood glucose levels are < 100 mg/dL.

---

[1]Mayo Clinic staff. (2009, March 19). *Diabetes and exercise: When to monitor your blood sugar.* Retrieved on May 1, 2009, from http://www.mayoclinic.com/health/diabetes-and-exercise/DA00105
[2]American College of Sports Medicine. (2006). *ACSM's guidelines for exercise testing and prescriptions* (7th ed.). Baltimore: Lippincott Williams & Wilkins.

- Check participant's layers of clothing.
- Perform stretches.

During Testing

During testing, complete the following activities:

- Perform warm-up exercises.
- Ensure that participants exercise with proper form.
- Provide spotting accordingly.
- Ensure that participants display proper breathing techniques.
- Assess participants' consciousness and alertness.
- Ensure that participants are maintaining their fluid intake.
- Perform cool-down exercises.

Measuring Heart Rate

Purpose:

- Measure number of heartbeats per minute

Equipment needed:

- Stethoscope (optional)
- Watch or a clock with a second hand
- Appropriate data sheet(s) and pen (*Note:* A Fitness Data Collection Form is included in this appendix.)

Test instructions:

- Three sites are typically used to measure a heartbeat:

  1. Radial pulse (wrist)
  2. Apical pulse (chest)
  3. Carotid pulse (neck)

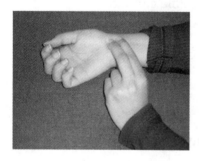 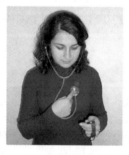 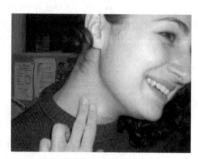

- If you have a stethoscope:

  1. Place it directly over participant's heart.
  2. Listen until you hear participant's heartbeat.
  3. Count heartbeats for 10 seconds (look at your watch and time 10 seconds).
  4. Multiply that number by six.
  5. This the number of heartbeats per minute.

- If you do not have a stethoscope:

    1. Use your index and middle fingers (not the thumb because it has a pulse of its own) and place them on one of the two most commonly used sites: the wrist or the neck. *Note:* When using the neck site, avoid applying too much pressure to the carotid artery. Using too much pressure could stimulate a reflex mechanism that could slow down the heart.
    2. Feel for the pulse.
    3. Count heartbeats for 10 seconds (look at your watch and time 10 seconds).
    4. Multiply that number by six.
    5. This is the number of heartbeats per minute.

Measuring Blood Pressure

We recommend using portable wrist blood pressure cuffs for the exercise classes. Using a wrist cuff is a fun way to engage participants in learning about their blood pressure. Taking their blood pressure with a portable wrist monitor gives people hands-on experience with seeing how exercise may improve their blood pressure.

Participants have a range of abilities and are able to actively participate in various parts of the blood pressure reading ranging from wrapping the cuff around the wrist, pressing "Start," and reading their blood pressure. The upper arm cuffs are sometimes difficult for people with various body sizes and do not allow for active engagement in the blood pressure measurement. Within seconds, each participant can see his or her blood pressure and pulse displayed on the digital panel. Many of the portable blood pressure cuffs on the market have been tested, evaluated, and proven to meet the rigorous safety and accuracy standards set by independent organizations.

Measuring Cholesterol

On-site collection of a fasting finger stick blood sample for a total cholesterol analysis using a portable cholesterol test device is another fun way to engage participants in learning about their health. By using a portable cholesterol test device, participants can have the opportunity to learn what their lipid profile is within 3–7 minutes prior to starting a health promotion program and see how their profile changes over time. This is one way of enhancing experiential learning by giving people the information they need to monitor their own health and make lifestyle changes. Many of the machines also test blood glucose. Refer to Lesson R in Appendix A for information on cholesterol.

Measuring Body Composition[3]

Height

Purpose:

- Determine participant's height

Equipment needed:

- Stadiometer (If one is not available, use a measuring stick and a right-angle headboard for reading the measurement.)
- Appropriate data sheet(s) and pen

---

[3]Lee, R.D., & Nieman, D.C. (1996). *Nutritional assessment* (2nd ed.). New York: McGraw-Hill.

Test set-up:

- If a wall is used, it should not have a thick baseboard as that could affect the accuracy of measurements.
- Participants should not stand on carpet as that could affect the accuracy of measurements.
- Instruct participants to remove shoes, any extra clothing (e.g., sweaters, jackets), and objects that would contribute to their circumference (e.g., backpacks, purses).

Test instructions:

1. Stand with heels together, arms to the side, legs straight, shoulders relaxed, and head facing forward.
2. Heels, buttocks, shoulder blades, and the back of the head should, if possible, be against the vertical surface of the stadiometer (wall).
3. Some participants may not be able to touch all four points against the stadiometer (wall).
4. Do not force anyone into a position. Instead, have participants touch two or three of the four points to the vertical surface.
5. Inhale deeply, hold breath, and maintain an erect posture ("stand up tall") while the headboard is lowered on the highest point of the head with enough pressure to compress the hair.
6. The measurement should be read to the nearest 0.1 cm or ⅛ inch and at eye level with the headboard to avoid errors.
7. Indicate whether you measured in centimeters (cm) or inches (in.).
8. Repeat three times.

Weight [4]

Purpose:

- Determine participant's weight

Equipment needed:

- Electronic scale or balance-beam scale with nondetachable weights. *Note:* Do not use a spring-type bathroom scale as it does not provide required accuracy.
- Appropriate data sheet(s) and pen

Test set-up:

- Instruct participant to remove any shoes, extra clothing (e.g., sweaters, jackets), and objects that would contribute to weight (e.g., backpacks, purses).

Test instructions:

1. Stand in the middle of the scale's platform without touching anything. Body weight should be equally distributed on both feet.
2. Record the weight to the nearest 100 g (or ¼ pound).
3. Indicate if you measured in pounds (lb) or kilograms (kg).
4. Repeat three times.

[4]American College of Sports Medicine. (2006). *ACSM's guidelines for exercise testing and prescriptions.* (7th ed.). Indianapolis, IN: Author.

Body Mass Index (BMI)

- Body mass index (BMI) is a measure of body fat based on height and weight that applies to both adult men and women.
- BMI measures your height/weight ratio. It is your weight in kilograms divided by the square of your height in meters. Too much body fat can be a problem because it can result in illnesses and other health problems.
- Use the following guidelines when calculating BMI[5]:

  < 18.5 underweight

  18.5–24.9 normal

  25.0–29.9 overweight

  30–39.9 obese

  40+ extremely obese

  BMI can also be calculate using the following formula:

  BMI = [weight in pounds/(height in inches x height in inches)] x 703

  or

  $$BMI = weight\ (kg)/height\ (meters)^2$$

Waist and Hip Circumference (Waist–Hip Ratio) [6]

Purpose:

- Basic anthropometric measurement used to help assess body fat composition

Equipment needed:

- Tape measure
- Appropriate data sheet(s) and pen

Test set-up:

- Instruct participant to remove any extra clothing (e.g., sweaters, jackets) and objects that would contribute to circumference (e.g., backpacks, purses).

Test instructions:

1. Stand upright with both feet together.
2. Hold the measuring tape snug against the skin without compressing the tissues.
3. The zero-end (beginning of the tape) is held below the value to be recorded.
4. Measure at the end of a normal expiration (breathing out).
5. To measure the waist, place the tape measure:
   - At the narrowest part of the torso
   - Between the xiphoid process (cartilage attached to the lower end of the breastbone or sternum) and the umbilicus (belly button) (usually at the level of the umbilicus)
   - In a horizontal plane

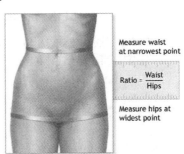

[5]National Heart Lung and Blood Institute. (n.d.) *Calculate your body mass index.* Retrieved May 4, 2009, from http://www.nhlbisupport.com/bmi

[6]American College of Sports Medicine. (2006). *ACSM's guidelines for exercise testing and prescriptions.* (7th ed.). Indianapolis, IN: Author.

6. To measure the hips, place the tape measure:
   - At the maximal circumference of the hips or buttocks region (whichever is larger)
   - Above the gluteal fold
7. Record each circumference on the appropriate data sheet(s).
8. Repeat the test three times.

Measuring Flexibility

Shoulder Flexibility Test [7]

Purpose:

- Measures shoulder flexibility and determines the range of motion or asymmetry of movements when comparing the two shoulders

Equipment needed:

- Tape measure
- Appropriate data sheet(s) and pen

Test set-up:

- Instruct participants to stretch as much as possible.

Test instructions:

1. Stand or sit upright. This test should be done with the person standing, if he or she is able to stand. Otherwise, if a person is unable to stand, the test can be done by having him or her sit in an upright position. Regardless of position, be consistent with the position for the person on pre- and posttesting.
2. To assess the left shoulder:
   - Bring the right arm behind the back by internally rotating and hyperextending the left shoulder and flexing the right arm to about 90°. The dorsal side of the right hand should be touching the back. Participants should appear as if they are scratching their middle/lower back (see Figure 1).

   - Bring the left arm behind the head by externally rotating and hyperflexing the left shoulder and flexing the left arm to about 90°. The palm of the left hand should be touching the back of the neck. Participants should appear as if they are scratching the lower part of the back of the neck (see Figure 1).

   - Try to touch or exceed touching the fingertips of both hands.

   - Hold the position until a measurement is taken.
3. To assess the right shoulder, perform Step 2 the opposite way.
4. Measure the space in between the fingertips (see Figure 2):
   - The fingertips touching equals a "0" measurement.

   - The fingers overlapping are recorded as a "negative" measurement (see Figure 3).

[7]Miotto, J.M., Chodzko-Zajko, W.J., Reich, J.L., & Supler, M.M. (1999). Reliabililty and validity of the Fullerton Functional Fitness Test: An independent replication study. *Journal of Aging and Physical Activity, 7,* 339–353.

Rikli, R.E., & Jones, C.J. (1999). Development and validation of a functional fitness test for community-residing older adults. *Journal of Aging and Physical Activity, 7,* 129–161.

5. Record each trial on the appropriate data sheet(s).

6. Repeat the test three times for each shoulder.

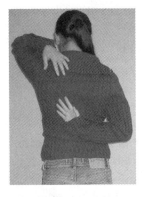
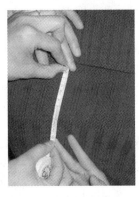
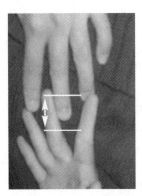
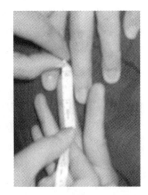

Figure 1. Behind the back. This position assesses the flexibility of the left shoulder.

Figure 2. Measure from the tip of one middle finger to the tip of the other middle finger.

Figure 3. Measure from the tip of one middle finger to the tip of the other. Record in negative (–) centimeters.

V (YMCA) Sit-and-Reach

Purpose:

- Flexibility test for the lower body[8]

Equipment needed:

- Tape (e.g., masking tape)
- Tape measure or a yardstick
- Appropriate data sheet(s) and pen

Test set-up:

- Place the tape measure or a yardstick on the floor.
- Put a 12-inch long piece of tape at a right angle to the tape measure/yardstick with the zero (0) mark.
- Put a second piece of tape longer than 12 inches at the 15-inch mark (see Figure 4).

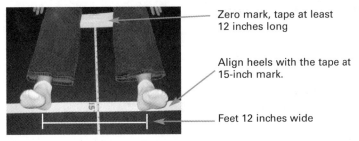

Zero mark, tape at least 12 inches long

Align heels with the tape at 15-inch mark.

Feet 12 inches wide

Figure 4. Sit-and-Reach positioning using tape measure.

[8]American College of Sports Medicine. (2006). *ACSM's guidelines for exercise testing and prescriptions* (7th ed.). Indianapolis, IN: Author. Heyward, V.H. (2006). *Advanced fitness assessment and exercise prescription* (5th ed., p. 254). Champaign, IL: Human Kinetics Publishers.

Test instructions:

1. Instruct participants to remove shoes and sit down facing the zero mark.
2. *Starting position:* Sit upright on the floor facing the zero mark with legs at least 12 inches apart.
3. Participants' feet should be approximately 12 inches apart and heels aligned with the tape at the 15-inch mark on the tape measure/yardstick.
4. Also, both arms should be fully extended in front of the chest with both hands on top of one another, with the tips of the fingers aligned (see Figure 5).
5. Take a deep breath.
6. Exhale and slowly lean forward by dropping the head toward or between the arms. Remind participants to avoid fast, jerky movements and not to hold their breath.
7. Participants' fingers should maintain contact with the tape measure/yardstick while you keep their knees straight. Do not force the knees down. Remind participants not to bend their knees.
8. Relax and then sit back upright.
9. Repeat the test three times. Record the farthest points reached with the highest tip of the aligned fingers (see Figure 6).

Note: There is a slight risk of muscle strain or pull if a forward movement is attempted that is too vigorous. Make sure that participants are warmed up with gentle stretching of the lower back and hamstrings.

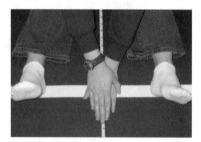

Figure 5. Hands on top of one another, with the tips of the fingers aligned.

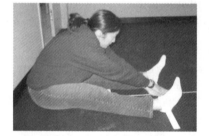

Figure 6. Fingers should maintain contact with the tape measure/yardstick. Knees should be straight at all times.

Measuring Aerobic/Cardiovascular Fitness

Six-Minute Walk Test [9]

Purpose:

*   To assess aerobic endurance

[9]American Thoracic Society Statement: Guidelines for the Six-Minute Walk Test (2002). *American Journal of Respiratory Critical Care Medicine, 166,* 111–117.

Enright, P.L. (2003). The Six-Minute Walk Test. *Respiratory Care, 48*(8), 783–785.

Kervio, G., Carre, F., & Ville, N. (2003). Reliability and intensity of the Six-Minute Walk Test. In *Healthy Elderly Subjects, Medicine & Science in Sports & Exercise.* Retrieved Sept. 9, 2009, from http://www.acsm-msse.org.

Oh-Park, M., Zohman, L.R., & Abrahams, C.A. (1997). A simple walk test to guide exercise programming of the elderly. *American Journal of Physical Medicine and Rehabilitation, 76*(3), pp 208–212.

O'Keefe, S.T., Lye, M., Donnellan, C., & Carmichael, D.N. (1998). *Reproducibility and responsiveness of quality of life assessment and Six-Minute Walk Test in elderly heart failure patients.* UK: Department of Geriatric Medicine, University of Liverpool.

Equipment needed:

- Stopwatch
- Long measuring tape
- Ten cones or ten 2-liter full bottles of water
- Stickers
- Masking tape, chalk, or some other type of marker
- Six chairs
- Appropriate data sheet(s) and pen

Test set-up:

- The test involves assessing the maximum distance that can be walked in 6 minutes along a 50-yard course marked in 5-yard segments.
- Mark the inside perimeter with cones or any other object previously listed in 5-yard segments (see Figure 7).
- The walking area can be indoors or outdoors, should be well lit, and should have a level surface that is not slippery.
- To keep track of the distance walked, stickers can be given to participants (or placed on their sleeve or a piece of paper) each time they round a cone, or a partner can mark a score card each time a lap is completed.
- Two or more participants should be tested at a time, with starting times staggered (10 seconds apart) so that participants do not walk in clusters or pairs.
- For safety purposes, chairs should be positioned at several points alongside the walkway.

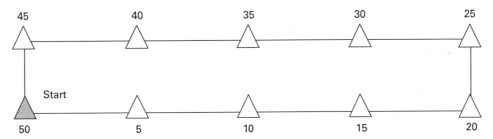

Figure 7. Fifty yards measured into five-yard segments.

Test instructions:

1. On the signal "Go," participants are instructed to walk (not run) as fast as possible around the course as many times as they can in 6 minutes.
2. If necessary, participants may stop and rest (on provided chairs), then resume walking.
3. The timer should move to the inside of the marked area after everyone has started.
4. To assist with pacing, elapsed time should be called out when participants are approximately half done (when 2 minutes are left, and when 1 minute is left).
5. Encouraging phrases, such as "You're doing well" and "Keep up the good work," should be called out at approximately 30-second intervals.
6. At the end of 6 minutes, participants should be instructed to stop and move to the right, where an assistant will record their score.
7. To assist with proper pacing and to improve scoring accuracy, a practice test should be given prior to the actual test day.
8. The score is the total number of yards walked in 6 minutes to the nearest 5-yard mark.

Measuring Balance

Timed Get-Up-and-Go Test[10]

Purpose:

- To assess gait and balance (agility and coordination); useful to measure risk of falls

Equipment needed:

- Tape measure
- Two sturdy chairs with backs (with no arms)
- Stopwatch
- Appropriate data sheet(s) and pen

Test set-up:

- Choose a smooth, nonslippery surface.
- Measure 10 feet (3 meters) for the test if a line has not already been set up.
- Place one chair at one end of the line to designate the starting point for participants. It is recommended to have a starting chair, where participants sit, placed against a wall to provide additional security.
- Instruct participants to perform the test as quickly and safely as possible and not to run.
- Practice before the test.
- Repeat the test three times. Use the best score (the lowest time).
- A normal score will be shorter than 10 seconds.

Test instructions:

1. Starting position: Sit upright against a chair.
2. Stand up from the chair and start the timer.
3. Move quickly along the line toward the opposite end (see Figure 8).
4. Touch the end and then turn around and walk back toward the chair.
5. Move quickly all the way back to the chair.
6. Pivot.
7. Sit back down and end the timer.
8. Record the time.

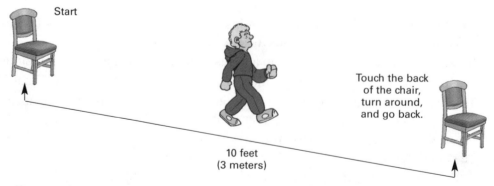

Start

Touch the back
of the chair,
turn around,
and go back.

10 feet
(3 meters)

Figure 8.　Timed Get-Up-and-Go (TGUG) Test

[10]Podsiadlo D., & Richardson, S. (1991). The timed "Up and Go" Test: A test of basic functional mobility for frail elderly persons. *Journal of American Geriatric Society, 39,* 142–148.

Measuring Strength and Endurance

Upper Body: One-Minute Timed Modified Pushup [11]

Purpose:

- Measures the endurance of the arms and shoulder girdle

Equipment needed:

- Mat for the floor or carpeted floor
- Any larger size book such as a textbook
- Stopwatch
- Appropriate data sheet(s) and pen

Test set-up:

- None

Test instructions:

1. Keep participant's knees bent at right angles (see Figure 9). To make sure that the knees are bent at right angles, you may want to use a large book and place it inside the knees.
2. Place hands on the floor directly under shoulders (see Figure 10).
3. Have participant lower his or her body to the floor until the chest touches the floor. You may want to place a small, folded towel or a sponge on the floor directly below the chest to serve as an indicator (see Figure 11).

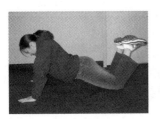 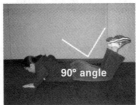 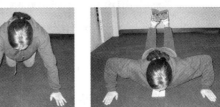

Figure 9. Starting position: Hands directly under shoulders and knees bent at 90° angle. A book can be placed inside the knees to make sure the angle is 90°.

Figure 10. Hands directly under the shoulders.

Figure 11. Lower the body to the floor. Chest must touch the floor on the indicator.

4. Push back to the starting position (see Figure 12).
5. Repeat as many times for 1 minute as possible without rest.
6. Participant's body must not sag but should maintain a straight line throughout the test (see Figure 13).
7. Count the number of correct pushups executed in 1 minute.
8. Scoring is terminated if participant stops to rest.
9. If the chest does not touch the mat or if the arms are not completely extended on an execution, the trial does not count (see Figure 13).

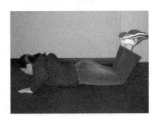

Figure 12. Push back to the starting position. Arms must be completely extended (as in Figure 9).

[11]American College of Sports Medicine. (2006). *ACSM's guidelines for exercise testing and prescriptions* (7th ed.). Indianapolis, IN: Author.

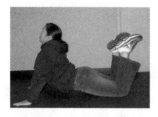 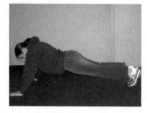 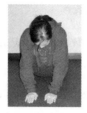 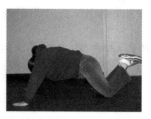

Back and head too arched   Knees not on floor   Hands too close   Head too low, back too curved

Figure 13.   Incorrect pushup positions for the One-Minute Timed Modified Pushup Test.

Upper Body: YMCA Bench Press [12]

1. Start metronome
2. Subject lies supine on bench
    —Knees bent flat on floor
3. Hand barbell to subject
4. Subject grips bar (overhand) shoulder width
5. Subject benches with pace of metronome
    —Subject pressed bar upward
    • Arm is fully extended
    —Subject returns bar to chest
6. Encourage subject to breath regularly and not strain during test
7. Stop test when subject no longer can keep pace of metronome
    —A little faster or a little slower rhythm is acceptable
8. Record successful number of repetitions

Lower Body: One-Minute Timed Sit-to-Stand Muscular Endurance [13]

Purpose:

• Measures muscle strength and endurance of large leg muscles

Equipment needed:

• Chair without arm rests
• Stopwatch
• Appropriate data sheet(s) and pen

Test set-up:

• Place a chair without arm rests against the wall in an unobstructed area.

Test instructions:

1. Sit in a chair with arms resting on the knees (see Figures 14.1 and 14.2).
2. Using leg muscles, stand up keeping back straight (see Figures 14.3–14.6).
3. Repeat as many times as possible for 1 minute without rest.
4. The body must not sag but maintain a straight line throughout the test.
5. Count the number of correct sit-to-stands executed in 1 minute.

[12]YMCA of the USA. (2000). *YMCA fitness testing and assessment manual* (4th ed.). Retrieved July 29, 2008, from http://www.exrx.net/Calculators/YBenchPress.html

[13]Bohannon, R.W. (1995). Sit-to-Stand Test for measuring performance of lower extremity muscles. *Perceptual Motor Skills,* 80, 163–166.
   Gross, M.M., Stevenson, P.J., Charette, S.L., Pyka, G., & Marcus, R. (1998). Effect of muscle strength and movement speed on the biomechanics of rising from a chair in healthy elderly and young women. *Gait & Posture,* 8(3), 175–185.

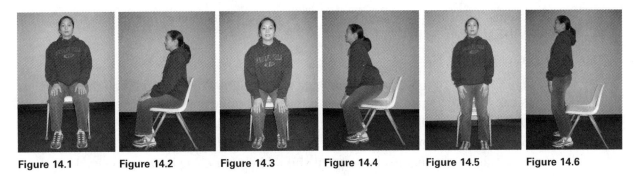

Figure 14.1   Figure 14.2   Figure 14.3   Figure 14.4   Figure 14.5   Figure 14.6

6. Scoring is terminated if participant stops to rest. Indicate the total number of sit-to-stands, which is the total score.

7. If participant does not have his or her back straight or is holding a chair, the trial does not count (see Figure 15).

8. At 1 minute, stop and record the number of sit-to-stands.

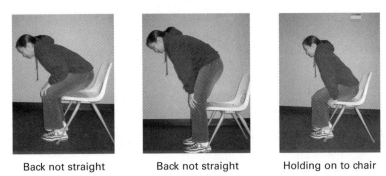

Back not straight   Back not straight   Holding on to chair

Figure 15. Incorrect positions for the One-Minute Timed Sit-to-Stand Muscular Endurance Test

Machine Testing: One-Repetition Maximum (1-RM) Test [14]

If you have exercise weight equipment, the one-repetition maximum (1-RM) test can be used to assess dynamic muscle strength. It measures the maximum amount of weight that can be lifted with good form. The machines that will be used determine which muscles will be tested.

Equipment needed:

• Selected piece of gym equipment
• Appropriate data sheet(s) and pen

Test set-up:

• You must be familiar with the equipment and the correct form positioning before any testing.
• Prepare the piece of equipment that participant will be using (e.g., adjust any knobs).
• Record the position of the seat, arm distance, or any placement that is unique to participant. This will ensure that participant gets tested with a proper form each time.

---

[14]American College of Sports Medicine. (2006). *ACSM's guidelines for exercise testing and prescriptions* (7th ed.). Indianapolis: Author.

- There must be at least one spotter for each participant. Have other spotters ready if a heavy 1-RM is perceived.

Test instructions:

1. Warm up with 5–10 repetitions at an easy weight (40%–60%) of what you think participants can lift. Participants will get used to the machine and learn the right form.
2. Rest for 1 minute while stretching.
3. Perform 3–5 repetitions at 60%–80% of the perceived maximum.
4. Increase the weight slightly. Participant should be at or close to the perceived 1-RM.
5. Increase the weight by increments (5–10 lbs) until participant feels he or she has reached the 1-RM. If participant's arms or legs start shaking and he or she is slowly lifting the weight, you have probably reached the maximum. Remember, the weight must be lifted with good form.
6. Record the 1-RM on the appropriate data sheet(s).

Fitness Data Collection Form

Participant's name: _____   ID number: _____

Interviewer's name: _____   ID number: _____

Date: _____

Test period (circle response):

Pretest (T1)   Posttest (T2)   6-month posttest (T3)   1-year posttest (T4)

Heart Rate, Blood Pressure, and Cholesterol Measurements

Heart rate: _____   Blood pressure: _____

Currently on high blood pressure medication?   Yes   No   Don't know

Currently on cholesterol lowering medication?   Yes   No   Don't know

Cholesterol results

    Total cholesterol (TC): _____

    Triglycerides: _____

    High density lipoprotein (HDL): "Good" cholesterol: _____

    Low density lipoprotein (LDL): "Bad" cholesterol: _____

    TC/HDL ratio (risk of heart disease): _____

Fitness Data Collection Form

Body Composition Measurements

Height, Weight, and Waist-to-Hip Circumference

Measurement   Circumference

Height: _____ _____ _____   Waist: _____ _____ _____

Weight: _____ _____ _____   Hip: _____ _____ _____

Body Mass Index (BMI): _____   Blood pressure: _____

Flexibility Measurements

Shoulder Flexibility Test   ### V (YMCA) Sit-and-Reach

Left side   Right side   Shoes (circle one):   On   Off

_____ cm   _____ cm   _____ inches

_____ cm   _____ cm   _____ inches

_____ cm   _____ cm   _____ inches

Aerobic/Cardiovascular Fitness Measurements

Six-Minute Walk Test

Lap tally (cross lap number after each lap):

1	2	3	4	5	6	7	8	9	10
11	12	13	14	15	16	17	18	19	20
21	22	23	24	25	26	27	28	29	30

Total number of laps = _____

End time (indicate if not exactly 6 minutes): _____ minutes

Calculate total number of yards = _____

Number of laps x 50 yards + extra yards (if less than a full lap of 50 yards, to the closest 5-yard segment)

Fitness Data Collection Form

Balance Measurements

Timed Get-Up-and-Go Test

_____ seconds   _____ seconds   _____ seconds

Strength and Endurance Measurements

***One-Minute Timed
Modified Pushup Test***   Number of pushups: _____

YMCA Bench Press Test   Number of repetitions: _____

***One-Minute Timed Sit-to-Stand
Muscular Endurance Test***   Number of repetitions: _____

One-Repetition Maximum (1-RM) Test   Maximum weight: _____ lbs

Equipment: _____ Maximum weight: _____ lbs

Equipment: _____ Maximum weight: _____ lbs

Equipment: _____ Maximum weight: _____ lbs

Equipment: _____ Maximum weight: _____ lbs

KNOWLEDGE AND PSYCHOSOCIAL ASSESSMENT PROTOCOL

People with disabilities have unique perspectives and opinions about their health, attitudes, and knowledge related to physical activity and nutrition. The Knowledge and Psychosocial Assessment can be used to evaluate individuals with DD before and after the health promotion program. The scales in this form have been tested for reliability and validity with people with DD.

Tips for Conducting Interviews with People with Disabilities

- Conduct your interview in a room that ensures privacy and confidentiality.
- Conduct an interview with individuals with DD alone. You do not need to speak through the accompanying parent or support staff person.
- Allow additional time for the interview process.
- Identify yourself clearly to the person being interviewed.
- Explain the purpose of the interview.
- Use your usual tone and volume of voice.
- Look at and speak directly to the person you are interviewing.
- If individuals have some communication limitations, do not correct them or complete their sentences. Avoid speaking for them.
- If you do not understand what a person is saying, ask him or her to repeat it. Do not pretend to understand. Repeat it to the person to confirm if you understood the response correctly.

Issues to Consider When Interviewing

Several considerations should be taken into account when interviewing people with DD. These include the following:

- *Acquiescence.* People with DD may want to please others perceived to be in power, including interviewers. Their answers may not be accurate and they may respond to questions in a certain manner or direction (e.g., all questions are answered with "yes" or "no") because they think that is the "expected" or "desired" response.
- *Processing time.* People with DD may need additional time to process the question and prepare their response. Ensure that there is enough time to respond and that they are not feeling pressed to answer.

Setting the Stage for an Interview

Use the following introduction to explain the purpose of the interview:

> "My name is _____. I am going to ask you questions about your health and how you are feeling. I will also be asking you questions about exercise and nutrition. You don't have to answer any question you don't want to, and I'll stop anytime you want. There are no right or wrong answers. I will not be telling anyone about what you say. Do you have any other questions for me? Let's begin."

Overview of the Sections of the Knowledge and Psychosocial Assessment

The following section explains the goals and objectives of the different parts of the protocol.

I. Health Status

Goal: To improve health status

Goals and objectives	Measures	Description
a. Improve overall health status	Overall health	A person's self-reported health status
b. Increase life satisfaction	Life Satisfaction Scale for adults with developmental disabilities	How people feel about work, home, free-time activities, and social support
c. Improve psychosocial well-being	Depression Scale	Assesses the number of depressive symptoms in adults with intellectual and developmental disabilities
d. Decreased level of pain	Pain Scale	A person's self-reported level of pain
e. Increased opportunities for making choices in daily activities	Choice-making Inventory Scale	A person's opportunities for making choices and who makes the choices in everyday activities
f. Improved health-promoting behaviors and decreased risk factors	Inventory of risk factors and health-promoting activities	An inventory of health-promoting and disease preventing behaviors
g. Increased level of energy	Energy Scale	Evaluates a person's level of energy/fatigue
h. Improved adaptive functioning	Activities of Daily Living (ADLs) and Instrumental ADLs (IADLs)	Assesses adaptive behavior

II. Physical Activity and Nutrition Knowledge and Supports

Goal: To improve physical activity and nutrition cognitions

Goals and objectives	Measures	Description
a. Improved knowledge of exercise and healthy food choices	Nutrition and Activity Knowledge Scale (NAKS)	Assesses knowledge of physical activity and healthy food choices
b. Increase outcome expectation for physical activity and nutrition	Exercise and Nutrition Outcome Expectation Scales	A person's perception of the benefits of physical activity and nutrition
c. Reduce perceived barriers for physical activity and nutrition	Barriers to Eating Fresh Fruits and Vegetables Scale Barriers to Exercise Scale	Assesses reasons that it might be difficult for a person to engage in physical activity and to eat fruits and vegetables
d. Increase in confidence (self-efficacy) to engage in physical activity	Self-efficacy Scale	A person's degree of certainty (or confidence) to engage in physical activity
e. Increase social/environmental supports	Social/Environmental Supports Scale for Exercise and Nutrition	Assesses things that might make it easier for a person to engage in physical activity and eat nutritious foods

III. Adherence to Physical Activity and Eating Fruits and Vegetables

Goal: To improve physical activity adherence and eating nutritious foods

Goals and objectives	Measures	Description
a. Increase in frequency and duration of physical activity	Physical Activity Participation Survey	Assesses the number of times people engage in physical activity per week
b. Improved dietary intake of fruits and vegetables	Daily Intake of Fruits and Vegetables	Assesses intake of fruits and vegetables

---

Knowledge and Psychosocial Assessment

Participant's name: _____   ID number: _____

Interviewer's name: _____   ID number: _____

Date: _____

Test period (circle response):

Pretest (T1)   Posttest (T2)   6-month posttest (T3)   1-year posttest (T4)

I. HEALTH STATUS

General Health Status [23]

"I am going to ask you questions about your health and how you are feeling. I will also be asking you questions about exercise and how you feel about it. You don't have to answer any question you don't want to, and I'll stop anytime you want me to. There are no right or wrong answers. I will not be telling anyone about what you say. Okay, let's get started. Let's start with some questions about your overall health."

1. In general, would you say your health is
    a. Excellent or very good
    b. Good
    c. Fair
    d. Poor

Psychosocial Well-Being

Several scales are available to measure psychosocial well-being, including the Children's Depression Inventory [13]. The Glasgow Depression Inventory [2] is available free of charge and has two versions: one for people with intellectual disabilities and another for caregivers.

Life Satisfaction Scale for Adults with Developmental Disabilities [4,11,14]

"Now, I will ask you questions about your life. I will ask about how you feel about your work, your home, things you do in your free time, and your friends. First we will talk about things you do for fun."

Free Time

1. What kind of things do you do for fun now?_____

_____

_____

_____

---

[23]SF-36® Health Survey© 1988, 2002 by Medical Outcomes Trust and QualityMetric Incorporated. All Rights Reserved. SF-26R is a registered trademark of Medical Outcomes Trust. (SF-36 Acute, US Version 1.0.).

Knowledge and Psychosocial Assessment

2. Are you happy with what you do in your free time or not happy with what you do in your free time?

   Happy   Not happy   Neither or both

3. Do you have enough things to do in your free time or not enough things to do in your free time?

   Enough things to do   Not enough things to do   Neither or both

Health and Wellness

"Let's talk about your health."

1. What do you do to be healthy (to keep your body feeling good and not sick)?

   _____

   _____

2. What do you eat to be healthy?

   _____

   _____

3. What do you not eat to be healthy?

   _____

   _____

4. Do you feel that the food you eat is healthy or not healthy?

   Healthy   Not healthy   Neither or both

5. Do you get as much exercise as you want or not enough?

   Enough exercise   Not enough exercise   Neither or both

Work and Retirement

"Now we will talk about your work."

1. What kind of work do you do now?

   _____

   _____

2. Do you want to keep doing this work or not keep doing this work?

   Keep doing work   Not keep doing work   Neither or both

Knowledge and Psychosocial Assessment

3. How happy are you with the amount of money you make?

    Happy   Not happy   Neither or both

4. How happy are you with the kind of work you do?

    Happy   Not happy   Neither or both

5. How happy are you with your boss or employer?

    Happy   Not happy   Neither or both

6. How happy are you with the people you work with?

    Happy   Not happy   Neither or both

Living Arrangement

"Now we will talk about where you live."

1. Where do you live now?
    a. With my family (own or foster)
    b. Supervised apartment (1–2 people, with staff to help)
    c. Small supervised residence (3–15 people, with staff to help)
    d. Large supervised residence (> 15 people; e.g., ICFDD, nursing home)
    e. On my own (with or without roommates)
    f. Other (please specify) _____

    _____

2. Do you like where you live or not like where you live?

    Like where I live   Do not like where I live   Neither or both

3. Would you like to live somewhere else, or would you like to stay where you are living?

    Live somewhere else   Like to stay   Neither or both

4. How happy are you where you live now with the food?

    Happy   Not happy   Neither or both

5. How happy are you where you live now with the neighborhood?

    Happy   Not happy   Neither or both

6. How happy are you where you live now with the people you live with?

    Happy   Not happy   Neither or both

Health Matters: The Exercise and Nutrition Health Education Curriculum for People with Developmental Disabilities
by Beth Marks, Jasmina Sisirak, and Tamar Heller
387

Knowledge and Psychosocial Assessment

7. How happy are you where you live now with the way it looks?

Happy   Not happy   Neither or both

8. How happy are you where you live now with rules (what you are allowed to do)?

Happy   Not happy   Neither or both

Social Support

"Now we are going to ask you how happy you are with the help you get from other people."

1a. Are your parents alive?

Yes   No   No response

1b. Are you happy or not happy with the help you get from parents?

Happy   Not happy   Neither or both

2. Are you happy or not happy with the help you get from other relatives?

Happy   Not happy   Neither or both

3. Are you happy or not happy with the help you get from friends?

Happy   Not happy   Neither or both

4. Are you happy or not happy with the help you get from staff?

Happy   Not happy   Neither or both

Pain [12]

"The next questions are about pain. How much do the following activities hurt?"

1. Walk inside

Doesn't hurt   Hurts a little   Hurts a lot

2. Climb stairs

Doesn't hurt   Hurts a little   Hurts a lot

3. Get in and out of chairs

Doesn't hurt   Hurts a little   Hurts a lot

Knowledge and Psychosocial Assessment

4. Wash all the parts of your body

    Doesn't hurt   Hurts a little   Hurts a lot

5. Put on pants

    Doesn't hurt   Hurts a little   Hurts a lot

6. Put on a shirt

    Doesn't hurt   Hurts a little   Hurts a lot

7. Do your feet hurt?

    Don't hurt   Hurt a little   Hurt a lot

Choice-Making Inventory[7]

"Do you or does someone else get to choose?" (If respondent says "someone else," then ask who chooses: a relative, a friend, or staff member. Remember, friends may include neighbors, coworkers, or peers, and staff members may include paraprofessionals or professionals. Circle the number for the person(s) they name. Circle all that apply.)

		Self	Someone else	Family	Friend	Staff
1.	What food you eat	☐	☐	1	2	3
2.	What food is cooked in your home	☐	☐	1	2	3
3.	How much you eat	☐	☐	1	2	3
4.	What clothes you wear	☐	☐	1	2	3
5.	When you exercise	☐	☐	1	2	3
6.	Who you spend your free time with	☐	☐	1	2	3
7.	Where you go in your free time	☐	☐	1	2	3
8.	What television shows you watch	☐	☐	1	2	3
9.	How you spend your money	☐	☐	1	2	3
10.	What time you go to bed	☐	☐	1	2	3
11.	How you decorate your room	☐	☐	1	2	3
12.	When you clean your room	☐	☐	1	2	3
13.	When you have guests visit in your room	☐	☐	1	2	3
14.	What job you have or what work you do at your workplace	☐	☐	1	2	3
15.	What type of exercise you do	☐	☐	1	2	3

Knowledge and Psychosocial Assessment

II. PHYSICAL ACTIVITY KNOWLEDGE AND SUPPORTS

Attitudes and Beliefs about Exercise [6,8]

"I am going to read you some possible reasons why you might want to exercise. Do you think that exercise would"

1. Help you lose/control your weight or not help you lose/control your weight?

    Help   Not help   Neither or both

2. Make you feel less tired or make you feel more tired?

    Less tired   More tired   Neither or both

3. Make your body feel good or not make your body feel good?

    Feel good   Not feel good   Neither or both

4. Make you feel happier or not make you feel happier?

    Feel happier   Not feel happier   Neither or both

5. Make you hurt less or not make you hurt less?

    Hurt less   Not hurt less   Neither or both

6. Help you meet new people or not help you meet new people?

    Help   Not help   Neither or both

7. Help you get in shape or not help you get in shape?

    Help   Not help   Neither or both

8. Make you look better or not make you look better?

    Look better   Not look better   Neither or both

9. Improve your health or not improve your health?

    Improve   Not improve   Neither or both

10. Make your cholesterol level better or not make your cholesterol level better?

    Lower   Not lower   Neither or both

11. Make your blood pressure better or not make your blood pressure better?

    Make better   Not make better   Neither or both

Knowledge and Psychosocial Assessment

12. Improve your strength or not improve your strength?

    Improve   Not improve   Neither or both

Barriers to Exercise [6,9]

"I am going to read you a list of things that might or might not make it hard for you to exercise. Do you think that"

1. Exercise costs too much money or does not cost too much money?

   It does   It doesn't   Neither or both

2. It's hard to find a way of getting to an exercise program or it is not hard to get to an exercise program?

   Hard   Not hard   Neither or both

3. You don't have enough time to exercise or that you do have enough time to exercise?

   Not enough   Enough   Neither or both

4. You feel like exercising or you don't feel like exercising?

   Feel like   Don't feel like   Neither or both

5. You get too tired to exercise or do not get too tired to exercise?

   Too tired   Not too tired   Neither or both

6. Exercise is boring or not boring?

   Boring   Not boring   Neither or both

7. Exercise will not make you healthier or that it will make you healthier?

   Not healthier   Healthier   Neither or both

8. Exercise will make you sick or that it will not make you sick?

   Sick   Not sick   Neither or both

9. Exercising is too hard or is not too hard?

   Hard   Not hard   Neither or both

10. You don't know how to exercise or do know how to exercise?

    Don't know how   Know how   Neither or both

Knowledge and Psychosocial Assessment

11. Your health keeps you from exercising or does not keep you from exercising?

    Keeps from exercising   Does not keep from exercising   Neither or both

12. You are too lazy to exercise or that you are not too lazy to exercise?

    Too lazy   Not too lazy   Neither or both

13. You don't have anyone to exercise with you or you do have someone to exercise with?

    Don't have   Do have   Neither or both

14. The equipment (like machines/weights) is hard for you to use or not hard for you to use?

    Hard   Not hard   Neither or both

15. You worry that people might make fun of you or you do not worry that people might make fun of you?

    Worry   Don't worry   Neither or both

16. You don't have anyone to show you how to exercise or you do have someone to show you how to exercise?

    Don't have   Do have   Neither or both

17. You would have a hard time using a fitness center (health club, YMCA, park district) or not have a hard time using a fitness center?

    Have hard time   Don't have hard time   Neither or both

Self-Efficacy (Confidence) to Exercise [5,6,15]

"I would like to know how sure you are that you can do certain activities. Do you think that you can:"

1. Do exercises to stretch your muscles?

   Not at all sure   A little sure   Totally sure

2. Do exercises to make your muscles stronger?

   Not at all sure   A little sure   Totally sure

3. Do an exercise that makes you sweat, breathe hard, or increase your heart rate such as walking or bicycling?

   Not at all sure   A little sure   Totally sure

Knowledge and Psychosocial Assessment

4. Do you think you can use an exercise machine (e.g., bike, treadmill, or stepper)?

    Not at all sure   A little sure   Totally sure

5. Do you think you can use an exercise machine to lift weights?

    Not at all sure   A little sure   Totally sure

Social/Environmental Supports for Exercise [4]

"Now I will ask you about things that might help you exercise." (First ask if anyone provides the following supports and then probe who.)

Does anyone (circle all that apply):

		No one	Family	Friends	Doctor/ nurse	Staff
1.	Tell you to exercise?	1	2	3	4	5
2.	Take you to an exercise program?	1	2	3	4	5
3.	Pay for an exercise program?	1	2	3	4	5
4.	Show you how to exercise?	1	2	3	4	5
5.	Exercise with you?	1	2	3	4	5
6.	Tell you not to exercise?	1	2	3	4	5

7. Do you prefer exercising by yourself, with another person, or with a group?

    By yourself   With another person   With a group

8. Do you have a place where you can exercise?

    Yes   No   Don't know

    If the answer to Question 8 is "yes," then ask where.

    a.   Room at day program

    b.   Room at home

    c.   In a fitness center (e.g., health club, YMCA, park district)

    d.   Other, please specify: _____

9. Do you have any exercise equipment that you can use?

    Yes   No   Don't know

Knowledge and Psychosocial Assessment

If the answer to Question 9 is "yes," then ask where.

a. At home

b. At work

c. At a fitness center (e.g., health club, YMCA, park district)

d. Other, please specify: _____

10. Is there an exercise group activity (e.g., class) that you can attend?

Yes   No   Don't know

If the answer to question 10 is "yes," then ask where.

a. At home

b. At work

c. At a fitness center (e.g., health club, YMCA, park district)

b. Other, please specify: _____

Attitudes and Beliefs About Eating Fruits and Vegetables [18,20,21,22]

"I would like to know the reasons why you would eat healthy. For each of these reasons, answer whether you agree or disagree."

If you eat fruits and vegetables every day, it would:

1. Help you lose or control your weight or not lose or control weight?

   Lose or control weight   Not lose/control weight   Neither or both

2. Give you more energy or less energy?

   More energy   Less energy   Neither or both

3. Make your body feel good or not feel good?

   Feel good   Not feel good   Neither or both

4. Make you feel stronger or not feel stronger?

   Feel stronger   Not feel stronger   Neither or both

5. Help you get in shape or not get in shape?

   Get in shape   Not get in shape   Neither or both

6. Help you look better or not look better?

   Look better   Not look better   Neither or both

Knowledge and Psychosocial Assessment

7. Improve your health or not improve your health?

    Improve my health   Not improve my health   Neither or both

8. Improve your cholesterol level or not improve your cholesterol level?

    Improve my cholesterol   Not improve my cholesterol   Neither or both

9. Improve your blood pressure or not improve your blood pressure?

    Improve blood pressure   Not improve blood pressure   Neither or both

10. Help you be healthier or not help you be healthier?

    Help me be healthier   Not help me be healthier   Neither or both

Barriers to Eating Fruits and Vegetables [18,20,21,22]

"I would like to know the reasons that keep you from eating fruits and vegetables. Please answer the following questions."

1. Do you cook at home?   Yes   No

2. Do you do grocery shopping?   Yes   No

3. Fruits and vegetables cost too much money or they do not cost too much money?

    Too much money   Not too much money   Neither or both

4. You don't have enough time to cook fruits and vegetables or you do have enough time to cook fruits and vegetables?

    Don't have enough time   Do have enough time   Neither or both

5. Fruits and vegetables will make you sick or they will not make you sick?

    Sick   Not sick   Neither or both

6. Fruits and vegetables are too hard to chew/swallow or they are not too hard to chew/swallow?

    Hard   Not hard   Neither or both

7. Eating fruits and vegetables is too hard or it is not too hard?

    Hard   Not hard   Neither or both

8. You do not know how to cook fruits and vegetables or you do know how to cook fruits and vegetables?

    Don't know how   Know how   Neither or both

Knowledge and Psychosocial Assessment

9. You are too lazy to make food with fruits and vegetables or you are not too lazy to make food with fruits and vegetables?

    Too lazy   Not too lazy   Neither or both

10. No one will show you how to make food with fruits and vegetables or someone will show you how to make food with fruits and vegetables?

    No one will show me   Someone will show me   Neither or both

11. Fruits and vegetables go bad too fast or they do not go bad too fast?

    Go bad too fast   Not go bad too fast   Neither or both

12. Fruits and vegetables do not taste good or they do taste good?

    Taste good   Not taste good   Neither or both

Social/Environmental Supports for Nutrition [17]

"Now I will ask you about things that might help you make healthy food choices." (First ask if anyone provides the following supports and then probe who.)

Does anyone (circle all that apply):

		No one	Family	Friends	Doctor/ nurse	Staff
1.	Tell you not to eat "junk foods" such as candy, cake, and chips?	1	2	3	4	5
2.	Remind you to eat more fruits and vegetables?	1	2	3	4	5
3.	Compliment you on trying to eat healthier (e.g., "Good job," "Keep it up," "We are proud of you")?	1	2	3	4	5
4.	Give you fruits and vegetables as a snack during the day?	1	2	3	4	5

III. NUTRITION KNOWLEDGE AND SUPPORTS

Nutrition and Activity Knowledge Scale [11,19,21]

The Nutrition and Activity Knowledge Scale (NAKS) is a picture-based instrument designed to assist with the assessment of nutrition and activity knowledge of people with DD. The scale focuses on assessing knowledge as it relates to weight gain and loss and the energy needs of people participating in different activities. The illustrations are designed to assist the assessor in ensuring the question is understood by the respondent.

Knowledge and Psychosocial Assessment

Nutrition and Activity Knowledge [16]

1. Before you exercise, should you stretch and do warm-ups or just start exercising?

   Stretch and warm up   Just start exercising   Don't know

2. While you are exercising, should you drink more water or drink more soda?

   Drink more water   Drink more soda   Don't know

3. While you are exercising, will your heart beat faster than usual or slower than usual?

   Faster than usual   Slower than usual   Don't know

4. Before you exercise, should you eat your breakfast (or lunch) or start exercising without eating any breakfast (or lunch)?

   Eat breakfast (or lunch)   Not eat breakfast (or lunch)   Don't know

5. Before you exercise, should you take your medications or start exercising without taking your medications?

   Take your medications   Not take your medications   Don't know

IV. ADHERENCE TO PHYSICAL ACTIVITY AND EATING NUTRITIOUS FOODS

Exercise/Activity Participation [1]

1. What do you do during the day?

   a. Mostly sitting or standing

   b. Mostly walking

   c. Mostly heavy work (e.g., lifting, moving boxes)

   d. Don't know/not sure

2. Do you do any exercises?

   Yes   No   Don't know

   If the answer to question 2 is "yes," then ask what types of exercise.

   _____

3. Are you in Special Olympics?

   Yes   No   Don't know

   Note: Additional information collected using the Information Outcome Evaluation Form.

Informant Outcome Evaluation Form

Test period (circle response):

Pretest (T1)   **Posttest (T2)**   **6-month posttest (T3)**   **1-year posttest (T4)**

This section will be completed by participant's informant.

Informant's ID number: _____   Date: _____

Participant's ID number: _____   Date (initial entered): _____

1. What is your relationship to the adult with a disability?
    a. Parent
    b. Other relative: _____
    c. Residential staff (specify position): _____
    d. Vocational/day program staff (specify position): _____
    e. Other: _____

Health Status [23]

Please circle one response for the following questions.

1. In general, would you say his or her health is
    a. Excellent
    b. Very good
    c. Good
    d. Fair
    e. Poor

Energy/Fatigue [23]

These questions are about how you think he or she has been feeling during the past month.

How much time during the past month

1. Did he or she feel worn out?

None of the time	A little of the time	Some of the time	A good bit of the time	Most of the time	All of the time
0	1	2	3	4	5

2. Did he or she have a lot of energy?

None of the time	A little of the time	Some of the time	A good bit of the time	Most of the time	All of the time
0	1	2	3	4	5

---

[23]SF-36® Health Survey© 1988, 2002 by Medical Outcomes Trust and QualityMetric Incorporated. All Rights Reserved. SF-26R is a registered trademark of Medical Outcomes Trust. (SF-36 Acute, US Version 1.0.).

Informant Outcome Evaluation Form

3. Did he or she feel tired?

None of the time	A little of the time	Some of the time	A good bit of the time	Most of the time	All of the time
0	1	2	3	4	5

4. Did he or she have enough energy to do the things he or she wanted to do?

None of the time	A little of the time	Some of the time	A good bit of the time	Most of the time	All of the time
0	1	2	3	4	5

5. Did he or she feel full of pep?

None of the time	A little of the time	Some of the time	A good bit of the time	Most of the time	All of the time
0	1	2	3	4	5

6. Did he or she have trouble sleeping at night?

None of the time	A little of the time	Some of the time	A good bit of the time	Most of the time	All of the time
0	1	2	3	4	5

Functional Status

Functional Limitations—Social/Role Activities Limitation [15]

1. Has the participant's health interfered with his or her normal social activities with family, friends, neighbors, or groups?

Not at all	Slightly	Moderately	Quite a bit	Almost totally
0	1	2	3	4

2. Has the participant's health interfered with his or her hobbies or recreational activities?

Not at all	Slightly	Moderately	Quite a bit	Almost totally
0	1	2	3	4

3. Has the participant's health interfered with his or her household chores?

Not at all	Slightly	Moderately	Quite a bit	Almost totally
0	1	2	3	4

4. Has the participant's health interfered with his or her errands and shopping?

Not at all	Slightly	Moderately	Quite a bit	Almost totally
0	1	2	3	4

Informant Outcome Evaluation Form

Current Medications

1. Currently on high blood pressure medication?   Yes   No   Don't know
2. Currently on cholesterol lowering medication?   Yes   No   Don't know
3. Current medications:

_____

History of Falls

1. Does he or she have a history of falls?   Yes   No

2. If yes, has he or she had one or more falls in the last 6 months?   Yes   No

3. Number of fall(s):   _____

4. Reasons of falls (please specify):   _____

5. Does he or she rush to the toilet or have incontinence?   Yes   No

6. Does he or she have trouble seeing (poor eyesight)?   Yes   No

7. Does he or she have foot pain when walking and/or swelling and/or deformity of feet?   Yes   No

Adherence to Healthy Behaviors

Physical Activity [1]

1. During a typical day, which of the following best describes what he or she does?
    a. Mostly sitting or standing
    b. Mostly walking
    c. Mostly heavy labor or physically demanding work
    d. Don't know/Not sure

Nutrition

1. How many servings of fruits and vegetables does he or she have each day (one serving is about the size of the palm of the hand)?
    a. 0–2
    b. 3–4
    c. 5–6
    d. 7–8
    e. 9–11
    f. 12 or more

Informant Outcome Evaluation Form

2. How many glasses of water (8 ounces) does he or she have each day?
   a. 0–2
   b. 3–5
   c. 6–8
   d. 7–8
   e. 9 or more

Healthy Behaviors [17]

1. In general, which of the following best describes his or her health behaviors?

How often does he or she...	Rarely	A few times	Often	Very often
Stick with his or her exercise program even when he or she has work demands?	1	2	3	4
Stick with his or her exercise program after a long, tiring day at work?	1	2	3	4
Pack his or her own lunch?	1	2	3	4
Choose fruits and/or vegetables as a snack instead of "junk food"?	1	2	3	4
Actively participate in his or her health care activities (e.g., occupational or physical therapy)?	1	2	3	4
Ask questions about his or her health care treatment plans	1	2	3	4

2. We would like to know how much total time he or she spends on each of the following activities during a 1-week period.[15]

	None	Less than 30 minutes per week	30–60 minutes per week	1–3 hours per week	More than 3 hours per week
Vigorous activities that cause large increases in breathing or heart rate (e.g., running, lifting heavy objects, participating in strenuous sports)	0	1	2	3	4
Moderate activities (e.g., moving a table, pushing a vacuum cleaner, bowling, playing golf)	0	1	2	3	4
Stretching	0	1	2	3	4
Strength training	0	1	2	3	4
Walking	0	1	2	3	4
Swimming	0	1	2	3	4
Using a treadmill or bicycle	0	1	2	3	4
Other	0	1	2	3	4

by Beth Marks, Jasmina Sisirak, and Tamar Heller

Informant Outcome Evaluation Form

Smoking

Does he or she currently smoke?   Yes   No

If yes, how many cigarettes per day?   _____

Alcohol

Does he or she currently drink alcohol?   Yes   No

If yes, how much per day?   _____

Health Conditions and Health Care Utilization

Health Conditions

Does he or she currently have any of the following conditions?

Conditions	Yes	No
1. Anemia	1	2
2. Arthritis or rheumatism	1	2
3. Asthma	1	2
4. Back pain	1	2
5. Cancer	1	2
6. Circulation trouble in arms/legs	1	2
7. Constipation	1	2
8. Diabetes	1	2
9. Down syndrome	1	2
10. Dizziness (vertigo)	1	2
11. Emphysema or chronic bronchitis	1	2
12. Glaucoma	1	2
13. Heart trouble	1	2
14. High blood pressure	1	2
15. High cholesterol	1	2
16. Incontinence	1	2
17. Osteoporosis	1	2
18. Sleeping problems	1	2
19. Stomach problems (e.g., diarrhea)	1	2
20. Stroke	1	2
21. Thyroid/other glandular disorders	1	2
22. Ulcers (of the digestive system)	1	2
23. Upper respiratory infection	1	2
24. Other: _____	1	2
25. Other: _____	1	2

Informant Outcome Evaluation Form

Health Care Utilization

Visits to Health Providers

During the past 6 months, did he or she visit any of the following health professionals? (Fill in the blank with a "0" or other number; do not include visits while in the hospital.)

How many visits?

Physician   _____

Nurse practitioner or physician's assistant   _____

Home health nurse   _____

Physical, occupational, or respiratory therapist   _____

Visits to Mental Health Providers

During the past 6 months, did he or she visit any of the following health professionals? (Fill in the blank with a "0" or other number; do not include visits while in the hospital.)

How many visits?

Psychiatrist   _____

Psychologist or other mental health counselor   _____

Visits to Emergency Room

How many times did he or she visit the emergency room in the past 6 months?

None   _____ times

Reasons for emergency room visit(s):_____

Number of Hospital Stays

How many different times did he or she stay in a hospital overnight or longer in the past 6 months?

None   _____ times

Nights in Hospital

How many total nights did he or she stay in a hospital overnight in the past 6 months?

None   _____ times

Reasons for hospitalization(s): _____

Outpatient Surgeries

In the past year, how many times did he or she have outpatient surgery (surgery where he or she did not stay overnight in the hospital)?

None   _____ times

FORMS ENDNOTES

[1]Centers for Disease Control and Prevention (CDC). (2007). *Behavioral Risk Factor Surveillance System Survey Questionnaire*. Atlanta, GA: Author; reprinted by permission.

[2]Cuthill, F.M., Espie, C.A., & Cooper, S. (2003). Development and psychometric properties of the Glasgow Depression Scale for people with a learning disability. *British Journal of Psychiatry, 182,* 347–353.

[3]Hawkins, B.A., Ardovino, P., & Hsieh, C. (1998). Validity and reliability of the Leisure Assessment Inventory. *Mental Retardation, 36*(4), 302–313.

[4]Heller, T. (2001a). Exercise: Social/Environmental Support Scale. In T. Heller, B.A. Marks, & S.H. Ailey (Eds.), *Exercise and Nutrition Education Curriculum for Adults with Developmental Disabilities* (1st ed., pp. A.11–A.12). Chicago: University of Illinois at Chicago, Rehabilitation Research and Training Center on Aging and Developmental Disabilities; reprinted by permission.

[5]Heller, T. (2001b). Self-efficacy scale. In T. Heller, B.A. Marks, & S.H. Ailey (Eds.), *Exercise and Nutrition Education Curriculum for Adults with Developmental Disabilities* (1st ed., p. A.12). Chicago: University of Illinois at Chicago, Rehabilitation Research and Training Center on Aging and Developmental Disabilities; reprinted by permission.

[6]Heller, T., Hsieh, K., & Rimmer, J. (2004). Attitudinal and psychological outcomes of a fitness and health education program on adults with Down syndrome. *American Journal on Mental Retardation, 109*(2), 175–188; reprinted by permission.

[7]Heller, T., Miller, A., Hsieh, K., & Sterns, H. (2000). Later life planning: Promoting knowledge of options and choice-making. *Mental Retardation, 38,* 395–406.

[8]Heller, T., & Prohaska, T.J. (2001). Exercise Perception Scale. In T. Heller, B.A. Marks, & S.H. Ailey (Eds.), *Exercise and Nutrition Education Curriculum for Adults with Developmental Disabilities* (1st ed., p. A.9). Chicago: University of Illinois at Chicago, Rehabilitation Research and Training Center on Aging and Developmental Disabilities; reprinted by permission.

[9]Heller, T., Rimmer, J., & Rubin, S. (2001). Barriers Scale. In T. Heller, B.A. Marks, & S.H. Ailey (Eds.), *Exercise and Nutrition Education Curriculum for Adults with Developmental Disabilities* (1st ed., pp. A.9–A.10). Chicago: University of Illinois at Chicago, Rehabilitation Research and Training Center on Aging and Developmental Disabilities; reprinted by permission.

[10]Heller, T., Sterns, H., Sutton, E., & Facor, A. (1996.) Impact of person-centered later life planning training program for older adults with mental retardation. *Journal of Rehabilitation, 62,* 77–83.

[11]Illingworth, K., Moore, K.A., & McGillivray, J. (2003). The development of the nutrition and activity knowledge scale for use with people with an intellectual disability. *Journal of Applied Research in Intellectual Disabilities, 16,* 159–166.

[12]Jette, A. (1980). Functional status index: Reliability of a chronic disease evaluation instrument. *Archives of Physical Medicine and Rehabilitation, 61,* 395-401.

[13]Kovacs, M. (1985.) The Children's Depression Inventory (CDI). *Psychopharmacology Bulletin, 21,* 995–1124.

[14]Lawton, M.P., Moss, M., Fulcomer, M., & Kleban, M.H. (1982). A research and service-oriented multilevel assessment instrument. *Journal of Gerontology, 37,* 91–99.

[15]Lorig, K., Stewart, A., Ritter, P., González, V., Laurent, D., & Lynch, J. (1996). *Outcome measures for health education and other health care interventions.* Thousand Oaks, CA: Sage Publications; reprinted by permission.

[16]Marks, B., & Sisirak, J. (2008). *Establishing community-based exercise and nutrition health promotion programs for adults with developmental disabilities: Train the trainer.* Chicago: University of Illinois at Chicago, Rehabilitation Research and Training Center on Aging and Developmental Disabilities; reprinted by permission.

[17]Sallis, J.F., Grossman, R.M., Pinski, R.B., Patterson, T.L., & Nader, P.R. (1987). The development of scales to measure social support for diet and exercise behaviors. *Preventive Medicine, 16,* 825–836.

[18]Sisirak, J., & Marks, B. (2008). *Fruit and Vegetable Outcome Expectations Scale for people with I/DD.* Rehabilitation Research and Training Center on Aging with Developmental Disabilities, University of Illinois at Chicago; reprinted by permission.

[19]Sisirak, J., Marks, B., & Heller, T. (2005, December 14). *Reliability of adapted Nutrition and Activity Knowledge Scale for people with intellectual disabilities.* American Public Health Association, 133rd Annual Meeting & Exposition, Philadelphia.

[20]Sisirak, J., Marks, B., Heller, T., & Riley, B. (2007, November 6). *Dietary habits of adults with intellectual and developmental disabilities residing in community-based settings.* American Public Health Association, 135th Annual Meeting & Exposition, Washington, DC; reprinted by permission.

[21]Sisirak, J., Marks, B., Riley, B., & Heller, T. (2006, November 7). *Learning through pictures: Nutrition and physical activity health literacy information for adults with I/DD.* Poster session presented at the American Public Health Association, 134th Meeting & Exposition, Boston.

[22]Sisirak, J., Marks, B., Riley, B., & Heller, T. (2008, August 28). *Factors associated with fruit and vegetable intake among adults with I/DD.* IASSID 13th World Congress, People with Intellectual Disabilities: Citizens of the World, Cape Town, South Africa.

[23]Ware, J.E., Jr., Kosinski, M., Gandek, B., (1993, 2000). *SF-36r Health survey: Manual & interpretation guide.* Lincoln, RI: QualityMetric Incorporated.

Resources

HEALTH AND HEALTH PROMOTION

Ailey, S., Marks, B.A., & Hahn, J.E. (2003). Promoting sexuality across the lifespan for individuals with intellectual and developmental disabilities. *Nursing Clinics of North America, 38*(2), 229–252.

Bagley, M., & Mascia, J. (1999). *Hearing changes in aging people with mental retardation.* Available online at http://www.people1.org/articles/aging_hearing_changes.htm

Braunschweig, C.L., Gomez, S., Sheean, P., Tomey, K.M., Rimmer, J.H., & Heller, T. (2004). High prevalence of obesity and low prevalence of cardiovascular and type 2 diabetes risk factors in adults with Down syndrome. *American Journal on Mental Retardation, 109*(2), 186–193.

Chicoine, B., & McGuire, D. (1996). *Promoting health in adults with Down syndrome.* Chicago: University of Illinois at Chicago, Rehabilitation Research and Training Center on Aging with Developmental Disabilities.

Chicoine, B., & McGuire, D. (1997). Longevity of a woman with Down syndrome: A case study. *Mental Retardation, 35*(5), 477–479.

Chicoine, B., Braddock, D., & McGuire, D.E. (1998). Overweight prevalence in persons with Down syndrome. *Mental Retardation, 36*(3), 175–181.

Fernhall, B., Pitetti, K.H., Rimmer, J.H., et al. (1996). Cardiorespiratory capacity of individuals with mental retardation including Down syndrome. *Medicine and Science in Sports and Exercise, 28,* 366–371.

Flax, M.E., & Luchterhand, C. (1996). *Aging with developmental disabilities: Changes in vision.* Chicago: The Arc and the University of Illinois at Chicago, Rehabilitation Research and Training Center on Aging with Developmental Disabilities.

Gill, C.J., & Brown, A.A. (2000). Overview of health issues of older women with intellectual disabilities. In J. Hammel & S. Nochajski (Eds.), Aging and developmental disability: Current research, programming, and practice implications (pp. 23–36). London: Haworth Press.

Hawkins, B.A., & Eklund, S.J. (1994). *Aging related changes for adults with mental retardation: Final report.* Chicago: University of Illinois at Chicago, Rehabilitation Research and Training Center on Aging with Developmental Disabilities.

Hawkins, B.A., Eklund, S., & Martz, B.L. (1992). *Detecting aging-related declines in adults with developmental disabilities: A research monograph.* Bloomington, IN: Indiana University Institute for the Study of Developmental Disabilities

Hawkins, B.A., & Freeman, P.A. (1993). Correlates of self-reported leisure among adults with mental retardation. *Leisure Sciences, 15*(2), 131–147.

Heller, T., Hsieh, K., & Rimmer, J. (2004). Attitudinal and psychological outcomes of a fitness and health education program on adults with Down syndrome. *American Journal on Mental Retardation, 109*(2), 175–185.

Heller, T., Miller, A., Sterns, H., & Hsieh, K. (2000). Later life planning: Promoting knowledge of options and choice-making. *Mental Retardation, 38,* 395–406.

Heller, T., Ying, G., Rimmer, J.H., & Marks, B.A. (2002). Determinants of exercise in adults with cerebral palsy. *Public Health Nursing, 19*(3), 223–231.

Hsieh, K., Heller, T., & Miller, A. (2001). Risk factors for injuries and falls among adults with developmental disabilities. *Journal of International Disability Research, 45*(Part 1), 76–82.

International Association for the Scientific Study of Intellectual Disability (IASSID), Ageing and Intellectual Disabilities Special Interest Research Group (SIRG). (2000). *Ageing and intellectual disabilities: Improving longevity and promoting healthy aging.* Available online at http://www.uic.edu/orgs/rrtcamr/

Janicki, M.P. (Ed.). (1994). *Alzheimer disease among persons with mental retardation: Report from an international colloquium.* Albany: New York State Office of Mental Retardation and Developmental Disabilities.

Janicki, M.P., & Dalton, A.J. (2000). Prevalence of dementia and impact on intellectual disability services. *Mental Retardation, 38,* 277–289.

Janicki, M.P., Dalton, A.J., Henderson, C.M., & Davidson, P.W. (1999). Mortality and morbidity among older adults with developmental disability: Health services considerations. *Disability and Rehabilitation, 21*(5–6), 284–294.

Janicki, M.P., Heller, T., Seltzer, G.B., & Hogg, J. (1995). Practice guidelines for the clinical assessment and care management of Alzheimer and other dementias among adults with mental retardation. *Journal of Intellectual Disability Research, 40*(4), 374–382.

Janicki, M.P., Heller, T., Seltzer, G.B., & Hogg, J. (1996). Practice guidelines for the clinical assessment and care management of Alzheimer's disease and other dementias among adults with developmental disability. *Journal of Intellectual Disability Research, 40*(4), 374–382.

Kunde, K., & Rimmer, J.H. (2000). Effects of pacing vs. nonpacing on a one-mile walk test in adults with mental retardation. *Adapted Physical Activity Quarterly, 17,* 413–420.

Marks, B.A., Brown, A., Hahn, J.E., & Heller, T. (2003). Nursing care resources for individuals with intellectual and developmental disabilities across the lifespan. *Nursing Clinics of North America, 38*(2), 373–393.

Marks, B.A., & Heller, T. (2003). Bridging the equity gap: Health promotion for adults with developmental disabilities. *Nursing Clinics of North America, 38*(2), 205–228.

Marks, B., & Sisirak, J. (2009). *Health matters assessments.* Rehabilitation Research and Training Center on Aging and Developmental Disabilities, Department of Disability and Human Development, University of Illinois at Chicago.

McCracken, A., & Lottman, T. (1997). *McCracken Intervention Matrix: Guidelines for careers to help older adults with mental retardation maintain optimal functioning.* Chicago: University of Illinois at Chicago, Rehabilitation Research and Training Center on Aging with Developmental Disabilities.

McGuire, D., & Chicoine, B. (1996). Depressive disorders in adults with Down syndrome. *The Habilitative Mental Healthcare Newsletter, 15*(1), 1–7.

Rimmer, J. (1997). *Aging, mental retardation and physical fitness: Fact sheet.* Chicago: University of Illinois at Chicago, Rehabilitation Research and Training Center on Aging with Developmental Disabilities.

Rimmer, J. (2000a). Achieving a beneficial fitness: A program and a philosophy in mental retardation. *Contemporary Issues in Health, 1*(1).

Rimmer, J.H. (2000b). *Disabilities and health limitations. In Group fitness instructor manual: ACE's guide for fitness professionals* (pp. 226–246). San Diego: American Council on Exercise.

Rimmer, J.H., Braddock, D., & Fujiura, G. (1994a). Cardiovascular risk factor levels in adults with mental retardation. *American Journal of Mental Retardation, 98*(4), 510–518.

Rimmer, J.H., Braddock, D., & Fujiura, G. (1994b). Congruence of three risk indices for obesity in a population of adults with mental retardation. *Adapted Physical Activity Quarterly, 11,* 396–403.

Rimmer, J.H., Braddock, D., & Marks, B. (1995). Health characteristics and behaviors of adults with mental retardation residing in three living arrangements. *Research in Developmental Disabilities, 16*(6), 489–499.

Rimmer, J.H., Braddock D., & Pitetti, K.H. (1996). Research on physical activity and disability: An emerging national priority. *Medicine and Science in Sports and Exercise, 28*(8), 1366–1372.

Rimmer, J.H., Goreczny, A.J., & Hersen, M. (Eds.). (1999). Mental retardation and physical health In Handbook of pediatric and adolescent health psychology (pp. 299–399). Boston: Allyn & Bacon.

Rimmer, J., Heller, T., Wang, E., & Valerio, I. (2004). Improvements in physical fitness in adults with Down syndrome. *American Journal on Mental Retardation, 109*(2), 165–174.

Rimmer, J.H., Rubin, S.S., Braddock, D., & Hedman, G. (1999). Physical activity patterns of African-American women with a severe physical disability. *Medicine and Science in Sports and Exercise, 31*, 613–618.

Seltzer, G.B., Schupf, N., & Wu, H.S. (2001). A prospective study of menopause in women with Down's syndrome. *Journal of Intellectual Disability Research, 45*, 1–7.

Sung, H., Hawkins, B.A., Eklund, S.J., Jim, K.A., Foose, A., May, M.E., et al. (1997). Depression and dementia in aging adults with Down Syndrome: A case study approach. *Mental Retardation, 35*(1), 27–38.

SELF-ADVOCACY

The Arc of the United States. (1994). *Learning about the Americans with Disabilities Act and working.* Silver Spring, MD: Author.

Berkobien, R. (1995). Learning about the Americans with Disabilities Act and Title II: Opening up government services and activities for people with disabilities. Silver Spring, MD: The Arc of the United States.

Berkobien, R. (1996). *Learning about the Americans with Disabilities Act and Title III: Public accommodations.* Silver Spring, MD: The Arc of the United States.

Hawkins, B.A. (1991). An exploration of adaptive skills and leisure activity of older adults with mental retardation. *Therapeutic Recreation Journal, 25*(4), 9–27.

Hawkins, B.A. (1993). An exploratory analysis of leisure and life satisfaction of aging adults with mental retardation. *Therapeutic Recreation Journal, 27*(2), 98–109.

Heller, T., Factor, A., Sterns, H., & Sutton, E. (1996). Impact of person-centered later life planning training program for older adults with mental retardation. *Journal of Rehabilitation, 62*(1), 77–83.

Heller, T., Miller, A., Nelis, T., & Pederson, E. (1995). *Getting involved in research and training projects: A guide for persons with disabilities.* Chicago: University of Illinois at Chicago, Rehabilitation Research and Training Center on Aging with Developmental Disabilities.

Heller, T., Miller, A., Sterns, H., & Hsieh, K. (2000). *Later life planning: Promoting knowledge of options and choice in mental retardation.* Chicago: University of Illinois at Chicago, Rehabilitation Research and Training Center on Aging with Developmental Disabilities.

Heller, T., Pederson, E., & Miller, A. (1996). Guidelines from the consumer: Improving consumer involvement in research and training for persons with mental retardation. *Mental Retardation, 34*(3), 141–148.

Heller, T., Preston, L., Nelis, T., Brown, A., & Pederson, E. (1996). *Making choices as we age: A peer training program.* Chicago: University of Illinois at Chicago, Rehabilitation Research and Training Center on Aging with Developmental Disabilities.

Pederson, E. (1997). Including self-advocates in community leadership. *Disability Solutions, 2*(4), 1, 3–9.

Pederson, E., & Chaikin, M. (1993). *Voices that count training package* (Videotape, Audio Cassette, Presenter's Guide). Chicago: University of Illinois at Chicago, Rehabilitation Research and Training Center on Aging with Developmental Disabilities.

Riemenschneider, S. (1997). *Down syndrome pioneer.* Chicago: University of Illinois at Chicago, Rehabilitation Research and Training Center on Aging with Developmental Disabilities.

Sutton, E., Heller, T., Sterns, H.L., Factor, A., & Miklos, S. (1993). *Person-Centered Planning for Later Life: A curriculum for adults with mental retardation.* Chicago: University of Illinois at Chicago, Rehabilitation Research and Training Center on Aging with Developmental Disabilities.

Sutton, E., Sterns, H.L., & Roberts, R.S. (1992). Retirement for older persons with developmental disabilities. *Generations, 16*, 63–64.

GENERAL AGING WITH DEVELOPMENTAL DISABILITIES

A/DDVantage. (Newsletter published by the University of Illinois at Chicago, Rehabilitation Research and Training Center on Aging with Developmental Disabilities.)

Anderson, D., Polister, B., Kloos, E., Heller, T., & Roberts, R. (1993, Spring). *IMPACT: Feature Issue on Aging and Developmental Disabilities*, *6*(1). Minneapolis: University of Minnesota.

Factor, A. (1997). *Aging with developmental disabilities: An information packet on understanding age-related changes and supporting successful aging.* Chicago: University of Illinois at Chicago, Rehabilitation Research and Training Center on Aging with Developmental Disabilities.

Hawkins, B., & Eklund, S. (1994). *Aging-related change in adults with mental retardation. Research brief.* Arlington, TX: The Arc of the United States.

Heller, T., (1997). Older adults with mental retardation and their families. In N.W. Bray (Ed.), *International review of research in mental retardation* (Vol. 20). San Diego: Academic Press.

Suttie, J., & Heller, T. (1997). *1997 International Roundtable on Aging and Intellectual Disabilities Conference Proceedings of the International Association for the Scientific Study of Intellectual Disability.* Chicago: University of Illinois at Chicago, Rehabilitation Research and Training Center on Aging with Developmental Disabilities.

Sutton, E., Factor, A., Hawkins, B., Heller, T., & Seltzer, G. (Eds.). (1993). *Older adults with developmental disabilities: Optimizing choice and change.* Baltimore: Paul H. Brookes Publishing Co.

POLICY/SERVICE DELIVERY

Braddock, D. (1999). Innovations in mental retardation services. In D. Biegel & A. Blum (Eds.), *Innovations in practice and service delivery with vulnerable populations across the lifespan* (pp. 169–196). New York: Oxford University Press.

Braddock, D., Hemp, R., Parish, S., & Westrich, J. (2000). *The state of the states in developmental disabilities: 2000 study summary.* Washington, DC: American Association on Mental Retardation.

Factor, A. (1996a). *Innovative internetwork service models serving older adults with developmental disabilities and older family caregivers: Final report.* Chicago: University of Illinois at Chicago, Rehabilitation Research and Training Center on Aging with Developmental Disabilities.

Factor, A. (1996b). *Project brief: Innovative internetwork service models serving older adults with developmental disabilities and older family caregivers.* Chicago: University of Illinois at Chicago, Rehabilitation Research and Training Center on Aging with Developmental Disabilities.

Gordon, R.M., Seltzer, M.M. & Krauss, M.W. (1996). The aftermath of parental death: Changes in the context and quality of life. In R.L. Schalock (Ed.), *Quality of life: Vol. II. Application to persons with disabilities.* Washington, DC: American Association on Mental Retardation.

Hawkins, B.A. (1996). Promoting quality of life through leisure and recreation. In R.L. Schalock (Ed.), *Quality of life: Vol. II. Applications to people with disabilities.* Washington, DC: American Association on Mental Retardation.

Hawkins, B.A. (1999). Rights, place of residence, and retirement: Lessons from case studies in aging. In S.S. Herr & G. Weber (Eds.), *Aging, rights, and quality of life: Prospects for older people with developmental disabilities.* Baltimore: Paul H. Brookes Publishing Co.

Hawkins, B.A., Eklund, S.J., Kim, K., Green, K., Foose, FA., & Ardovino, P. (1997). *Five Dimensional Life Satisfaction Index* (2nd ed.). Chicago: University of Illinois at Chicago, Rehabilitation Research and Training Center on Aging with Developmental Disabilities.

Hawkins, B.A., May, M.E., & Brittain Rogers, N. (1996). *Therapeutic activity intervention with the elderly: Foundations and practices.* State College, PA: Venture Publishing.

Heller, T. (1999). Emerging models. In S.S. Herr & G. Weber (Eds.), *Aging, rights, and quality of life: Prospects for older people with developmental disabilities.* Baltimore: Paul H. Brookes Publishing Co.

Janicki, M.P. (1999). Public policy and service design. In S.S. Herr & G. Weber (Eds.), *Aging, rights, and quality of life: Prospects for older people with developmental disabilities.* Baltimore: Paul H. Brookes Publishing Co.

Janicki, M., & Ansello, E. (Eds.). *Community supports for aging adults with lifelong disabilities.* Baltimore: Paul H. Brookes Publishing Co.

Janicki, M.P., & Dalton, A.J. (1999). Mental retardation. In American Geriatrics Society (Eds.), *Geriatrics Review Syllabus: A core curriculum in geriatric medicine* (4th ed.). New York: Blackwell Science Publishing Co.

Jones, R. & Factor, A. (1996). *Opening all the doors under the ADA: Making your programs accessible to older adults with cognitive disabilities.* Chicago: University of Illinois at Chicago, Rehabilitation Research and Training Center on Aging with Developmental Disabilities.

King, M., & Wright, B. (1999, January). *State legislative report: Personal assistance services for people with disabilities* (Vol. 24, No. 2). Chicago: University of Illinois at Chicago, Rehabilitation Research and Training Center on Aging with Developmental Disabilities.

Roberts, R., Sutton, E., & Caramela-Miller, S. (1992). *Peer companion model implementing community integration for older persons with developmental disabilities.* Chicago: University of Illinois at Chicago, Rehabilitation Research and Training Center on Aging with Developmental Disabilities.

Wright, B., & King, M. (1999, January). NCSL Legisbrief: Developmental Disabilities and Aging (Vol. 7, No. 15). Chicago: University of Illinois at Chicago, Rehabilitation Research and Training Center on Aging with Developmental Disabilities.

RESOURCES FOR EXERCISE

- *Chimes Exercise Manual*—Tom Prohaska, Ph.D., University of Illinois at Chicago, School of Public Health, Center for Health Interventions with Minority Elderly, Prohaska@uic.edu.
- DynaBands (resistive fitness bands)—The Hygenic Corporation, http://www.hygenic.com
- Heart rate monitors—We have used heart rate monitor watches with of our community groups, and they are really easy to use. We recommend Polar Heart Rate Monitors B1 Type.
- Local community-based recreation programs
- National Center on Physical Activity and Disability (NCPAD), http://www.ncpad.org/.
- Pep Up Your Life with Exercises: The Key to The Good Life—AARP, http://library.monterey.edu/instruction/icmodules/evaluate/aarp.html.
- Wrist blood pressure monitors—Wrist blood pressure monitors are very easy to use, and many participants can use them on their own. We recommend the Mark of Fitness MF 77 Wrist Blood Pressure Monitor with IQ System & PC Compatibility.
- YMCA/YWCA

RESOURCES FOR SELF-ADVOCACY AND LEADERSHIP

Advocating Change Together (ACT), http://www.selfadvocacy.com—ACT is a nonprofit, organization formed in 1979 to promote self-advocacy by people with developmental disabilities. ACT is managed by a board of directors comprised primarily of persons with disabilities.

People First of Oregon, http://www.people1.org—People First is people with developmental disabilities joining together to learn how to speak for themselves.

Self Advocates Becoming Empowered (SABE), http://www.sabeusa.org/—A primary goal of SABE is to make self-advocacy available in every state including institutions, high schools, rural areas and people living with families with local support and advisors to help.

Index